OXFORD MEDICAL PUBLICATIONS

Why We Sleep

Why We Sleep

The Functions of Sleep in Humans and Other Mammals

JAMES HORNE

Professor, Department of Human Sciences,
Loughborough University

OXFORD NEW YORK TOKYO
OXFORD UNIVERSITY PRESS

Oxford University Press, Walton Street, Oxford OX2 6DP
Oxford New York Toronto
Delhi Bombay Calcutta Madras Karachi
Petaling Jaya Singapore Hong Kong Tokyo
Nairobi Dar es Salaam Cape Town
Melbourne Auckland
and associated companies in
Berlin Ibadan

Oxford is a trade mark of Oxford University Press

Published in the United States
by Oxford University Press, New York

First published 1988
Reprinted 1989
First published in paperback 1989
Reprinted 1990

British Library Cataloguing in Publication Data
Horne, James
Why we sleep: the function of sleep
in humans and other mammals.
1. Sleep
I. Title
599.01'88   QP425
ISBN 0-19-261682-X
ISBN 0-19-261892-X (Pbk)

Library of Congress Cataloguing in Publication Data
Horne, James (James A.)
Why we sleep.
(Oxford medical publications).
Includes bibliographies and index.
1. Sleep—Physiological aspects.   I. Title
II. Series   [DNLM: 1. Sleep—physiology.   WL 108 H815w]
QP426.H67   1988   599'.0188   87-22084
ISBN 0-19-261682-X
ISBN 0-19-261892-X (Pbk)

Printed in Great Britain by
Courier International Ltd
Tiptree, Essex

To my most critical but devoted reader,
my wife, Helen, who diligently read
through three complete versions of the
manuscript, making innumerable
comments each time.

Acknowledgements

I am indebted to the following people for their time and much valued comments in reading through various drafts of this book: David Dinges, Jake Empson, Rainer Goldsmith, Shojiro Inoué, Adrian Morrison, Paul Naitoh, John Normanton, and Allan Rechtschaffen. Harriet Thistlethwaite's advice on publishing matters was very helpful. My pictorial skills are poor, and many of the diagrams were drawn by David Easom, to whom I am most grateful. For help in typing the manuscript, and being unfailingly available at an instant's notice, I am thankful to my word processor, but no thanks to the manufacturers of its badly designed VDT screen for my eyestrain.

I came into sleep research from obscure beginnings. In finding my feet certain people in the field have given me much support and guidance, and for this I would like to make a special acknowledgement of their kindness, again to Paul Naitoh, Allan Rechtschaffen, and lastly to Bob Wilkinson, whose work and person inspired me in the first place, and who has been a good friend ever since.

Loughborough   J.A.H.
1987

Contents

Abbreviations

ACTH	adrenocorticotrophic hormone
ADP	adenosine diphosphate
AER	averaged evoked response
AMP	adenosine monophosphate
ATP	adenosine triphosphate
BAT	brown adipose tissue
CBR	cerebral blow flow
CEC	cell energy charge
CMR	cerebral metabolic rate
CNV	contingent negative variation
DSIP	delta sleep-inducing peptide
ECG	electrocardiogram
ECoG	electrocorticogram
EEG	electroencephalogram
EQ	encephalization quotient
FSH	follicle-stimulating hormone
GH	growth hormone
GP	general practitioner
H	high intensity
hGH	human growth hormone
IL-1	interleukin-1
IQ	intelligence quotient
L	low intensity
LH	Luteinizing hormone
MDP	muramyl dipeptide
MIMA	middle ear muscle activity
MMPI	Minnesota multiphasic personality inventory
P	passive heating
PET	positron emission tomography
PGO	ponto-geniculo-occipital
REM	rapid eye movement
SPS	sleep-promoting substance
SUSOP	sustained operation
SWS	slow wave sleep
TSH	thyroid-stimulating hormone

1. Introduction

This is a book about the purpose of sleep in mammals, particularly in humans. My approach has been to take a broad biological perspective, looking at sleep in relation to the natural lifestyles and behaviour of mammals, and making what I hope is a series of informed opinions about what sleep means to them, and especially to us. Of course, I do not have the answer to why we sleep, as too much is still unknown. What I have attempted to do is clear away many misconceptions and try and make some sense of what is left. This book is not meant to be a comprehensive text on sleep, but a selective and personal account giving several hypotheses about a variety of aspects of sleep. Many of my conclusions may well turn out to be wrong, as that is the way of most theories. However, I hope that before they fall they prove to be of use in stimulating other ideas.

I have tried to make the book readable, and present my case within an unfurling story about sleep. Technicalities have been kept to a minimum, although at times, and of necessity, I go into some detail. Wherever possible, I have tried to make it understandable, as the book is aimed not only at sleep researchers, but at a readership having more of a passing interest in sleep, with only a basic background in biology and psychology. Little coverage is given to the brain's neurophysiological and neurochemical mechanisms regulating sleep. Whilst they help explain how sleep occurs, the fundamental questions about what they are doing there in the first place, that is the function of sleep, still have to be answered. Besides, there are already excellent texts describing these mechanisms (e.g. ref. 1).

Many people feel that, despite 50 years of research, all we can conclude about the function of sleep is that it overcomes sleepiness, and that the only reliable finding from sleep deprivation experiments is that sleep loss makes us sleepy. Such a forlorn outlook has been partly responsible for many sleep researchers turning away from basic research to the more stimulating field of sleep disorders. Besides, is knowing why we sleep such a vital question after all? Employment prospects are far better in the area of sleep disorders, and there is the satisfaction of being able to help or cure many patients. Numerous sleep disorders centres have been established in the United States and Europe over the last decade (alas, not in the UK), and this is by far the greatest growth area in sleep research.

Whilst it could rightly be argued that the study of sleep disorders is a far more worthwhile area for sleep research, unfortunately, like the neuro-

1

physiological mechanisms of sleep, it still does not tell us much about why we sleep. Certainly, it has provided valuable information about the neurophysiological mechanisms, and about the association between sleep and breathing (which is not really related to the function of sleep either). This is why the book contains little about sleep disorders. Again, there are already several excellent accounts available (e.g. refs. 2–4).

The aim of this book is to show that we have not reached a dead-end in our understanding about the functions of sleep, but rather that we may have taken too much for granted. As will be seen, this topic is still an unknown and exciting entity, with many avenues still to follow, and there is much work to be done.

Writings about why we sleep date back to before the days of Aristotle. Most couch the purpose of sleep in terms of rest and recovery from the 'wear and tear' of wakefulness. One cannot really argue with this idea as it makes so much sense, and besides, we all know that we feel the 'worse for wear' without sleep, and so much better after sleep. Nevertheless it is a vague idea—what exactly is recovered? This is still a matter for considerable debate, as will be seen throughout the book.

It is commonly thought that 7–8 hours sleep a night is necessary. This idea is reinforced from many quarters, for example by the popular press ('you must get your beauty sleep') and by many GPs. Asking a patient 'how are you sleeping?', may only be a stock phrase for helping the GP to establish rapport, but it still emphasizes the need for a 'good night's sleep'. The key symptom of insuffient or disturbed sleep is excessive sleepiness in the daytime. But many insomniacs do not experience this, and a major concern is about 'not getting enough sleep', and what may happen to their health as a consequence. However, we probably do not really need the last few hours of a typical night's sleep, and sleep loss is far less harmful than most would think.

Most of the theories about the function of sleep concentrate on dreams or dreaming sleep, nowadays called 'rapid eye movement' sleep (REM sleep). Few look at the remaining sleep. Many people believe that we only go to sleep for the purpose of dreaming or having REM sleep. Clearly, dreams are the most enjoyable and noticeable part of sleep, but the importance of this sleep is probably overrated. As will be seen, a large portion of REM sleep is dispensable, without ill-effect. REM sleep only occupies about one-quarter of our nightly sleep, and to call the rest of sleep 'non-REM' sleep, by describing it in terms of an absence of REM sleep, not only debases the majority of sleep but overlooks what may losely be described as the 'deeper' part of non-REM sleep, called 'slow wave sleep' (SWS) in humans. This form of sleep may well turn out to be the most crucial for us. Nevertheless, despite the fact that no one really knows what REM sleep does, or whether it is 'good' for us, there is concern if it is diminished. For example, if a sleeping tablet leaves REM sleep unchanged, or even increases it, then this is often seen to be a selling point for the drug, and little concern is usually expressed if the drug impairs or alters non-REM sleep, which, by the way, many of these tablets do to a noticeable extent. This is not meant as a criticism of drug companies, as they have only been following the climate of opinion in sleep research.

REM sleep has traditionally been viewed to be essential for the normal functioning of the brain during wakefulness, while non-REM sleep, particularly SWS, is for the rest of the body. Rightly or wrongly so, the old idea of 'dualism', the body versus mind controversy in biology, has strongly influenced perspectives on sleep. However, as will be seen, this is too simple an explanation, as apart from anything else the functions of sleep have probably changed with mammalian evolution. For example, whereas sleep may well provide generalized body tissue repair for the mouse, it is unlikely that this is the case for humans, where sleep seems particularly beneficial to the cerebrum. On the other hand, for us, and perhaps even the mouse, REM sleep may partly be some form of substitute for wakefulness, keeping the brain stimulated without having to awaken the sleeper. Perhaps dreams themselves are just a 'cinema of the mind'—the brain's great entertainer to while away the night-time hours! However, it is important not to fall into the trap of thinking about each type of sleep in isolation, each having its own distinct function, separate from whatever the other types of sleep are doing. Sleep is a complex process and it is likely that different types of sleep interact with one another to promote a variety of functions, even though one type of sleep may be associated more with one function than another.

The last three paragraphs are introductions to most of the key themes of this book, which are developed a little more at the end of the next section. Each chapter expands these themes further, and there are summaries at the end of most chapters. Each chapter is a fairly self-contained unit, and does not have to be read in sequence, although this is recommended. A grand summary of all the main themes is given in the last chapter, 'Why Do We Sleep?', and the reader might like to take a preview of it.

1.1 Early sleep theories

Apart from viewing sleep as some sort of recovery process, most of the early theories only looked at the mechanisms that produce sleep, rather than what exactly sleep does. For example believing it to be the result of a build-up of some substance in the brain during wakefulness, that is dissipated during sleep. Even Aristotle thought along these lines 2000 years ago, and considered that sleep resulted from warm vapours rising from within the stomach:

The evaporation attendant upon the process of nutrition . . . naturally tends to move upward. This explains why fits of drowsiness are especially apt to come after meals. It also follows certain forms of fatigue; for fatigue operates as a solvent, and the dissolved (warm) matter acts like food prior to digestion.

In the last century, with more advancements in the understanding of the brain, heart, and vascular system, one school of thought considered sleep to be caused by the 'congestion of the brain' by blood. This contrasted with another popular theory at the time, of 'cerebral anaemia', due to blood being drawn away from the brain and diverted elsewhere in the body, especially to the gut. Such ideas even led to opposing beliefs about how to induce 'better' sleep. Some people propounded sleeping without pillows to encourage blood flow to the head, and others encouraged the opposite—using plenty of pillows to drain the blood away.

'Behavioural' theories were also common in the nineteenth-century, particularly that sleep was due to an absence of external stimulation, with wakefulness only being possible if the organism was constantly stimulated. Take the stimulation away and the animal will fall asleep. To some extent this notion is true, as we can all testify, but it is not the answer. At the turn of the century another behavioural theory became very popular, proposed by a Frenchman, Dr Eduard Claparède. He considered that sleep was not so much a passive response, but an active process like an instinct, to avoid fatigue occurring—'we sleep not because we are intoxicated or exhausted, but in order to prevent our becoming intoxicated or exhausted'. For him, sleep ends when we have had enough. This is an interesting idea initially, but it has as much depth of understanding as saying that we eat in order to prevent ourselves from starving. The real purpose of eating is to provide nutrients that undergo complex processes which allow the body to live, grow, and repair itself.

The beginning of the twentieth century also produced many of what are termed 'humoral' theories, whereby various sleep-inducing substances accumulated in the brain. These ranged from known chemicals like lactic acid, carbon dioxide and cholesterol, to the vaguely described 'leucomaines' and 'urotoxins'. Nevertheless, by 1907 some headway began to be made when two French researchers, Drs Rene Legendre and Henri Piéron, claimed to have obtained a substance they called 'hypnotoxin' from sleep-deprived animals. This gave a large boost to the humoral theories for the next 20 years or so, with much activity by several groups of researchers. However, success was hard to come by and interest dwindled, that is until the 1960s, when great headway has since been made into 'sleep substances' (see Section 5.12).

In those interim years most of the excitement came from advances in neurophysiology that could be related to sleep, and a spate of different neural 'inhibition' theories for sleep appeared. Many had had their early impetus from Pavlov's views on 'cortical inhibition'—that sleep originated from a form of blocking within the cerebral hemispheres. Although Pavlov vehemently dismissed the alternative, of sleep-inducing 'centres' in more basic parts of the brain below the cortex, these have since been found to exist, and have become the centre of one of the prominent fields of sleep research, especially, after the discovery in the late 1940s, of arousal centres in the reticular formation. Unfortunately though, sleep centres and humoral theories still do not tell us much about the purpose of sleep, in the same way that knowing about centres in the brain that regulate eating behaviour explain little about the purpose of eating.

Hypotheses about the function of sleep have centred on various types of recovery following the wear and tear of wakefulness, and come under the heading of 'restorative' theories. In contrast, there are alternatives that reject this standpoint and claim that sleep is non-restorative—simply a form of instinct or 'non-behaviour' for keeping us, as well as other mammals, out of harm's way, and occupying the otherwise tedious and unproductive hours of darkness. Through this immobility, sleep will also prevent any waste of energy through needlessly moving about. Hence sleep is often seen as an 'energy conserver'.

Whilst I believe that these restitutional and instinctive theories have their merits, they seem to fail because each is usually applied universally to all mammals. Why should the functions of sleep for a small nocturnal mammal like the mouse, with a poorly developed cerebral cortex, unable to relax during wakefulness, continually having to forage for food and be on the lookout for predators, be exactly the same as that for humans, who are usually the opposite in all these respects?

One theme I shall be developing in this book is that these three aspects of sleep function—restoration, energy conservation, and as an occupier of time, will alter as the evolutionary scale is ascended, depending on various inter-related circumstances of the mammal, particularly body size, level of cerebral development, amount of relaxed wakefulness, and type of diet.

Furthermore, for most mammals including ourselves, the functions of sleep may well alter as each night's sleep progresses, initially serving more important purposes, then changing to those of less benefit. Not only does this idea break with the traditional division of sleep into REM and non-REM sleep, but also means that the last part of sleep may be 'superfluous' in many mammals. For humans, this applies to the last 2 hours or so of the typical 8 hours of nightly sleep. This is similar to eating and drinking, where we can easily consume more than we really need, or do with a little less, without any ill-effects, apart from some harmless adjustment of body weight, for example.

My standpoints on sleep are somewhat heretical, and argue against many commonly held ideas. But before entering this controversy, let me provide a little background about some of the more common phenomena of sleep and how they are measured.

1.2   Daily sleep and wakefulness

The lives of all mammals are very much influenced by internal biological clocks under the control of centres within the brain that regulate not only the level of alertness over the day, but the timing of sleep, wakefulness, and most other physiological functions. There is much debate about whether these rhythms come under the control of one, two or more central clocks. At the moment it is thought that there may be two—one controlling sleep and wakefulness, the other body temperature and various aspects of general physiology. On the other hand, it is possible that both are part of some less well understood 'master clock'. However, assuming there to be two clocks, it seems that neither runs precisely at 24 hours, and the term 'circadian', from the latin *circa diem* ('about a day') has been adopted to describe them.

Human circadian rhythms are inclined to run a little slower than 24 hours, more like 24.5 hours, but they are restrained to 24 hours through the brain being aware of regular daily events in the environment. Such events are called 'zeitgebers', a German word loosely translated as 'time giver'. For many mammals sunrise and sunset are the main *zeitgebers*. If the *zeitgebers* are removed, for example by keeping an animal in an artificial environment under constant light, then the body temperature clock 'free runs' at its natural period (i.e. 24.5 hours in humans). But in the modern world of electric lighting, our internal clocks can no longer rely on daylight and darkness as a *zeitgeber*, and instead somehow use other regular cues such as mealtimes, and perhaps morning wakening by an alarm clock.

Under normal everyday conditions our internal clocks are linked together, with body temperature and most physiological activities increasing during wakefulness and declining during sleep. This is not simply an effect of different levels of physical activity. For example, if sleep is lost at night and taken in the day instead, as happens in shift work, the temperature rhythm remains the same for several days, still falling at night and rising by day. Then it flattens out, and eventually begins to reshape itself to rise at night and fall by day. Full adaptation of the temperature rhythm may take over 2 weeks and until this occurs, with the sleep–wakefulness rhythm completely resynchronized with it, the shift worker experiences various discomforts such as sleepiness at work, indigestion, loss of appetite, and headaches. These are not harmful, just annoying, and are in effect a worse form of 'jet lag', where the timing of sleep and wakefulness is also suddenly shifted in relation to body temperature and local time.

Why Nature has given animals these circadian clocks is not exactly clear, and the reason may vary somewhat from species to species. However, most animals are very much at the mercy of daylight and darkness, irrespective of whether they live diurnal or nocturnal lifestyles. One view of the function of the circadian clocks is that they preempt each part of the day by ensuring that sleep, wakefulness, alertness, and various physiological changes will be at their most suitable levels. Such preempting may be necessary as there is a time lag for these changes to occur, which might be too long if they did not begin until the external event arrived. For example, a warm brain works better than a cool one, but during the sleep period body and brain temperature fall a little. Some time is required for the brain to warm up, and if this did not begin until wakefulness then behaviour could be impaired for a while. The circadian clock seems to anticipate wakefulness and starts the warm-up process a few hours beforehand, ensuring that the brain is at a good working temperature when wakefulness begins.

1.3 Measuring sleep

If one simply watches a sleeping mammal, including humans, certain common features are seen:

- A typical body posture.
- A specific site or nest for this behaviour.
- Physical inactivity.
- A regular daily occurrence influenced by a circadian clock.
- More stimulation is required to rouse the animal than during wakefulness.

However, advanced mammals like ourselves can feign some of these characteristics during wakefulness by resting with the eyes shut, and a more accurate method for measuring sleep is needed. Furthermore, as it is tedious to watch an animal sleeping for many hours at a time, some form of automatic recording is desirable. The organ that shows the clearest changes during sleep compared with relaxed wakefulness is the brain, and this is particularly obvious in its electrical activity. Concentrating on the brain in this way is appropriate in other respects, as not only does it contain the control mechanisms of sleep, but out of all the body's organs it is for the brain and behaviour (i.e. mainly the cerebral cortex) that sleep seems to be the most vital. Monitoring this electrical activity in animals involves surgery and the placing of minute electrodes in the brain and other parts of the head. These are normally connected by flexible wires to a junction box above the cage. This can restrict the animal's movement, and if more freedom is wanted then a miniature radio transmitter can be fixed to the head instead.

In humans, electrodes are just fixed to the surface of the scalp with a quick-drying sterile glue, which is easily removed by a solvent. Wires from the electrodes are plugged into a junction box, and the signals amplified by a machine similar to that used for animals. Such amplifiers are technically very sophisticated as they have to boost the brain's signals by about a million-fold, because the electrical activity of the brain is only at a few millionths of a volt.

After amplification, the signals can be written out by mechanical ink pens on paper, or recorded on magnetic tape.

The human brain largely consists of the cerebral cortex (sometimes called the 'encephalon') surrounding the rest of the brain like the canopy of a mushroom around its stalk. As the electrodes are located above the cortex, the electrical activity they pick up is that of the cortex, rather than of deeper brain areas. Hence the term 'electroencephalography' (EEG for short) is used to describe this technique of scalp recording. The paper write-out is called an 'electroencephalogram' (also called the EEG), and the machine containing the amplifiers and pens, an 'electroencephalograph'. When electrodes are placed on the cortex itself, as with animals, the electrical activity should strictly be called the 'electrocorticogram' (ECoG). However, for simplicity, many people including myself, also refer to it as the EEG, even though this is incorrect.

Much of sleep can be assessed from the EEG alone, but for the measurement of REM sleep additional electrodes have to be placed around the eyes, to detect the rapid eye movements, and over muscles in the chin or neck. For reasons that are not understood, in REM sleep these muscles profoundly relax ('tonus' is lost), and this can be used as a further guide to REM sleep. Although muscles in the rest of the body do not lose their tonus, they are unable to move as there is also a type of paralysis going on during REM sleep that prevents voluntary movement. For many mammals the EEG of REM sleep is very much like that of aroused wakefulness, which is why REM sleep used to be called 'paradoxical' sleep—the animal is behaviourally asleep but the brain seems to be awake. So without knowing about the activities of the eyes and neck muscles, we could easily mistake REM sleep for wakefulness. For humans the EEG of REM sleep is very much like that of light non-REM sleep (stage 1 sleep), and consequently was once called 'stage 1-REM sleep'. Again, eye and neck muscle recordings are essential to separate REM sleep from stage 1 sleep.

The EEG consists of waves that can be measured in terms of:

- *Amplitude*: the voltage between the peak and the trough of a wave, measured in millionths of a volt (microvolts—μV). Amplitude rises as consciousness falls—from alert wakefulness, through drowsiness to deep sleep.
- *Frequency:* the number of complete waves or cycles occurring in one second, expressed as hertz (Hz—cycles per second). The effective range in the human EEG is from about 0.5 Hz to 25 Hz. Generally speaking, frequencies above about 15 Hz are 'fast waves', and frequencies of under about 3.5 Hz are 'slow waves'—these are the waves of slow wave sleep (SWS). Whereas amplitude rises as sleep deepens, frequency falls. With the very advanced mammals, especially apes and humans, the EEG of both wakefulness and sleep is more complex, and enables further specific

types of EEG to be identified according to certain frequency bands. These are given Greek letters, and, going from high to low frequencies, the *main* divisions are as follows (there are some gaps):

Beta—is usually above 15 Hz and consists of fast waves of low amplitude (under 10 μV) that occur when the cerebrum is alert or even anxious.
Alpha—is normally the range 8–11 Hz, and is typical of relaxed wakefulness and when there is little input to the eyes, especially when they are shut or staring at a blank wall.
Theta—is in the range of 3.5–7.5 Hz and it reflects drowsiness and light sleep.
Delta—these are the slow waves of SWS, and have the lowest EEG frequency, of under 3.5 Hz. They are of a high amplitude, often over 100 μV, and increase in appearance as sleep becomes 'deeper'.

There are some other, more transient EEG activities found only during sleep, such as 'vertex sharp waves' occurring with theta activity at sleep onset, and spindles and 'K complexes' that are most prominent in stage 2 sleep (see Section 6.9). All these EEG characteristics allow human non-REM sleep to be broken down further, and there are standard reference works for this purpose, one for infants[5] and the other for adults[6], describing in detail the EEG and other characteristics of REM sleep and of the four increasingly 'deeper' EEG stages of non-REM sleep—stages 1, 2, 3, and 4 sleep. However, the staging of non-REM sleep is arbitarily defined and still a matter for debate, particularly in the case of the elderly[7]. Nevertheless, this sleep staging is generally accepted. Wakefulness is called stage 0, and is typified by alpha or beta activities. Stage 1 is really a transition stage from wakefulness or drowsiness to true sleep (stage 2 sleep or deeper), and usually occupies only about 5 per cent of the night. Stage 1 is typified by theta activity, a loss of alpha, and often some vertex sharp waves. There is also much 'eye rolling', as the eyelids slowly open and shut a few times, with the eyes rolling upwards and downwards. If one watches someone falling asleep, especially if they are also struggling to remain awake, then these movements of the eyes and eyelids can be clearly seen.

The bulk of human sleep, around 45 per cent of it, is made up of stage 2 sleep, containing a mixture of theta activity, sleep spindles, K complexes, and a few delta waves. Stage 3 is more of a transition phase from stage 2 to stage 4, and constitutes only about 7 per cent of sleep in the young adult. It contains 20–50 per cent delta activity of a certain amplitude. When this activity goes beyond 50 per cent then the 'deepest' sleep, stage 4, is reached. This makes up about 13 per cent of sleep in the young adult. SWS is the collective term for stages 3 and 4 sleep, where delta activity increasingly predominates. The EEG characteristics of the various sleep stages are shown in Fig. 1.1.

REM sleep occurs regularly throughout sleep in nearly all mammals. The

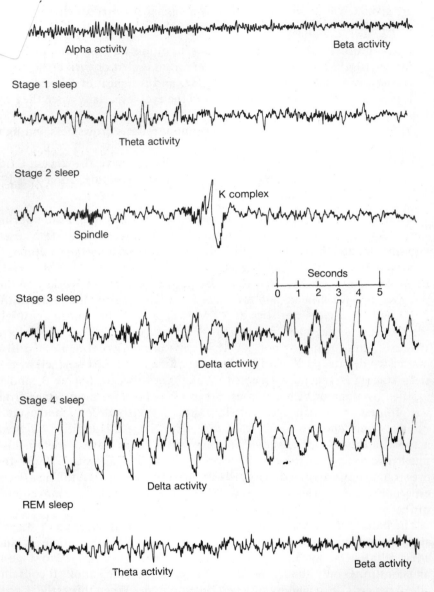

Alpha activity · Beta activity

Stage 1 sleep

Theta activity

Stage 2 sleep

K complex

Spindle

Seconds
0 1 2 3 4 5

Stage 3 sleep

Delta activity

Stage 4 sleep

Delta activity

REM sleep

Theta activity · Beta activity

Fig. 1.1 EEG of human sleep stages. Wakefulness shows alpha activity (subject relaxed) and beta activity (alert). Theta activity can be seen in Stage 1 sleep. Stage 2 sleep shows spindles and a K complex. Note the large slow waves (delta activity) of stage 4, also apparent to some extent in stage 3 sleep. Stages 3 and 4 together are 'slow wave sleep' (SWS). The EEG of REM sleep resembles that of stage 1, and contains a mixture of beta and theta activities. To avoid mistaking these two stages, recordings are made of eye movements and chin muscle tonus (see text).

time from the beginning of one episode of REM sleep to the beginning of the following is remarkably regular within any species, and seems to depend on the brain size of that species.[8] The larger the brain, the longer is this time interval. Whilst in humans it is about 90 minutes, for the rat it is only about 12 minutes. Interestingly, although REM sleep makes up only a small portion of total sleep in most mammal species, normally about 10–15 per cent, humans have roughly double this value. However, for all of them, including humans, this declines with age (Fig. 5.4), and, as I have already mentioned, is much more evident in the newborn. REM sleep is discussed in detail in Chapter 8.

Usually, for humans each minute or half-minute of sleep is broken down into the sleep stages, and the results can be plotted out as a 'hypnogram'. A simplified version is seen in Fig. 1.2, and shows certain key features of sleep:

1. A rapid descent to stage 4 sleep soon after sleep onset.
2. A regular 90-minute cycling of REM sleep and other stages.
3. The prevalence of stages 3 and 4 sleep (SWS) in the first cycle, less in the second cycle, and only some stage 3 sleep in the third cycle. SWS is largely confined to the first half of sleep.
4. A greater predominance of REM sleep and stage 2 sleep in the second half of the night.

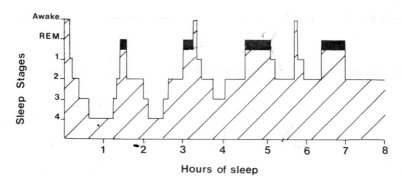

Fig. 1.2 A simplified 'hypnogram' of sleep stage changes over the night in young human adults.

References

1. McGinty, D.J., Drucker-Colin, R., Morrison, A. and Parmeggiani P-L. (ed.) (1985). *Brain Mechanisms of Sleep*. Raven Press, New York.
2. Williams, R.L. and Karacan I. (ed.) (1978). *Sleep Disorders, Diagnosis and Treatment*. Wiley and Sons, New York.

3. Chase, M. and Weitzman, E. (ed.) (1983). *Sleep Disorders: Basic and Clinical Research*. MTP Press, New York.
4. Parkes, J.D. (1985). *Sleep and its Disorders*. W.B. Saunders Co, London.
5. Anders, T., Emde, R. and Parmelee, A. (1971). *A Manual of Standardised Terminology, Techniques and Criteria for Scoring States of Sleep and Wakefulness in the Newborn Infant*. UCLA Brain Information Service, Los Angeles.
6. Rechtschaffen, A. and Kales, A. (1968). *A Manual of Standardised Terminology, Techniques and Scoring System of Sleep Stages in Human Subjects*. UCLA Brain Information Services, Los Angeles.
7. Webb, W.B. and Drebelow, L.M. (1982). A modified method for scoring slow wave sleep of older subjects. *Sleep*, **5**, 195–199.
8. Zepelin, H. and Rechtschaffen, A. (1974). Mammalian sleep, longevity and energy metabolism. *Brain and Behavioural Evolution*, **10**, 425–470.

2. Sleep deprivation

2.1 Problems with animal experiments

One way of finding out about the functions of sleep is through sleep
deprivation, and there have been many such investigations on animals and
humans since the turn of the century. The general findings are that although
humans appear to cope fairly well, other mammals tend to come off worse.
This does not necessarily mean that humans have different sleep functions to
those of animals, but that most of the animal experiments have introduced
additional stresses which have been more eventful. With humans, we can ask
for volunteers to go without sleep for a few days, and impress on them that
they are free to withdraw whenever they want. Also, these volunteers are
carefully looked after, their safety is ensured, and nothing harmful will be
allowed to happen to them. However, none of these factors really apply to
animals, as, for example, we cannot communicate these assurances to them
and so to speak put their minds at rest and allay apprehension. Their natural
lifestyle is totally disrupted, as they are kept awake at times of the day when
they expect to sleep, through methods they do not understand and have no
control over. Although sleep deprivation in animals can be given for a longer
time than for humans, implying that more interesting findings might be
forthcoming, we can still be more confident that the results from human sleep
deprivation studies are less affected by additional stresses.
   The first well-documented experiment of this type on animals was carried
out in France during 1894 by a Dr M. de Manacéine, who kept puppies awake
for 4–6 days by walking or handling them continually. By the end of this time
their body temperatures had fallen by about 4°C, and there was a drop in the
number of red blood cells. Autopsies revealed many small haemorrhages in
the cerebral cortex. These findings stimulated much interest and soon led to
further studies by other laboratories, also on puppies. Again, falls in body
temperature were found, and, although changes in the cerebral cortex were
also reported, these were more variable and of a different nature to those of
Manacéine's puppies. However, few of these experiments used a control
group of animals, and it is likely that some of the changes attributed to sleep
deprivation may have been due simply to laboratory techniques unrelated to

the deprivation itself. Ideally a control group would consist of littermates allowed to sleep normally, so that comparisons could be made with the deprived animals. Such a method was subsequently used in the substantive studies carried out by an American, Dr Nathaniel Kleitman, in the 1920s. Over the next 40 years he performed many more investigations into sleep in both animals and humans, and for these efforts he is usually regarded as the 'father' of sleep research. His great work, *Sleep and Wakefulness*[1], was for many years *the* textbook on sleep.

In Kleitman's early experiments, puppies were kept awake for 2–7 days by groups of assistants walking or playing with the animals. This technique was successful for up to 3–4 days of continued wakefulness, with most of the animals feeding and drinking normally. Thereafter though, they would lose all interest in the surroundings. However, when they were compared with littermate control animals that were not sleep deprived, there was no greater fall in body temperature, nor any important change to vital functions. The only real finding was a confirmation of the earlier reports of a drop in the number of red blood cells in the sleep-deprived animals. Examination of the brains of all the animals showed similar and clear abnormalities for both the groups. Whilst the true reasons for these latter effects are unknown, it is likely that the damage was done during autopsy, as the techniques used for preparing the brains for analysis were crude by today's standards.

Other sleep deprivation experiments of this era used rabbits, but again few used control groups. Probably the best known was by another American, Dr W.G. Crile, who kept rabbits awake for 4–5 days. A slight rise in body temperature and a slowing of respiration were found, but no fall in red blood cells. Autopsies revealed changes to the liver and adrenal gland, as well as to the cerebral cortex. Although Crile could not explain these findings, again it is likely that the autopsy procedure was to blame.

These early studies simply relied on the experimenters' claims that their animals remained awake, and it was not until the 1950s that advances in EEG recording techniques made it possible to measure whether the animal was truly asleep or awake. So until recent times about the only way of making sure that the animal remained awake was to keep it continually moving, but this meant that one was now looking at the effects of physical activity plus sleep deprivation. To some extent the influence of the physical activity alone could be 'subtracted' by giving the same amount of exercise to a control group allowed to sleep. However, it is possible that exercise interacts with sleep deprivation in a way not found in the control group, as, for example, forced exercise when wanting to sleep may be more stressful to a sleep-deprived animal than to a refreshed control animal. This is a problem that Kleitman readily acknowledged, even though he did use control groups. Nevertheless, this questioning about the impact of exercise may be rather theoretical, as it will be remembered that few of the early deprivation experiments which used exercise found any serious abnormality anyway—at least up to 7 days of wakefulness (although using limited and rather crude methods for determining an animal's state of health).

There is one more of the early sleep deprivation experiments that I must mention, carried out in 1946 by Drs J.C. R. Licklider and M.E. Bunch, from Harvard and Washington Universities[2]. Their first aim was to determine the least amount of sleep that laboratory rats could survive on, as usually these animals slept around 12 hours a day. Animals were kept awake by forced walking on a treadmill. Very much to the experimenters' credit, a variety of control groups were used. In an initial pilot experiment, animals were divided into four groups: no sleep, normal sleep, 8 hours sleep, and 4 hours sleep. They were kept like this for several weeks, or, as was to be the case for the totally sleep-deprived group, until they died. This usually occurred after 3–14 days. To Licklider and Bunch's surprise, the 4-hour group seemed to survive 'indefinitely'. The only finding of note was that these animals were extremely irritable and had to be handled with caution.

Licklider and Bunch's next experiment, their major one, now looked in more detail at the effects of 4 hours sleep per day, but this time on young (adolescent) animals, particularly at their rate of growth and learning ability. Control groups were again used, this time in order to try and clarify the effects of the exercise itself, and other potential problems. Animals from the experimental and control groups were still growing, and all had access to food all of the time. Measurements were taken for 10–18 weeks. However, within a few days from the start, the growth rates of the 4-hour sleepers began to fall behind those of the control groups, and after a further 50 days their body weights just levelled off whilst the others continued to grow. But according to the investigators the shortened sleepers seemed healthy enough, apart from irritability. Of great interest was that learning in these rats was certainly no worse than that of the control groups—it was even marginally better.

The most sophisticated studies of sleep deprivation using EEG methods also pair together sleep-deprived and control animals, so that when sleep onset occurs in the EEG of the sleep-deprived animal, it is stimulated into wakefulness. The control animal is similarly stimulated irrespective of whether it is awake or asleep. Because both animals have similar circadian sleep and wake patterns, the likelihood of sleep is greater at certain times of the day, so whenever the sleep-deprived animal is stimulated its partner may also be asleep. Consequently, the control animal also loses some sleep, but only about 20–30 per cent of it, and is certainly not totally sleep deprived. For both animals these laboratory procedures are stressful, and it is assumed that because one animal has total sleep deprivation plus these stresses, and the other only partial sleep deprivation plus the stresses, any greater effects on the first animal are due to the larger sleep loss.

These sophisticated studies are a great improvement on earlier ones where there was little or no control, but there is still the problem that the sleep-deprived animal has a greater disruption to its lifestyle as well as to its sleep. *To be stimulated into wakefulness from drowsiness or sleep, as is the case for the sleep-deprived animal, may be more stressing than to be stimulated whilst already awake*, as is the likelihood for the control animal. Although none of these animal experiments can be perfect of course, they do have the great advantage over the human studies in that more searching measurements can be done, and autopsies carried out afterwards.

Apart from changes in behaviour, one of the best signs of stress in both animals and humans is a marked increase in the output of certain hormones from the adrenal glands, particularly adrenaline and the corticosteroids, with the most notable example of the latter being cortisol. Adrenaline (otherwise called 'epinephrine') is the main hormone produced in the core of the adrenals, the 'medulla', whereas the corticosteroids come from the outer layer, the 'cortex'. Hence the more correct term for these latter hormones is the 'adrenocorticosteroids'. Cortisol helps the body withstand stress by protecting various tissues against excess damage, for example, by reducing inflammation. It combats shock by making body energy reserves more available, and trying to ensure that the volume of the blood and blood pressure can be maintained. The number of red cells in the blood falls as more are switched to a reserve store so that fewer cells would be lost during any bleeding. For reasons that are not clear, it also depresses the immune system. Cortisol can affect the central nervous system and behaviour.

Under non-stressful conditions cortisol is released in small amounts throughout the day, and has an obvious circadian rhythm, troughing at the beginning of a mammal's daily sleep period, and peaking around the start of wakefulness. However, rapid increases can occur within a short while of a stressor occurring, and may be maintained for many days as the adrenal gland can soon grow in size to produce more of the hormone. Eventually though, the gland becomes exhausted and the animal's ability to combat the stressing event fails. Death usually soon ensues. Whilst cortisol helps the organisms to endure stress, especially if the animal is helpless and unable to avoid the underlying cause, adrenaline has a more rapid alerting effect, commonly called the 'fight or flight' response, designed to help the animal quickly avoid the danger one way or another. Of the two hormones, adrenaline and cortisol, the sleep deprivation researcher usually prefers to measure the latter, because deprivation generally lasts for days, and this hormone is much easier to measure than is adrenaline.

In the 1950s a Canadian, Dr Hans Selye, identified three phases in the cortisol response to stress: alarm, resistance, and exhaustion[3], with the last one not usually occurring until many days have elapsed. Although Selye's interpretation is now thought to be too simple an explanation for what is clearly a complex response, his approach is still reasonable for our purposes. Whilst injury and illness are major causes for the intial alarm response, it will also occur whenever the body is pushed to extremes, for example during heavy exercise or in very hot or cold environments. More importantly, psychological factors such as apprehension and fear are potent triggers for this hormone. These can substantially add to the effects of more physical stimuli such as injury. Whilst animals usually show rises in cortisol during sleep deprivation, this tends not to be the case with humans. We can be sleepy, irritable, and have a great desire to sleep, but providing we know that no harm will be allowed to come to us, and that we can pull out of the experiment if necessary, then the deprivation will not necessarily be stressful. This suggests that some psychological factor in animals, such as fear, may be influencing their cortisol response to deprivation. It must be borne in mind that illness and tissue damage will also activate the alarm responses. So I cannot be clear about how much of the raised cortisol levels in sleep-deprived animals is due to physical illness, fear alone, or fear as a result of the illness.

2.2 Recent animal experiments

The most elaborate sleep deprivation studies ever performed on animals are being run at the Chicago University Sleep Laboratory—a premier sleep laboratory established 25 years ago by Dr Allan Rechtschaffen, and still under his direction. Kleitman was also at Chicago University, but in another department. He retired soon after Rechtschaffen's arrival, and his sleep laboratory closed down. Rechtschaffen's pioneering work along so many lines of sleep research has brought him a level of respect from sleep researchers that equals that accorded to Kleitman.

Rechtschaffen and his team began their sleep deprivation experiments on rats in the early 1980s[4-8]. Two main types of study were performed: (1) total sleep deprivation, and (2) deprivation of REM sleep only. For each of these there were impressive control procedures using control animals. The centrepiece of this laboratory's equipment was the apparatus for sleep deprivation —a horizontal, circular rotating platform 45 centimetres in diameter, surrounded by shallow water. A vertical barrier divided the platform into halves, allowing a sleep-deprived animal to be confined to one side and a control animal to the other. The platform could rotate slowly under the barrier. When this occurred, both animals had to move to avoid being gently propelled into the surrounding water. As rats dislike getting wet they would do their best to avoid falling in.

Each animal had its EEG continuously monitored by a computer. When sleep was detected in the rat to be deprived of sleep, the platform would promptly rotate, causing the animal to rouse and move along the platform. Its partner, which might be awake or asleep at the time, had to move likewise, and to the same extent. Generally, control animals lost about 25 per cent of their sleep, compared with about 92 per cent for the experimental group. Although this procedure was indeed stressful to sleep-deprived animals, as shown by increases in adrenal gland weights and cortisol secretion, the control animals seemed to experience a similar amount of stress for most of the experimental period, as both these indices rose to similar extents in them as well. For REM sleep deprivation alone, the platform only moved when REM sleep was detected. The technique was quite effective, as virtually all of REM sleep (99 per cent) could be eliminated, whereas the control partner only lost about 4 per cent of its REM sleep. Although the experimental animals were still able to take most of their non-REM sleep (which makes up about 88 per cent of sleep in the rat), there was some unavoidable loss of the 'deeper' form of non-REM sleep. This was a problem of some concern to the investigators, and I will come back to this later.

For both types of sleep deprivation, experimental and control animals were under constant light, and food was always available. The environmental temperature was set at what is neutral for the rat. Total sleep deprivation caused general debility, weight loss, and death by about the 21st day. The control rats all survived the experience, although they became debilitated and lost weight to some extent. Post mortem examinations were performed on all the animals. Examinations were carried out on the brain, liver, kidneys, spleen, lungs, duodenum, stomach, thyroid, and thymus, with the pathologists not being told from which group each animal had come. Surprisingly, no significant differences were found between the two groups for any of these organs. As the investigators pointed out, one of the remaining possibilities was that death may have been due to undetected biochemical abnormalities. So far though, there is no sign of what, if any, these might be.

In the total sleep deprivation procedure, both experimental and control animals ate much more food, whilst also losing weight. However, these effects were far more apparent in the experimental group. Calculations by the investigators on the energy obtained from digested food and from breakdown of the animals' own body tissues showed a very large rise in the energy usage, to around 2.5 times the baseline levels for the experimental group, and to 1.7 times these values for the control group. It seemed that such increases were being used to fuel a large rise in metabolism. Although most of this energy need was coming from voracious eating, particularly in the experimental animals, the fall in body weight showed that the animals' own energy stores were being depleted. But this weight loss was probably not the cause of death in the sleep-deprived animals, as at death their weight had only fallen to about 80 per cent of the starting value. The investigators have shown that starved rats that were not sleep deprived can still survive at 70 per cent of their original body weight.

Sleep-deprived animals were digesting their food normally, and there was no sign of diabetes or other illnesses that could account for weight loss and voracious eating. So what was happening to all this energy, and was it all going to fuel increased metabolism? The gland that has a major effect on metabolic rate is the thyroid, but its hormones showed no changes. Could 'stress' still be the answer? There were no noticeable differences in the size of the adrenal glands between the two groups for most of the time, from the start of the deprivation until the death of the sleep-deprived animal. However, there was a rise in adrenal weight a few days before death.

· To try and determine the stress responses further, the investigators made more detailed analyses of blood samples from both groups of animals, every few days. Apart from the measurement of cortisol and other blood con-stituents, assessments were also made of the hormone that controls cortisol release—adrenocorticotrophic hormone (ACTH). Both the sleep-deprived and control groups showed similar rises in these two hormones, with no significant differences between the two groups for either substance. Except of course, for the few days prior to the death of the experimental animals, when there was a greater rise in cortisol. The other blood constituents showed no notable differences between the groups, except that the hormone noradrenaline (norepinephrine) was far higher in the experimental animals. The exact reasons for this were not really known. This hormone has many interesting actions, with several relating to metabolism and the regulation of heat loss from the body. For example, it limits heat loss from the skin by restricting blood flow to skin capillaries; also, it makes body fat supplies more easily available as an energy source for other tissues. One important role for noradrenaline is to stimulate special heat-producing organs called 'brown adipose tissue' (BAT or 'brown fat') to burn up more energy for heat. However, this tissue is usually only found in infant animals and is gone by adulthood. It is not known if the rats used in the Chicago studies had any brown fat reserves. I shall cover the role of this tissue in more detail, in Section 8.13.

An important finding with the totally sleep-deprived group was that body temperature fell during their last days, and this, together with the earlier increases in feeding and raised metabolism, suggests that something serious happens to the ability of the animal to conserve its body heat—that is its thermoregulation becomes impaired. This state of affairs was not so appa-rent in the control animals. What seems to be happening, although we cannot be certain, is that soon after sleep deprivation begins the experimental animals increasingly lose body heat, presumably through the skin, and com-pensate by burning more energy to increase metabolism and create more body heat. More and more food has to be eaten, but even this is not enough, as body energy reserves also have to be sacrificed on this metabolic fire. For the first 2 weeks, heat production matches heat loss, as body temperature stays normal. But then there is a deterioration, with heat loss exceeding heat production, and body temperature falls. Although death follows a few days later, it is not yet known whether this is due directly to the collapse of thermoregulation, or just that this collapse is a symptom of something more subtle but nevertheless catastrophic which is not yet understood. The control group did not reach this state, as their body temperature never fell, at least up to the time they were killed, when their experimental partners died.

The physical appearances of the sleep-deprived animals changed in a characteristic way, apart from the weight loss. After about a week of total sleep deprivation their hair developed a yellowish tinge and became matted. The skin of the tail and paws developed small red inflamed areas that eventually developed into often quite large lesions, very much like ulcers, but containing only a minor infection. These got worse as the deprivation progressed, and also began to appear in the control group, but at a slower rate of development. Surprisingly, all the animals seemed unconcerned about these sores and paid little attention to them. The lesions were only on the bare skin of the tail and feet, and were not found under the fur. Careful examinations by specialists in skin diseases were made of the lesions, and it was concluded that these were not due to wetness or pressure on the skin. They remain a puzzle. Although there are suspicions that a biochemical change in the skin may be the cause, perhaps even a vitamin deficiency, there is no evidence of this, despite careful chemical analyses.

To see whether the animals were becoming debilitated from infections, blood was analysed to find out if the immune system was functioning normally. Immunology is a highly complex area (see Section 3.8), and only a few tests could be performed. Nevertheless, such tests would have been discerning enough to pick up anything unusual going on, but nothing remarkable was found. In fact, the remarkable finding was that there was nothing unusual, given the animals' circumstances.

What is happening to the sleep-deprived rat? So many blanks have been drawn. All that we apparently have so far is what seems to be a problem with thermoregulation, and the skin lesions. Neither of these seemed to be due to the animals getting wet through falling in the water, as this was also investigated. As far as can be seen, little else seems to be going wrong. Rechtschaffen and colleagues are cautious about speculating over their findings. Although they believe that heat loss and thermoregulation lie at the crux of the demise of their animals, they emphasize that more proof is required. This would, for example, come from careful measurements of metabolic rate, which so far have been difficult to carry out in the sleep deprivation apparatus. Usually, animals would be put inside a calorimeter (a chamber for measuring body heat production), but a sleep-deprived animal quickly falls asleep there, and sleep alters metabolic rate.

Nevertheless, I would like to concentrate on thermoregulation a little more as I believe it to be a crucial factor. Firstly, let me give some more background, because even the normal and healthy rat has potential problems with its thermoregulation. Like other small mammals it has a relatively large body surface area in proportion to its weight. Simple geometry shows that, as body weight doubles, surface area only increases by about 60 per cent. If you keep on doubling size in this way until something of the mass of a human is produced, the body surface becomes quite small in proportion to its weight. If there is any deterioration in the ability of the body surface to keep heat in, then this will become an increasing problem the smaller the mammal is, with less body mass to generate heat in proportion to surface area.

Body heat loss is less of a concern to humans than it is to rats, mainly because of our relatively large mass in proportion to surface area. But the animal usually has effective countermeasures, both physiological and behavioural. Both are mostly aimed at protecting its more exposed body areas, the paws, and especially the large tail. Physiologically, blood flow to the skin is reduced here and, behaviourally, the animal can sit on its tail or curl up into a ball.

Now, it seems to be fairly certain that sleep-deprived rats are losing a large amount of body heat; presumably, a major potential route for this loss is through the tail and paws. Even though these animals are in a neutral environmental temperature, this is still below that of their body, and body heat can still be lost. Since food intake rises and weight falls as soon as deprivation begins, the apparent increase in heat loss seems to begin immediately. I suspect that a sleepy rat is less aware of this loss, and the animal may 'forget' to sit on its tail to conserve body heat. It cannot curl up for long, as the inevitable sleep and prompt movement of the platform makes it wake up and walk. From what I have seen of sleep-deprived rats, their tails are almost always exposed. If too much heat is being lost here, then one would expect the animal to protect its tail as much as possible—but sleep-deprived rats are not doing this. They still have the physiological counter-measure, of reducing the blood flow to the skin of the tail and feet. Whether or not the eventual appearance of ulcers in these areas is related to the problems of thermoregulation, or is just a coincidence, is an open question. Perhaps a prolonged restricted blood supply to the skin of the tail and feet, lasting for a week or so, promotes skin ulcers?

Enough of this speculation of mine, and let us return to some other fascinating findings from the Chicago Group. They had suspicions that the inevitable REM sleep loss during total sleep deprivation might have been a key factor in the deterioration of their animals, as REM sleep deprivation alone also led to death. But, as the investigators noted, the difficulty with this idea is that death occurred much later during REM sleep deprivation, after an average of 37 days—almost twice as long as for totally sleep-deprived animals. REM sleep deprivation produced very similar effects to total sleep deprivation, including the skin lesions, except that the course of events was spread over a longer time. Stress seemed slightly higher in the REM sleep-deprived animals than in their control partners, as cortisol and ACTH levels were somewhat higher, but this was not really apparent until about the week before death. The most dramatic difference was again a large increase in food intake, which began soon after the REM sleep deprivation started. Calculations of the energy used by the REM-sleep-deprived animals showed a massive 3.2 times rise over that of the predeprivation levels, against a 1.9 rise for the control group. Body temperature stayed normal for the first 2 weeks of REM sleep deprivation and then fell, but always remained stable for the control animals.

If REM sleep deprivation was the key to the death of the totally sleep-deprived animals, why would REM sleep deprivation alone allow them to survive for twice as long? Maybe REM sleep deprivation is of little relevance after all! Instead, perhaps the fatal factor is not the type of sleep that is lost but the amount, of whatever type. Returning to my earlier line of thinking—the greater is the sleep loss the more the sleepiness, and the greater the impairment to the behavioural countermeasures, etc. Remember, as REM sleep deprivation allows animals most of their non-REM sleep, they had about as much sleep as did the control animals for the total sleep deprivation experiment. Although these latter animals were not allowed to survive for as long as the REM-sleep-deprived rats (they were killed off after about 3 weeks when their partner died), they were showing the same rate of decline and debility as the REM-sleep-deprived animals.

Interestingly, there is another line of argument that returns to the type of sleep that is lost—not REM sleep, but something else. This is a view that Rechtschaffen's group was inclined to take—cautiously though. It stems from an unwanted effect of REM sleep deprivation—the unavoidable loss of about half of the high amplitude variety of non-REM sleep, which might be the equivalent of SWS in humans (i.e. stages 3 and 4 sleep). To see whether this particular sleep is crucial, the Chicago group ran another experiment, depriving rats of it by using the standard procedure, with control animals also stimulated at the appropriate time.

However, survival time rose back up to an average of 41 days, close to that of REM sleep deprivation. Again animals showed the characteristic signs, almost a doubling of food intake, weight loss, and skin lesions. Unfortunately, there was a problem as this type of sleep deprivation also reduced REM sleep by about 60 per cent. It seems that one cannot deprive a rat of purely REM sleep or purely the 'deeper' non-REM sleep, as the two types depend on each other in some way. Totally deprive the animal of one and the other is seriously affected.

We still cannot be sure if loss of both these types of sleep, as happens in total deprivation, is *the* cause of death, or whether there are more vital aspects of sleep. Certainly, complete removal of one type and the inevitable loss of about half of the other does not produce such rapid death, but delays it by about another 2 weeks, despite retention of much of the 'lighter' sleep. Is this 'lighter' sleep helping to sustain the animal for these extra 2 weeks, or is it the presence of what is left of either REM sleep or the 'deeper' sleep? Or are both these factors important? These are unanswered questions I'm afraid, as we must wait and see what else comes out of this remarkable laboratory over the years.

Let me quickly summarize what is known about total sleep deprivation in animals. It is lethal, but we can still only make informed guesses as to why this is so, as most organs seem to function normally—except that is the skin on exposed body surfaces, which develops lesions, and perhaps the brain (in as much that its behaviour is impaired). Stress produced by the sleep deprivation method rather than the deprivation itself must have some impact. Nevertheless monitoring this stress via similarly disturbed control animals, as the Chicago Laboratory has done, still points to a fatal effect of sleep loss. Two types of sleep may be particularly crucial to survival: REM sleep and what I have loosely called the 'deeper' form of non-REM sleep. These interact with each other in some way. Surprisingly though, rats seem to survive quite well on much less than their normal sleep, even on as little as one-third and, of course, this was the main finding from Licklider and Bunch's study (Section 2.1). Presumably what sleep is left contains vital components, which may be the two types of sleep just mentioned. However, little is really known about this topic. So far, it seems that the debilitating effects of sleep deprivation are most noticeable through voracious eating, a fall in body weight, and what seems to be a large increase in the production of body heat, coupled with a similar body heat loss. Eventually body temperature falls, thermoregulation collapses and the animal dies. However, we do not know whether this collapse is just a symptom or is the cause of death. Neither do we know the explanation for the changes associated with body heat. Perhaps the energy exchange and metabolic processes within cells go awry, or maybe the thermoregulation control centres in the brain go 'out of tune'. Obviously the animals become very sleepy, and I have suggested that they are probably less 'aware' of heat loss, and 'forget' to behave in the appropriate way, for example by keeping their tails less exposed. This would worsen problems related to the physiological changes I have just mentioned, or it might even be the central problem.

2.3 Some problems with human experiments

The longest studies of sleep deprivation in humans were carried out in California during the late 1960s, where volunteers were deprived of sleep for 8 to 11 days[9-11]. These are discussed in detail in Sections 2.5–2.7. Surprisingly, little seemed to go wrong with the subjects physically. The main effects lay with sleepiness and impaired brain functioning, but even these were no great cause for concern. On the other hand, the Chicago Sleep Laboratory findings clearly showed that their rats were becoming seriously debilitated well within 8 days of total sleep loss. Why this difference between humans and rats? Perhaps it is because life and death go more quickly for a rat, with its higher metabolism and lifespan of only a few years. Of the doubtless numerous other alternatives, the following one may be particularly important.

Whilst the methods for keeping animals awake are stressful in their own right, requiring careful control and measurement, there is much less of a problem in this respect with human subjects. They are much more cossetted by their experimenters, perhaps too much so in some instances, with the subjects inadvertantly protected from the full effects of sleep loss. Apart from the deprivation, subjects usually lead a tranquil existence, are fed well, and, except for having periodically to undergo batteries of physiological and psychological tests throughout the day, they have plenty of time for relaxation. Usually, for their safety, and so that they can be observed closely, they have to stay within the vicinity of the laboratory. Although this rather unrealistic existence could counteract sleep deprivation effects, the alternative, to let them loose in a sleepy state into the outside world, would be unwise, as even crossing the road is dangerous. I am not claiming that this rather serene existence would totally counteract any debilitating or even fatal effect of sleep deprivation, only lessen it somewhat. More to the point, I do not believe that such an existence could have offset potentially harmful effects of sleep deprivation for as long as 8 to 11 days. The most plausable reason for the uneventful physical findings with these human subjects is that, in contrast with the rats, sleep loss is not particularly harmful.

More lifelike and real-world investigations of sleep deprivation in humans have been carried out by various military research groups throughout the world, mostly using male soldiers. Such enterprises are referred to by the military as a 'sustained operation'—'SUSOP' for short. Some of the ethical and safety factors applied to the civilian subject can be put aside, and typically sleep loss is for 3 days of continuously simulated battle. Unfortunately, from my perspective, this usually also includes heavy exercise and food restriction. So whilst the outcomes are more eventful, we still do not know to what extent the findings are due to sleep loss or the other factors. When more serious effects do emerge, the investigators tend to attribute these to the exercise etc. rather than to the sleep loss[12]. Such effects are generally stress responses of one sort or another.

Unlike the civilian subjects in the laboratory studies who can pull out of the experiment whenever they want to, the soldier cannot do this so easily, and is under pressure to see the manouevre through. Any anxiety he has about what may happen to him and whether he will be able to cope will add to the stress. On the more positive side of these studies, though, is the consant stimulation and physical activity of military maneouvres which help to counteract sleepiness. So, although I may have implied that safety is being jeopardized for the sleep-deprived soldier, in fact the alerting effect of the situation may result in greater safety in the longer run. Sleepiness is much more of a problem for the laboratory-bound subjects, who can be very bored after a day or so of sleep deprivation. Cossetting and tranquility, then, are perhaps the last things they want.

Another issue with human studies is that many of the measurements carried out are not really relevant to the understanding of sleep function. Investigators using civilian subjects in the laboratory have tended to assume that sleep deprivation will be be very stressful. For example, some believe that sleep rebuilds tissues after the 'wear and tear' of wakefulness, whilst others consider that sleep resolves 'inner emotional conflicts'. If these notions are true, then loss of sleep would presumably be stressful, for example, because of a lack of tissue repair, or through rising emotional conflicts. Such stresses would be in addition to those produced by more psychological factors such as the subject's apprehension. Consequently but reasonably, most of the measures carried out on these subjects are oriented towards stress, and not so much towards sleep function, particularly as stress is much easier to measure than are tissue repair processes. This is not meant as a criticism, as many investigators have not really been interested in sleep function, but in more practical aspects such as how subjects cope with sleep loss. Disappointingly for these researchers perhaps, is the fact that such stress measures have not produced very much.

If sleep were an essential tissue repair process for most of the human body, and sleep deprivation caused impairments to various organs, then there is little evidence of this. Although part of the reason may be the lack of appropriate measurements, so that potential troubles would not have been detected anyway, if any organ was ailing to any appreciable extent, then it would set off an alarm response and cortisol output would rise. This does not seem to be happening to the laboratory-bound subject. Even with the sleep-deprived soldier the alarm response is usually only minor, and is best explained not by organ malfunction but by anxiety and other psychological reasons.

When assessing how well subjects cope with sleep deprivation, comparisons are often made with the 'baseline' condition, that is the levels of the various measures taken before the deprivation begins. But often subjects have shown more signs of stress before the experiment than during it! This rather odd finding is easily explained as subjects may be excited by the challenge of sleep deprivation, or may be apprehensive about bad things that could happen to them during the deprivation. After all, so many of us are brought up on the idea that we need a good 7 hours or so sleep each night otherwise something bad will happen, even though few know what this might be. Such a notion makes good grounds for worrying about what might happen during deprivation. The experimenters themselves are often agitated at the beginning of these experiments, worrying about whether the equipment will work and whether the subjects will stay the course. This feeling of concern can be passed on unwittingly to the subjects, and further add to their apprehension and lead to rises in the subjects' cortisol levels. However, after the first night of sleep loss everyone begins to relax and settle into the routine, as subjects begin to see that things are not so bad as they may have thought and experimenters become more confident. Stress subsides. Several sleep deprivation studies have certainly been affected in this way, and sometimes without the experimenters realizing it. Consequently, the distorted findings lead to confusion about what exactly sleep deprivation does. Even though a few of these studies have run control groups of subjects who were not sleep deprived, it will not necessarily resolve this particular issue. Here is one advantage of animal studies, as during baseline measurements the animals have not the slightest idea of what is about to happen to them.

Finally, I have been and for the time being will be concentrating on total sleep deprivation in humans, and not on the effects of partial sleep loss over many days—such as curtailed sleep, or disturbed sleep periods containing much wakefulness. It could be argued that partial sleep loss is of far greater relevance to real life, found for example, with the insomniac, the shift worker, and the mother of a young baby. However, as I am concerning myself with the functions of sleep, the effects of total sleep deprivation will give more insight than would the findings of long-term partial sleep loss where many other unwanted factors creep in. The insomniac is usually an anxious person anyway, and often so is the mother of a new baby, who has many other pressures on her in coping with a new member of the family. The shift worker is sleeping at the 'wrong' time of the day, and may still have to look after certain household and family activities that normally occur in the daytime. In many of these cases it is not so much a lack of sleep but sleep disturbance, and this causes daytime sleepiness. As I will be describing in Section 6.8, if such sleepiness is not present, then despite what seems to the sufferer to be 'not enough sleep', sufficient sleep has usually been obtained. Besides, as will be seen in Chapter 6, most of us may not really need all of 7–8 hours sleep a night, and can 'learn' to take 1–2 hours less sleep per day without encountering increased daytime sleepiness, or difficulty in getting up in the mornings.

2.4 1896—The first real sleep deprivation experiment on humans

Nowadays, most of the scientific experiments carried out in the last century are seen to be just of historical interest, and all too easily dismissed because of crude techniques and equipment. Some though, are still impressive for their discoveries and careful experimentation, and amongst these is the sleep deprivation study run in 1896 at the Iowa University Psychological Laboratory, by Professor G. T. W. Patrick and his junior colleague, Dr Allen Gilbert[15]. These investigators showed remarkable powers of observation and still, nearly a century later, most of their original findings remain sound despite the volume of sleep deprivation research conducted since then. Several of the more recent studies have even fallen below the standards set by Patrick and Gilbert. Because their work is so impressive, let me describe it in more detail.

The experiment began with a preliminary pilot study on one subject, namely Allen Gilbert, who remained awake continuously for 90 hours. He is described as, 'a young man of 28 years, unmarried, of perfect health, of nervous temperament, of very great vitality and activity, who is accustomed to about 8 hours of sound sleep from 10 p.m. to 6 a.m.'.

Sleep loss ran from the night of Wednesday 27 November 1885 to midnight the following Saturday. When he was eventually allowed to sleep, the study was still not over, as the hapless Gilbert was awakened at 1-hourly intervals to see how deep his sleep was. Patrick wisely noted that a sound stimulus would not be practicable as the subject would soon get used to it. So an 'electric garter' was fixed around Gilbert's ankle. The current could be increased steadily until he awoke and pressed an 'electrical button' by his bedside. The level the current reached indicated the depth of sleep.

The second hour of his recovery sleep seemed to be the deepest as Gilbert could not be aroused until the current went well beyond expectation, and he 'responded with a cry of pain'. The next deepest period was in the very first hour of sleep, followed by the third hour. Even at these times the current was three times greater than what he could tolerate during wakefulness. The hourly procedure continued until he woke spontaneously at 10.30 a.m. next morning, and it was claimed that he was 'wholly refreshed, felt quite as well as ever, and did not feel sleepy the following evening'. The next night he slept for only 2 extra hours. If the extra sleep taken on these two recovery nights is added up, it comes to only 25 per cent of the total sleep lost. To account for this, Patrick and Gilbert concluded that it was the increased depth of sleep that held the key to recovery—an observation borne out many times since then.

During the deprivation Gilbert coped relatively well, although, 'on the second night he did not feel well and suffered severely from sleepiness. The third night he suffered less. The fourth day and following evening he felt well and was able to pass his time in his usual occupations'.

Over the last 50 hours he had to be watched closely and could not be left alone, as despite his best efforts he would lapse into sleep. In particular, Patrick noted that, 'the daily rhythm was well marked . . . during the afternoon and evening the subject was less troubled with sleepiness. The sleepy period was from midnight until noon, of which the worse part was about dawn'.

Gilbert experienced several visual illusions, especially after the second night; for example, 'the floor was covered with a greasy-looking molecular layer of rapidly moving or oscillating particles'. Often this layer was a foot above the floor, which caused some problem as he would try to step on to it when walking. Later, the air was full of these dancing particles that developed into what appeared to be swarms of coloured gnats, gathering around the gaslight. He even got up on a chair in an attempt to swat them away. Fortunately, this problem disappeared after his first night of recovery sleep.

Systematically, every 6 hours during the deprivation, and once on the day following the first recovery sleep, Gilbert was given a 2-hour series of 14 tests, mostly of a psychological nature. Because repetition at these latter tests improves performance, he had to practise them thoroughly before the study. This was a prudent move, which even some recent sleep deprivation studies have neglected. The extent and variety of this testing is impressive, even by today's standards. Measurements included:

- Body temperature and heart rate, body weight, grip and pull strengths.
- The average of 15 reaction times at a morse key to 'click' sounds.
- A vigilance test using the morse key, with the subject only required to respond to loud clicks and not to soft ones.
- Muscle fatigue, as shown by the decline in finger tapping over a minute.
- Sensitivity to pain, monitored systematically by increasing pressure on the fingertip using a 'specially prepared alogmeter'.
- Acuteness of vision, by reading with a candle placed 25 cm away.
- Memorizing nonsense syllables, and adding lists of numbers to see how many could be done in 3 minutes.

Patrick paid special attention to several of these findings, starting with Gilbert's body weight, as this increased by 27 oz over the deprivation, and then, perplexingly for them, fell 38 oz during the first recovery sleep (it is now known that sweating generally increases during sleep, and such a water loss would have accounted for some of the fall in weight, but not for all of it). Gilbert's grip and pull strength weakened, but when the end of the deprivation was in sight he regained his strength. Reaction time dropped, and so did vigilance, but both returned to normal after the first night of sleep. Surprisingly, acuteness of vision improved during deprivation, only to return to normal levels on recovery. Remember though that this was only the 'pilot study'. So let us go on to the main experiment, carried out a few weeks later.

This experiment was similar, and used two more volunteers from the University staff, who were men aged 24 and 27 years, 'accustomed to 8-9 hours sound sleep'. Both underwent 90 hours of deprivation. Neither experienced any illness, hallucinations, nor discomfort throughout the proceedings. One had more trouble keeping awake than the other, and could not have gone on beyond the 90 hours. Jogging in the streets was found to be good for livening up one subject, especially during the 5.00 a.m. sleepy period. On the first recovery night both slept from 11.15 p.m. to 10.30 a.m. the next morning, and this time their sleep was not interrupted like Gilbert's. They then dozed, one for a further 45 minutes and the other for 4 hours. Surprisingly, it was the subject who had coped better during the deprivation who slept for longer. Both then declared that they felt quite refreshed. By extending their recovery sleep to beyond their usual amounts, one subject regained 16 per cent of his lost sleep, and the other 35 per cent. This small recovery of lost sleep is a finding that has been noted many times by subsequent researchers.

A similar series of measurements was given as before, and in addition there were tests for: remembering shapes, speed in reading letters backwards, and discriminating between two sounds. Even the urine of these two subjects was chemically analysed for nitrogen and phosphoric acid, with both substances showing increased output during deprivation. The experimenters could not explain this, but we know now that the most likely reason is through increased eating, which is commonly found during sleep deprivation. Although Patrick and Gilbert made no mention of what or how much the subjects ate, this was probably the cause of the weight increases that were also found. Again, weight fell during the recovery sleep.

The new memory test caused problems for one subject who became thoroughly confused at one point. The reaction times, addition, and letter-reading tasks were all greatly impaired in both subjects. All subjects, including Gilbert, were seen to have frequent very short 'naps' lasting for only seconds, which are nowadays called 'microsleeps' (see Section 2.8). Daydreaming also commonly occurred. Several times the experimenters noted that if a subject put more effort and enthusiasm into various tasks then sleepiness could be countered somewhat, at least until about 60 hours of deprivation. This is exactly what has been concluded much more recently in reviews of modern sleep deprivation research[14,15]. Finally, Patrick and Gilbert noticed that body temperature fell 0.2–0.4°C in all subjects during deprivation, but that the daily rhythmicity of this temperature remained. In one subject, the one who had the greatest difficulty with the deprivation, the fall in body temperature was more eventful and dropped by 1.5°C for a short while. A fall in body temperature has subsequently been found to be a common outcome of sleep deprivation in humans (see Section 3.5), although it is still not clear whether this indicates a problem with thermoregulation, as seems to be the case for the sleep-deprived rat.

2.5 The longest study—264 hours without sleep

In January 1964 Randy Gardner, a 17-year-old schoolboy from California, was determined to beat the world record of 260 hours without sleep—4 hours

short of 11 days. Since his early youth he had been fascinated by 'extremes'
and enjoyed the challenge of difficult projects, especially if he had been told
that they could not be done. He was physically and mentally healthy, with no
history of psychiatric disorder. He was a self-assured and confident individual who described himself as 'a little on the egotistical side'. A local science
fair was to be held near his home in San Diego, and this seemed to be a good
opportunity for the marathon. Also, as it happened, not far away was a well-
known sleep laboratory, run by the US Navy. He set as his target 264 hours
without sleep, and enlisted the aid of two friends who worked shifts to keep
him awake, which they succeeded in doing successfully until his goal was
reached. His record still remains unbroken as the longest documented
account of continuous sleep loss, although there are other questionable
claims. At no time did he take any stimulant drugs, or even coffee. His
parents were apprehensive but encouraging, and as the news media got more
interested as the enterprise progressed, he and his supporters became even
more motivated to succeed.

   After 150 hours of wakefulness, to the relief of his parents, he was
supervised by a local Navy doctor and thereafter increasingly by researchers
associated with the sleep laboratory. These included other physicians, and he
underwent several physical, neurological, and psychiatric examinations
towards the end of the vigil, which I will come to shortly. However, no cause
was found for any serious concern about his health, which remained remarkably good throughout. Several reports have been written on these
findings[9,16,17].

   During the second deprivation day he began to notice difficulty in focusing
his eyes, which became extremely heavy and tired, and, for example, he had
to stop watching television for the rest of the experiment. By the third day he
had begun to develop mood changes, minor ataxia (impairment to co-
ordinated body movements), and some difficulty with speech, particularly in
repeating tongue twisters. Also, he felt nauseous. During the fourth day he
became irritable and unco-operative, and developed lapses of memory.
Difficulty in concentration became obvious, and he had the feeling of a tight
band around the head. He began to see 'fog' around street lamps, and on the
following night he had an illusion that a street sign was a person. Shortly
afterwards he imagined that he was a great football player, and became
resentful when people disputed this.

   By the fifth day things began to settle down and improve somewhat,
although daydreams, such as non-existent plants in a garden, were still
present. On the sixth day the ataxia returned together with the speech difficulties, memory lapses, some irritability and unco-operativeness, and the
inability to concentrate. These effects continued for the next 2 days, with his
speech becoming more impeded, and deteriorating to a slow, soft, and
slurred incoherence. By day nine his thoughts were fragmented and often he

did not complete sentences. Blurred vision became much of a problem during the last 2 days he believed that certain people were trying to make him seem foolish because he kept forgetting things. Throughout the 11 days, the early morning hours were the most difficult when Randy Gardner's sleepiness and all the associated problems were worse. At no time did he show true psychotic behaviour or lose contact with reality.

After having reached his goal, he went to bed and slept for 14.75 hours, waking up spontaneously and feeling well, but somewhat sleepy. All of the difficulties he experienced with speech, memory, daydreaming, etc. had disappeared. Over the next two nights he took a total of an extra 6.5 hours sleep on top of the normal amounts (4 hours the second night and 2.5 on the third). Although we do not know exactly how much more sleep he took over subsequent nights, apparently this was not much. Overall, he regained about 24 per cent of the lost sleep, a figure like that seen by Patrick and Gilbert so many years earlier, and a theme that I shall be focusing on later.

Before I go on to describe this recovery sleep in more detail, let me continue a little further with what happened to Randy Gardner during the deprivation, and describe the result of a full medical examination carried out on him 12 hours before the end of the vigil. His blood pressure and pulse were normal, although his body temperature was about 1.0°C under the norm. Nothing is known about his metabolic rate. The more clinically significant, although not serious findings, were dry eyes, nasal and throat congestion with swelling of the associated lymph nodes. A heart murmur was detected, but this was no cause for alarm and disappeared by the second recovery day. The electrical activity of his heart shown by an electrocardiogram (ECG) was quite normal. Blood and urine samples were taken and numerous tests were carried out on these, for example various blood cell counts (useful signs of many illnesses) and measures of liver and kidney function.

Tests were also carried out on the responsiveness of his autonomic nervous system (this looks after the control of most physiological processes—i.e. homeostasis). There were some signs of increased general activity, with the system's responsiveness to external stimuli reduced somewhat. The most noticeable finding was a large 10°C fall in skin temperature due to a pronounced constriction of the skin capillaries, indicating that body heat loss was being cut down. This effect, which may have something in common with the Chicago Sleep Laboratory findings with rats, returned to normal after the first night of recovery sleep. Unfortunately, little information is available about what happened to Randy Gardener's body temperature throughout the study.

Neurological tests showed a severe decline in attention, and speech and memory were clearly affected. These were obvious signs that cerebral function was affected. Eye movement control deteriorated, and a squint developed together with nystagmus (an involuntary and jerky movement of the eyes). A squint usually causes double vision, but he denied experiencing this. He showed severely drooping eyelids (ptosis), and under normal circumstances this would be of neurological concern, but of course this is a natural process of sleepiness. He generally lacked any facial expression, and although this might also have suggested some disorder, he could with effort still muster up the energy to show facial emotions, which was a more healthy sign. There was hand tremor, and occasional involuntary jerks occurred in his upper arms. However, co-ordination of the hands was hardly affected, and neither were his balance nor walking ability impaired, although some of the leg reflexes were more responsive. The conclusion[16] from this neurological examination was that the effects of sleep loss were relatively minor, except in the case of the cerebral cortex which seemed more affected. An EEG was taken, but this simply indicated extreme sleepiness and nothing particularly abnormal. However, it must be remembered that the EEG is only a rough guide to cerebral functioning. Neurological tests carried out 10 days after the deprivation showed that everything was almost back to normal.

The key to Randy Gardner's ability to stay awake was his determination to succeed, coupled with all the support and encouragement of those around him. The best methods for achieving this end were cold showers, physical activity, particularly walking, and having something interesting or exciting to do. These brought him back almost to normality for a while, and this is illustrated by what happened on the final night of deprivation. He and two of the experimenters went for a walk in San Diego, and one of them wrote[9], 'there was little in his behaviour during this period (midnight to 5 a.m. and 230 hours of sleep loss) to suggest that he had been awake longer than his companions. At one point, in an all-night restaurant, the three companions engaged in competition on a complicated pinball machine with the subject holding his own in every way'. (p. 31).

Randy Gardner's recovery sleep was recorded on an EEG for three successive nights in the nearby sleep laboratory. On each occasion he was allowed to sleep for as long as he wanted to. His sleep was not monitored before the deprivation began, and all the sleep laboratory had for comparison were further nights of recordings, at 6 and 10 weeks after the deprivation, when any 'carry-over' effects would have disappeared. In Table 2.1 I have averaged together these later nights, and show the amounts of the various sleep stages (see Section 1.3). If we can assume that these values are typical for a normal night of his sleep, then multiplying them by the 11 nights of deprivation gives us an idea of the totals lost. Below this row are the respective amounts for the three recorded recovery nights, but with the usual baseline value subtracted out. So they now show what is over and above the usual nightly value. For example, 90 minutes are given for stage 4 sleep on recovery night one. The full amount on that night would be 90 plus the 23 minutes

Table 2.1 Randy Gardner's recovery sleep—over three nights following 11 nights of total sleep deprivation. Note that recovery was incomplete by the third night, and that high priority was given to the return of the lost stage 4 sleep. See text for explanations. (Adapted from Gulevich et al.[9])

	Sleep stages (minutes)				
	1 + 2	3	4	REM	Total sleep
Baseline*	234	42	23	65	364
Total lost	2574	462	253	715	4004
Recovery sleep nights: amount in excess of baseline					
Recovery 1	164	91	90	171	516
Recovery 2	27	67	44	123	261
Recovery 3	− 9	56	37	87	171
Total	182	214	171	381	948
% regained	7%	46%	68%	53%	24%

*Average of 6 and 10 week post-sleep deprivation follow-up nights

baseline value taken from the row above. I have added the excesses across the three recovery nights and have given these as a percentage of the total lost.

What can now be seen is that about two-thirds of the lost stage 4 sleep was reclaimed, together with about half of the lost REM sleep. Only a very small portion of the lighter sleep stages, 1 and 2, was reclaimed. All together, this makes up only 24 per cent of the total sleep lost. Of special interest is the first recovery night, after which Randy Gardner felt almost back to normal. This contained five times the usual amount of stage 4 sleep and over three times the usual REM sleep, suggesting that these are the more crucial sleep stages. Stage 4 sleep, the 'deepest' sleep, occupied much of the first few hours of sleep, and this again bears out the observations of Patrick and Gilbert. In the next deprivation studies I will be describing, the evidence indicates that stage 4 sleep may be of greater importance than REM sleep to the subjects for their feeling of recovery, with, at best, only about half of our REM sleep being crucial in this respect.

What has this famous study to tell us about sleep? Some say very little, because only one subject was used, and what he showed may be the exception rather than the rule. A fair point, so I will go on to some other notable studies using more subjects. But these fall short of 264 hours in their length of deprivation. The findings with Randy Gardner certainly give us important clues about sleep, and these can be quickly summarized: (1) adverse effects were confined to the cerebrum and behaviour, with the rest of the body coping remarkably well; (2) body temperature fell, and there were signs that body heat loss was being cut down; however, there were no indications of large rises in his heat production; (3) a marked circadian rhythm in sleepiness was very evident; (4) much of the recovery from the deprivation occurred during one extended period of sleep, which contained relatively high amounts of stage 4 and REM sleep; (5) over the recovery nights, only specific portions of the lost sleep were reclaimed, particularly most of the lost stage 4 sleep and about half of the REM sleep.

2.6 Abnormal behaviour

Randy Gardner showed little sign of psychotic behaviour, and neither did the subjects of Patrick and Gilbert, nor for that matter do most other subjects undergoing sleep deprivation. This is an important point because some textbooks have claimed that sleep deprivation produces artificial psychoses that can be used as 'models' for the real illnesses. So it is reasoned that we could learn more about psychotic illness by studying normally healthy sleep-deprived subjects. Such a notion has arisen mostly through a misunderstanding of various behaviours in sleep-deprived subjects, and perhaps an unwarranted interest in the rare subject who does show strong psychotic tendencies. In these cases it is usually found that the individual had some sort of psychological problem already. One sleep deprivation study actually used hospitalized schizophrenic patients, and it is perhaps not surprising that the deprivation caused a psychotic flare-up. In two other often-mentioned studies claiming that florid psychoses develop, each case had a previous history of psychiatric disorder, for example obsession and pyromania. In my own work, where we usually sleep deprive subjects for 72 hours, we have only ever encountered difficulties, albeit minor, in a few people with more extremes of personality, for example those who are very introverted and withdrawn, or very excitable and extroverted. These people make up only a minority of the population. Now we screen them out as potential subjects because they can be disruptive and upset everybody else. Since this precaution has been taken, we have never had any problems of this kind.

It is common for subjects to experience visual misperceptions, such as those reported by Patrick and Gilbert, and by Randy Gardner. An excellent example of the range of these is given by the five-point rating scale, shown in Table 2.2. This was developed by researchers at the Walter Reed Medical Centre in Washington, renowned in the 1960s for its work into sleep loss[18]. The scale goes from minor visual difficulties, with a rating of 1, to simple hallucinations at a rating of 5. At this latter level, subjects believe in what they see, and such beliefs can be more a sign of psychotic-like behaviour than the visual experience itself. It is a more healthy sign if a subject knows that the misperceptions are not real. Studies at the Walter Reed Centre, which I shall be coming to in Section 2.8, found that 90 hours of deprivation seldom brought scale ratings beyond 2 or 3. And it can be seen in Fig. 2.2 that even in

Table 2.2 Visual misperception scale for sleep deprivation. (From Morris et al.[18]. Reproduced by permission of American Medical Association—*Archives of General Psychiatry*)

---

1. Eye itching, burning or tired; difficulty seeing, blurred vision or diplopia.
2. Visual illusions: changes in or loss of shape, size, movement, colour or texture constancies; disturbed depth perception.
   Examples: 'The floor seems wavy.'
   'The light seems to flicker.'
   'The size and colour of the chairs seems to change.'
3. Labelling of illusions, but with no doubt concerning their illusory character.
   Examples: 'Looks like fog around the light.'
   'That black mark looked like it was changing into different rock formations.'
4. Labelling of illusions with some doubt concerning their reality.
   Example: 'I thought there was fuzz around the bottle.'
   'I thought steam was rising from the floor, so I tested my eyes to check whether it was real.'
5. Labelling of illusions (hallucinations) with, for a time at least, belief in their reality.
   Example: 'I saw hair in my milk. The others said there wasn't any, but I still felt there was and would not drink it.'
   'That (Rorschach card) looked like an envelope, I turned it over to check, and it had my name and address on it.'

---

the 8-day deprivation experiment, covered in the next section, the average rating only rose to 4.

Some experimenters refer to all the misperceptions experienced by sleep-deprived subjects as hallucinations, which is a gross overstatement as this should only apply to experiences comparable to scale point 5 and worse. Remember, point 5 is still relatively trivial as hallucinations go. Nevertheless, because psychotic patients hallucinate, especially those with schizophrenia, parallels have been drawn between this disorder and sleep deprivation effects in normal people. Not only is there a great contrast in the magnitude of these experiences, but more importantly the types of hallucination these patients have are mostly auditory and not visual. Hearing voices and believing in what these say is the commonest example. Very few sleep deprivation studies have reported such auditory hallucinations, or even anything minor in this respect, like auditory misperceptions.

I would like to make two final cautionary remarks about visual misperceptions. First, sleep-deprived subjects are usually kept within the confines of a laboratory environment, and this produces a form of visual monotony which by itself can also lead to visual misperceptions, especially if the lighting is poor. Consequently, we do not really know to what extent the misperceptions of sleep deprivation are due to monotony, sleep deprivation, or both. Second, sleep deprivation can have a peculiar effect of heightening suggestability, as the sleepy and confused state of subjects may easily lead them to believe something which they would be less credulous about under normal circumstances. A night of recovery sleep soon brings them back to their normal reasoning. During sleep deprivation the experimenters can unwittingly lead subjects to expect that certain things may happen to them, including experiencing misperceptions. This is a self-fulfilling prophesy as the misperceptions will appear more readily, owing to the subjects' heightened suggestability. Another aspect of this suggestability relates to something I mentioned in Section 2.3, that subjects sometimes become worried about what might happen to them during sleep deprivation, which may be the basis for a stress response. Because of the heightening of suggestability during sleep deprivation, such beliefs can occasionally get out of all proportion.

Before leaving the topic, I must emphasize that this suggestability is not the same as hypnotic suggestability, and there is no evidence to show that sleep-deprived subjects are more hypnotizable. 'Brainwashing', an appalling practice known to have been carried out on prisoners of war, builds on the confused state produced by sleep loss, plus prolonged isolation and depersonalization.

Irritability, aggression, and suspiciousness can also occur in subjects. Although these could be more symptoms of psychosis, and supporting the 'model of psychosis' idea for sleep deprivation, some degree of irritability is natural with extreme sleepiness. The monotony and confinement of the experiment, with repetition of what can seem to the subject to be senseless tests, will be aggravating, and worsened by sleep loss. Experimenters can be under pressure and may be socially inept with the subjects, and subjects may fall out with each other. So, any irritability shown by subjects has to be taken within the context of the actual study, and this is often overlooked by the experimenter in their subsequent reports. A similar argument applies to suspiciousness. Whilst this behaviour can sometimes be largely attributed to the loss of sleep itself, alternatively and understandably it happens because the experimenter has decided not to tell subjects exactly what is going on, so as not to prejudice the outcome of a test. In these circumstances the subjects may have grounds for being suspicious, and this feeling can be worsened by loss of attention through sleepiness, and the subject forgetting how to do the test.

There have certainly been great differences between studies in their approach to subjects. For example, one (that shall remain nameless), involved 5 days without sleep, and incorporated strict military-type discipline, with vigorous sports, tactical problems, night marches, etc. On the other hand there was the friendly, everybody-is-equal approach of the Walter Reed experiments (see Section 2.8). Coincidentally or otherwise, chaos broke out in the former study, with widespread irritability amongst subjects, several unprovoked fights, gross feelings of persecution, and a 22 per cent drop-out rate. None of this happened to the Walter Reed subjects, who were deprived of sleep for almost as long. Now it could be argued, of course, that the first study paints a more realistic picture of what happens during sleep loss, whereas in the other the subjects were so cosseted that their behaviour was artificial.

Overall, the evidence is not strong that sleep deprivation produces psychosis, or leads to such disorders in the weeks afterwards. In the second longest study, of 205 hours without sleep, to be described next, the experimenters were quite definite about the absence of psychotic signs in their subjects. Interestingly, one or more nights of total or partial sleep loss, especially REM sleep deprivation, or restricting sleep to the first half of the night, may even be beneficial to those people suffering from the more severe ('endogenous') type of depression. Mood improvement is often found, even euphoria, and such forms of sleep deprivation have been used as a therapy[19,20]. These effects though, only seem to occur in depressed patients, and are seldom found with normal subjects. I will be covering this area more in Chapters 6 and 8.

2.7 The longest study with more than one subject—205 hours

The study on Randy Gardner not only involved a single subject, but was largely unplanned as the experimenters were not at first aware that the marathon was taking place. Word only got to them when it was well under way, and the circumstances were not ideal. Nevertheless, they responded quickly and obtained valuable findings. The longest planned study using more that one subject was run in September 1966, at the Neuropsychiatric Institute at the University of California at Los Angeles. Participants were to be paid quite well, and an advert at a student employment bureau brought forward seven volunteers all in their early twenties. Two were rejected on health grounds and one other pulled out when he clearly understood what was involved. The remaining four, all men, were in excellent physical health, and seemingly in good mental health, although it turned out that one was a troubled man. He became progressively withdrawn during the study and needed much support from the others. He had 'led an extremely unstable existence' in childhood, and not long after successfully completing the study he was arrested for being a naval deserter—a complete surprise to the investigators.

A large and impressive variety of measures was incorporated into the experiment, covering physiology, hormones, neurology, EEG, psychology, and behaviour[10,11,21,22], together with recovery sleep[23]. The subjects were initially studied for 3 days beforehand, with baseline measurements taken every 6 hours. This 6-hourly assessment continued throughout the deprivation period and into 3 recovery days. The laboratory was spacious, comfortable, air conditioned, brightly lit, with a TV, table tennis, and a record player. Experimenters were always around. To help keep awake, the subjects had alcohol rubs, and periodically immersed their faces in bowls of ice cubes and water. Meal times were every 6 hours.

They ate very well, in fact remarkably well, as at their request the daily Calorie intake had to be increased to beyond 5000 per 24 hours. This was at least 50 per cent more than they should have needed, even taking into consideration the extra food at night for being awake rather than asleep. Why these subjects wanted to eat so much is not clear. Boredom may have been a factor, but they were kept fairly busy. I have also noticed from my own experiments that subjects want much more food than seems necessary, and I am struck by the similarities here with the voracious eating of the sleep-deprived rats from the Chicago Sleep Laboratory.

The plan was for the subjects to go without sleep for 9 days (eight nights), which they all accomplished. At that point, at the end of their endurance, all thought that a further 24 hours could still be just possible—if they were paid enough. The offer was declined by the experimenters, who were themselves worn out. Extreme sleepiness did not set in until the third day, when, for example, reading became impossible. Keeping awake was particularly difficult between 02.00 h and 04.00 h each day, and this can be seen in Fig. 2.1, which shows their self-ratings of sleepiness. By the fourth day irritability was more common, and by the fifth day social interactions within the group had reached the lowest point, and misperceptions and general levels of coping were at their worst. Changes in their visual misperception ratings on the Walter Reed Scale (see last Section and Table 2.2) are shown in Fig. 2.2.

As I have already mentioned, this did not reach the level of true hallucinations, although an interesting experience was recorded with one subject (not the deserter), who temporarily went 'beserk' during a tedious task of tracking a spot of light across an oscilloscope screen. He suddenly screamed in terror and fell to the floor sobbing and muttering incoherently about a gorilla. It seems that he began to fall asleep during the task, and a nightmare or night terror rapidly came on. The investigators were obviously very concerned about this, and one of them, a psychiatrist, interviewed him when he had gathered his senses shortly afterwards. He confessed to having a similar experience in his sleep when a child, with the recurrent theme of Humpty Dumpty being attacked by a gorilla. When staring at the oscilloscope the screen changed into this scene, and this had already happened several times during the experiment, but he had felt too embarrassed to mention it. Having talked about the problem, he was able to return to the task, and after another similar episode, it seemed to disappear.

At the end of the fifth day, various improvements began to occur amongst

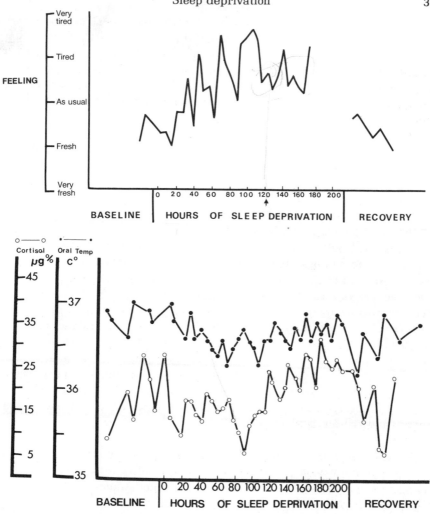

Fig. 2.1 205 hours of sleep deprivation—average changes for four men. (Upper) subjects' ratings of fatique; (Lower) oral temperature and blood cortisol (a measure of stress). Note the 'fifth-day turning point' (see text). (From Naitoh et al.[22]. Reproduced by permission of Elsvier Scientific Publishing.)

the subjects, and this is evident in their sleepiness ratings in Fig. 2.1. Other investigators have noticed this phenomenon and have called it the 'fifth-day turning point'. It is not really understood and it may be more psychological than 'organic'. For example, the end of the experiment comes in sight and morale improves, or the experimenters may inadvertently lead the suggestable subjects to believe in this turning point.

Although lapses of attention ('microsleeps'—see next section) were common, particularly in the early hours of the morning, it was reported that no subject exhibited 'psychosis, loosening of thoughts, flattening of emotions, delusions or paranoid ideas' (ref. 11—p. 502). Apart from defects in cerebral function, repeated neurological examinations showed nothing else of great clinical interest—only minor changes similar to those of Randy Gardner that I have already described.

Despite the battery of physiological and biochemical tests, there was nothing of clinical relevance to show that any subject suffered from physical illness. Again, the significant outcome of this investigation lay with the feeling of sleepiness, behavioural changes, and impaired performance at psychological tasks. These results further support the findings from earlier studies, that it is the cerebrum that is affected most by sleep loss, with the rest of the body coping remarkably well. To emphasize this lack of physical effect, let me briefly describe the various physiological measures that were taken, and the findings. Regular blood samples were taken and determined for cortisol, and urine was measured for metabolites of cortisol and adrenaline. The metabolites of the latter hormone showed great variation over the sleep deprivation period, but no overall trend. Fig. 2.1 shows that blood cortisol values decreased a little over the first days, and then showed a small rise up to the seventh day, to level off at a slightly higher value than that of the baseline. However, these baseline values are greater than what would normally be expected. One possible reason is that the subjects were apprehensive beforehand—an example of what I mentioned earlier in Section 2.3. Nevertheless, these baseline cortisol values still indicate that this anxiety was minor, and the levels at the end of deprivation point to little of clinical concern.

Heart and respiration rates, the ECG trace itself, blood pressure, and various psychophysiological tests of autonomic function all showed no changes of note during the deprivation. Like other studies, however, there was a fall in body temperature, this time up to the 'fifth day turning point', followed by a notional rise (see Fig. 2.1). EEGs were taken 6 hourly, and all that these revealed was a progressive change in brain activity towards increased sleepiness until the fifth day, when there was some improvement—as in the trends for the other measures. No abnormalities of brain function were found in the EEG, although it should be noted that measurements were not frequent enough to detect any spasmodic and short-lived phenomena, had they occurred.

All the subjects spent three recovery nights in the sleep laboratory and had their EEGs monitored continuously throughout sleep. Unlike Randy Gardner, they were not allowed to sleep for as long as they liked, but were only permitted 12 hours for the first night and 9 hours on each of the next two nights. Nevertheless, after the first night there was a considerable improvement in their well-being, and as can be seen from Fig. 2.1 their subjective ratings of tiredness show them to be feeling almost back to normal the next day. Although their performance at various psychological tests returned to baseline levels after this first recovery night, it is possible that increased motivation from feelings of success etc. and an overnight rest from the tasks, may have enhanced this effect.

In Table 2.3, I have given the sleep stage findings over the three recovery nights in the same way as before (Table 2.1), with the values shown as changes from the baseline levels. The baseline nights were recorded before the deprivation began. Again it can be seen that whilst all of the lighter stages 1 and 2 seem to have been lost for good, most (79 per cent) of the lost stage 4 sleep was recovered during these three nights, particularly on the first night, when over four times the baseline value was recorded. From the trends over the three nights it is likely that more stage 4 sleep recovery would have occurred over the subsequent unrecorded nights, indicating its almost total return. Partly as a result of the sleep restriction, only a third of the lost REM sleep was recovered on the recorded nights, with most of this return happening on the first night. But despite the lost two-thirds of REM sleep the subjects were behaviourally back to normal. More REM sleep recovery probably occurred on the unrecorded fourth night and beyond, although if one looks at the rapidly falling values in the return of REM sleep over the three recorded nights, halving each night (154, 81, and 39 minutes respectively), then it seems unlikely that the total return would have exceeded 50 per cent of that lost. Such findings again show that only a part of lost sleep needs to be recovered, with much of stage 4 sleep and about half of REM sleep

Table 2.3 Recovery sleep after 8 days sleep deprivation—sleep stage characteristics for three recovery nights, averaged for four young adults. Recovery was still incomplete after the third night. As in Table 2.1, the greatest return was in stage 4 sleep. Note that sleep length was limited, and that this may have curtailed the return of REM sleep. See text for details. (Adapted from Kales et al.[23])

	Sleep stages (minutes)				
	1 + 2	3	4	REM	Total sleep
Baseline	276	63	38	104	481
Amount lost	2208	504	304	832	3848
Recovery sleep nights: amount excess of baseline					
Recovery 1	− 78	37	126	154	239
Recovery 2	− 116	24	70	81	59
Recovery 3	− 46	23	43	39	59
Total	− 240	84	239	274	357
% regained	− 11%	17%	79%	33%	9%

Note: Total sleep times limited to 12, 9 and 9 h on the three recovery nights.

appearing to be crucial in this respect.

This experiment and that on Randy Gardner have produced so little of significance with general body physiology. Is this really so, or were the measures too crude to detect subtle changes? In the 20–25 years since these studies were completed there have been many technological advances in physiology and biochemistry, which have since been utilized in further sleep deprivation experiments. However, I am not going to deal with them now but in the next chapter—suffice it to say that the outcome is largely the same as these two classic investigations. For the moment I want to stay with some other pioneering work in sleep deprivation, albeit only 30 years ago. These were exciting times from the perspectives of what was happening to behaviour and performance at psychological tests. After all, it is in this field where the effects of sleep loss are really noticeable, and perhaps where the major functions of sleep may lie—seemingly in the cerebral cortex.

2.8 The Walter Reed experiments

In the 1950s and early 1960s most sleep deprivation investigations centred on the Walter Reed Army Institute of Research in Washington. Many experiments were run under the leadership of Dr Hal Williams. Several important findings were made with psychological performance and behaviour. Generally, deprivation lasted for 72–98 hours. Most of the published reports were based on results from relatively large numbers of subjects, using 20–60 young men at a time. I have already mentioned some of the work of this group in relation to the Visual Misperception Scale (Table 2.2). This was compiled by Drs Gary Morris, Ardie Lubin, and Hal Williams[18]. They also produced two other five-point scales for observers to rate sleep-deprived subjects—assessing 'Cognitive Disorganization' (Table

Table 2.4 Cognitive Disorganization Scale. (See text for explanation) (From Morris et al.[18]. Reproduced by permission of the American Medical Association—*Archives of General Psychiatry*)

1. Slowing of mental processes, some difficulty thinking of words (no undue interference with normal communication).
2. Occasional mistakes or failures in thinking and speech which can be corrected easily.
3. Loses train of thought, forgetting what he was thinking or talking about, leaving statements incomplete, etc. Sudden unexplained shifts in trend of thought or speech; can correct with effort if challenged.
4. Some thoughts or statements become completely incoherent. Clarification is not altogether possible. Some confusion of fantasies, dreams, or intrusive thoughts, with reality.
5. Rambling, incoherent speech for brief periods, with failure to recognize errors. Unable to straighten out jumble of incoherent thoughts when challenged.

Table 2.5 Temporal Disorientation Scale. (See text for explanation.) (From Morris et al.[18]. Reproduced by permission of the American Medical Association—*Archives of General Psychiatry*)

1. Time seems to pass slowly, or to be 'different' in duration.
2. Occasional mistakes in thinking about time with spontaneous correction.
3. Occasional mistakes as above, but does not recognize error until questioned.
4. More frequent mistakes which subject believes to be correct. Uncertain when confronted.
5. Gross disorientation in time, or unshaken belief in mistaken concept of time.

2.4) and 'Temporal Disorientation' (Table 2.5). The former scale concerns thinking and speech, and determines to what extent a chain of mental operations can be sustained. At a rating of 4, daydreams become incorporated into waking thought processes, and this ties in with a scale value of 4 for the 'Misperception Scale' described earlier. Both scales show similar trends during sleep loss, and relate to the general decline in cerebral functioning. Morris and colleagues reported that cognitive disorganization remained at a value of 1 up to the second night of deprivation, and then went up about one point daily, to reach a value of 3 at 90 hours of deprivation.

The awareness of time is something we take for granted. Most of us know about time and how it passes from our watches, clocks, etc. However, even without these aids we are quite good at estimating down to a fraction of an hour, how long ago a particular event occurred. It may seem surprising, but the ability to perceive time is an advanced form of mammalian behaviour requiring a high level of cerebral functioning. The Walter Reed researchers found that sleep deprivation distorts this perception in interesting ways, hence their 'Temporal Disorientation Scale'. Sleep researchers tend to underrate this phenomenon, and it is seldom explored systematically. Morris and colleagues noted that by the third night of deprivation a value of 1 on this scale was typical, rising to 2 after 90 hours.

All three scales were subsequently used in the 205-hour sleep loss study (Section 2.7), up to the sixth or seventh day of deprivation, and the results can be seen in Fig. 2.2. I have already described the findings with the Misperception Scale in the previous section. Changes in the Temporal and Cognitive Disorganization Scales were very similar to those of the Walter Reed studies, up to the 90-hour point. They then rose a little more to level off at the 'fifth day turning point'.

One of the most famous reports from the Walter Reed laboratory introduced the topic of 'microsleeps'[24], following a remarkably detailed account of the decline in psychological performance for a total of 49 subjects who were sleep deprived for 72–90 hours. A variety of tasks was given, for example, several types of reaction time test, vigilance, and memory tasks. Although performance declined in most of them, it was the way by which

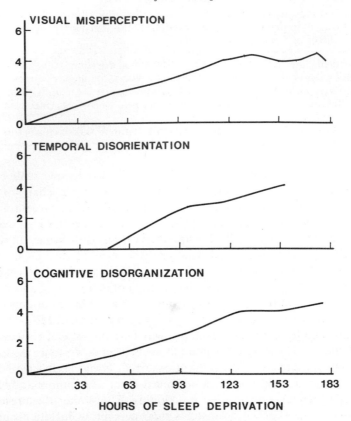

Fig. 2.2 Findings with the three Walter Reed rating scales (Tables 2.2, 2.4 and 2.5): changes in misperceptions, time estimation, and thinking, averaged over subjects during the 205-hour deprivation study. (From Pasnau *et al.*[11]. Reproduced with permission of the American Medical Association—*Archives of General Psychiatry.*)

performance fell that held great interest for the authors, as this seemed to take the form of lapses or 'microsleeps' lasting for a few seconds. These were defined as brief periods of no response, accompanied by extreme drowsiness and a change in the EEG, approaching that of light sleep. It will be remembered that something similar was described by Patrick and Gilbert (Section 2.4).

It is doubtful whether subjects obtain much benefit from these lapses as they are too short, and real sleep beyond stage 1 is thwarted. Even if all the microsleeps over a 24-hour period are added up, on say the third day of sleep loss, it is unlikely that the total will come to more than 20 minutes. The Walter Reed group noted that lapses not only increased in frequency and duration as sleep deprivation progressed, but were strongly affected by the monotony of the task—the duller and more monotonous this was, the more frequent were the lapses. In tasks where the subject had full control over the test, going at his or her own speed ('subject paced'), the time taken by the subject to complete the exercise lengthened due to the lapses, but errors were few. On the other hand, if the timing of the task was solely controlled by the experimenter, the test duration was unaltered, and errors were much more evident. Although this conclusion seems rather obvious, what Williams and colleagues did was to describe these effects in a systematic way.

They also measured how long sleep-deprived subjects could maintain a good standard at a simple and monotonous vigilance test. Under normal conditions, 10 minutes at this task presented no problem, but following one night of deprivation performance began to fall after about 7 minutes, and after 3 minutes following two nights deprivation. However, if the task became more interesting by telling subjects how well they were doing, then performance would greatly improve. At least, this was so for the second and perhaps third night of deprivation, and shows that subjects still had the capacity to do relatively well during the first few days of deprivation—it was their motivation which was affected initially. This is a theme that has been developed further by Dr Bob Wilkinson, a leading researcher in England, from the Applied Psychology Unit in Cambridge, whose work I will be coming to shortly.

Williams and coworkers believed that their lapse hypothesis could acount for impairments to other aspects of psychological performance during sleep deprivation, including memory. So it was thought that the reason for the noticeable decline in the recall of events presented only a short while before-hand (i.e. 'short-term' memory), was because of lapses during the original presentation of the material. However, further experiments by his group to test this idea failed to confirm it[25], but instead showed that the memory trace itself was affected in some way, independent of lapses. Nevertheless, with certain qualifications, the lapse hypothesis still seems to hold true, for several other aspects of performance decline during sleep deprivation. Needless to say, at the time of their investigations the Walter Reed group were very enthusiastic about the hypothesis. This was understandable, as other researchers were thinking along the same lines, and Williams and colleagues ended their famous paper of 1959 with the lucid description given a few years earlier by their English contemporary, Dr Donald Broadbent[26], also from the Applied Psychology Unit in Cambridge:

Crudely speaking, a (sleep deprived) man is not like a child's mechanical toy which goes slower as it runs down. Nor is he like a car engine which continues normally until its fuel is exhausted and then stops dead. He is like a motor which after much use misfires, runs normally for a while, then falters, again, and so on. (p. 2)

2.9 Motivation and cerebral 'impairment'

But not everyone agrees with the lapse hypothesis, especially Dr Anders Kjellberg[27]. He pointed out that sleep deprivation by itself cannot be the sole cause of sleepiness and lapses—we should also consider the environment and other circumstances that may encourage sleepiness. Often, these can promote sleepiness in their own right, particularly tedious tasks like vigilance tests. He sees lapses as the culmination of periods where there has been a progressive lowering of arousal, and not as sudden 'misfirings' as Broadbent suggests. In Kjellberg's terms, Broadbent's car begins to run slowly before it misfires. To continue this car analogy, a tedious task is as if the car was running uphill, and more likely to run slowly and misfire. A stimulating task can be compared with a downhill run with less misfiring.

A question that Dr Bob Wilkinson has been asking, which I have also been very interested in, relates to whether this downhill run can counteract the misfiring completely? That is, could the effect of sleep deprivation on cerebral functioning wholly be due to problems of motivation, rather than to some fundamental impairment of the brain through, for example, a lack of repair to neural networks? If motivation was the sole answer, then it would be possible to overcome sleepiness just by the sleep-deprived subject applying more compensatory effort. However, the incentive for the subject to do this would have to be very attractive and involve an exciting task.

I can put this issue into other terms. Sleepiness may not be a sign of necessary repair to neurones, etc. but simply the result of a build-up of some behavioural drive to sleep, designed to keep mammals occupied during tedious and unproductive times—the hours of darkness in the case of humans. If this was so, then conceivably a drug or chemical antidote might be found to remove sleepiness, leaving the brain to function normally without sleep for a very long time. Whilst this might be true, I believe that it is only part of the answer, as I shall be arguing in this book that both alternatives are operating. In other words, some sleep is probably necessary for essential repair to neurones, etc. and the rest of sleep is maintained beyond this point by a behavioural drive to sleep, occupying the remaining or unproductive hours of the night.

Therefore, during sleep loss, part of the behavioural and psychological changes could be due to cerebral impairment (because the essential repair and restitutive processes of sleep have been prevented), with the remainder being due to an accumulation of a non-restitutive sleep drive. I must emphasize however, that this *cerebral impairment is not to be viewed as brain damage, but a reversible state, analogous to the impairment and recovery of muscle after exercise.* However, unlike exercise recovery, which takes place during the physical rest of wakefulness, this cerebral restitution can only take place during sleep. Returning to the analogy for sleep deprivation of the misfiring car, I propose that the misfiring occurs not only because the engine is becoming worn, needing to be switched off, and serviced for a while (i.e. cerebral restitution), but also because the accelerator is sticking (i.e. a build-up of the sleep drive). Let me develop these ideas further, beginning with the work of Wilkinson.

2.10 Tasks sensitive to sleep deprivation

At the time the Walter Reed studies were in progress, the Applied Psychology Unit in Cambridge was also carrying out pioneering work into sleep loss, initiated by Broadbent but continued to considerable lengths by Wilkinson. In the late 1950s to mid 1960s Wilkinson ran a series of carefully conducted studies, several of which complement the Walter Reed experiments. His work led him to write an often quoted and succinct review covering the state of the art[14]. His views relating to the psychological aspects of sleep deprivation are still very much in vogue today, and I will summarize the key points. Of the main factors affecting how a sleep-deprived subject will cope with a psychological performance task, such as the length of deprivation, circadian rhythms, etc., Wilkinson highlighted two in particular:

Duration of the task—impairments worsen with the longer the task. Performance can be maintained at normal levels for a few minutes, even after a few days of deprivation. Therefore, if testing is only given for a minute of two, little effect may be found.

Type of task—Wilkinson noted in his review paper of 1965 that since the time of Patrick and Gilbert there had been over 40 experiments looking at the effects of sleep deprivation on psychological performance, using a wide variety of tasks. One would have thought that we could make fair comparisons of the vulnerability of these tests to deprivation. Sadly this was not to be, because, firstly, until the 1940s most of the tests were given for too short a duration to find anything worthwhile. Secondly, although some refinements have been made since then, only broad comparisons could still be made, owing to a lack of uniformity between laboratories in the way they administered the tests. However, Wilkinson could make some conclusions as it was clear that certain types of test nearly always show the effects of deprivation, and others do not. A category of sensitive tests is typified by 'reaction time'. This comes in various forms, but usually consists of a series of stimuli, given at a rate of around 12 per minute, to which the subject has to respond as quickly as possible by pushing a key. If there is only one type of stimulus and one response key, then the test is 'simple' reaction time. More complicated versions come with a greater array of stimuli and keys, and are called 'choice' reaction times. Another task that is sensitive to sleep loss is the vigilance test, where a subject has to watch a monotonous display, for example a radar screen, and try and spot an occasional small change. In his characteristic practical outlook to sleep deprivation, Wilkinson developed several performance tests that were sensitive to sleepiness. His reaction time and vigilance tests were purposely designed to be long, dull, and uninteresting, and it is not surprising that they are so sensitive to sleep loss. They are reminiscent of certain everyday tasks like motorway driving, and monitoring a production line in a factory.

. On the other hand, tasks involving plenty of visual stimulation and movement of the hands are more stimulating, and can maintain a subject's interest. Such tasks are remarkably resilient for up to 2 days of sleep deprivation, even when given for an hour or so at a time. One example is a computer-TV 'battle game', reminiscent of the fighter pilot in action, or even a car driver driving along a complex route at speed. Wilkinson demonstrated this resilience in one of his best-known studies of 20 years ago[28]. He used a battle-game task, not so elaborate as the modern computer versions, but good enough to keep subjects excited. It was comparable to what the soldier or pilot in the field might be doing, and showed no detriment in performance, even when given for an hour at a time after 60 hours without sleep. On the other hand, an equally difficult task that was much more abstract and less stimulating was severely impaired even after one night of sleep loss. It simulated what a battle commander at headquarters might be doing, that is, making a series of decisions on how to deploy one's defences after having been given information from coded signals. The main mistake made was to miss certain key signals and fail to act on them.

Although complex tasks are liable to be severely impaired by sleep deprivation, the return of near-normal performance when motivation is increased presents a problem for a cerebral restitution hypothesis for sleep. Such tasks are remarkably complex and require a high degree of cerebral involvement. So one might well ask, if the cerebrum needs sleep for essential repair processes, why then does sleep loss not rapidly impair performance here? Surely these findings only support a purely motivational hypothesis for sleep loss? That is, going back to the car analogy, are there just problems with the accelerator, not with the engine itself?

Further support for this latter interpretation seems to come from what happens to another highly 'cerebral' task, IQ (Intelligence Quotient) performance. This is also usually unaffected by two nights of sleep deprivation, although beyond this time IQ performance does fall. But for the moment I do not want to get sidetracked about IQ testing, as such tests do have a certain shortcoming (that I will come to later); I want to stay with the issue of motivation. The crucial question is, can performance really go back to normal if the incentive is high enough?

Let us return to the work of Wilkinson, as he became very involved with this theme in his other sleep deprivation experiments. Subjects would be given incentives to put extra effort into the tests, through competing with one another and by his giving them clear feedback on how they were doing ('knowledge of results'). He found that after one or two nights of deprivation the usual decline in performance at reaction time tests and at a monotonous vigilance task, the renowned 'Wilkinson Auditory Vigilance Test' (see below), could largely be avoided when this incentive was added. Interestingly, a reliable guide to whether or not the subject was actually applying extra effort came from measuring muscle tension in the forearm. Increased tension meant more effort and better performance.

Now it could easily be thought that such simple tests have little relevance to higher cerebral functioning. But this is not necessarily so, as the data from them can be analysed in more complex ways. Take for example Wilkinson's vigilance test, where the subject listens to a series of monotones given at a rate of one every 2 seconds. Interspersed among these background signals is another monotone, the target signal, which is slightly different from the others. As the two types of tone sound very alike, careful concentration is required to detect the difference. Subjects can make four types of response: (1) correctly identify a target signal (a hit), (2) miss this signal, (3) wrongly respond to a background signal (a false response), and (4) correctly identify this background signal and ignore it. Scores on these dimensions can be integrated in various ways, with one of the most interesting using the 'Theory of Signal Detection'[29]. Here, two values can be calculated, which have complex terms, but it is reasonable to call one '*detection*', and the other '*caution*'.

Within the context of sleep deprivation the former is a guide to certain aspects of cerebral function, whereas the latter is to some extent an indicator of motivation and how willing subjects are prepared to make a false response. These two values are separate entities. So, for example, a subject may not be sure if he or she detected a signal, and wonder whether to respond with a yes or no. Here is where caution comes in. If subjects are highly motivated to do well (and they are not 'punished' in any way for making a mistake) then they will be less cautious and say yes. Detection can be used as a guide to cerebral impairment, but there is some controversy about using caution as a measure of motivation. So, I will concentrate on detection, particularly as it is of greater interest to me anyway.

2.11 Higher levels of cerebral function

From Wilkinson's findings it is apparent that without additional incentives the sleep-deprived subject shows a steady fall in detection over two nights of sleeplessness. When incentives are added though, detection remains at normal baseline levels for at least one night and the following day of deprivation, but by the second night it falls. However, the types of incentive given by

Wilkinson may have lost some of their novelty and interest by this second night, and maybe his subjects could have done better if they had been more inspired. Consequently, we still do not know whether the eventual fall in detection reflected a real decline in the subjects' capacity to perform, or whether we are back to the problem of motivation again. I was intrigued by this issue and decided to follow up Wilkinson's work.

Money is an excellent incentive, particularly if the amount is relatively high, and this formed the basis of a 72-hour sleep deprivation experiment in my laboratory at Loughborough[30]. It ran over weekends, starting with a base-line day on a Friday, and continuing through from Friday night to the Monday lunchtime without sleep. A total of 15 volunteer male and female young graduate students were recruited, who were all physically and mentally healthy. All were paid well for doing the experiment, in addition to the 'rewards' that I will be coming to in a moment. They were carefully briefed about the study forehand, and were free to withdraw at any point; none did. They were divided into three groups and assessed regularly at Wilkinson's Auditory Vigilance Task. Two groups were sleep deprived, and the third acted as a control, allowed to sleep normally. The role of the control group was for us to see if they improved with practice over the 3 days. Had this happened, then we would have had to assume that the same would be likely for the sleep deprivation groups, and this would have at least partly countered any fall in performance due to sleep loss. As things turned out, no such 'practice effect' appeared in the control group, probably because all groups were well trained on the test on the Thursday beforehand.

Wilkinson's test was given for half an hour at a time, at 6-hour intervals during wakefulness. During the baseline Friday, all the groups were told to do their best at the test. This instruction continued into sleep deprivation (i.e the Friday night and beyond) for the control subjects and for one of the sleep-deprived groups, without any further incentives being added. However, the second deprivation group was more fortunate as they were also given a cash reward for every target signal they correctly identified, and were 'fined' a similar amount for each error. The total possible reward was quite generous on the Saturday, even better on the Sunday as the stakes were doubled, and on the Monday, the subjects could potentially get quite rich as it was doubled again. On the Monday it was possible for each of these subjects to win £12 per half-hour session. To add further to the incentive, a competition was run between these subjects, with the best scorer for each session getting an extra cash bonus.

We risked paying out several hundred pounds on the Monday, but to our great relief and surprise the total only came to £7! Despite each subject's keenness to become wealthy, and the great effort they put into trying to do well, they just could not manage the task that day. However, despite the smaller possible rewards for Sunday we did lose about £40 then, and a similar

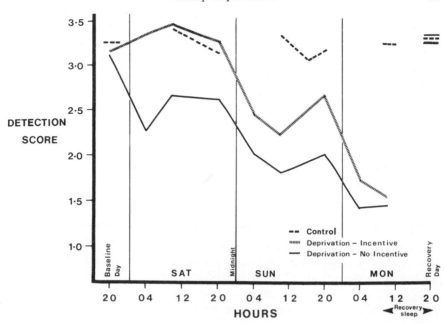

Fig. 2.3 Fall in performance during sleep deprivation and the effects of incentive. Deprivation lasted for three days (from Friday night to Monday morning). Changes in detection performance are shown for three conditions: with (hatched line) and without (solid line) an attractive incentive to do well, and for a control group sleeping normally at night (dashed line). The incentive kept performance up to normal levels until the second night (Saturday). It was still effective to some extent on the Sunday, but failed on the Monday. Following only 8 hours of recovery sleep on the Monday (from midday), performance was back to normal by that night, even without the incentives. See text for further details.

amount for the Saturday. Consequently, for the first 36 hours of sleep loss, that is, just into the Saturday night, this monetary incentive kept this group's detection scores up to the baseline level, and up to that of the control group. These findings can be seen in Fig. 2.3. However, a few hours later, at 4.00 a.m. on Sunday morning, detection fell noticeably, but then levelled off, and even picked up somewhat for the rest of the day. As can be seen, the scores were still much better than those of the other deprivation group, and the incentive was still having effect.

The real collapse in performance came at 4.00 a.m. on the Monday, leaving little difference between the two deprivation groups for detection scores—both groups were very bad. Meanwhile, the control group maintained level performance over all the days—it should be remembered that they missed early morning measurements as they were asleep. Note also, that usually during sleep deprivation it is the night-time that brings the greatest daily decline in performance, with a levelling off during the ensuing day.

So, despite the apparently poorer incentives Wilkinson used for his study, our findings were similar to his. In as much that detection is assessing cerebral impairment, incentive can successfully counteract these sleep deprivation effects until the second night of sleep loss. Beyond this point in time performance begins to fail as something more fundamental seems to be happening to the cerebrum.

Both of our deprivation groups were allowed 8 hours recovery sleep from midday until 8 p.m. on the Monday, in the laboratory. This was one-third of the amount of sleep they had lost. Following another hour to freshen up, they were then given a further go at the vigilance test, but this time, with no incentives for any group. Fig. 2.3 shows how detection returned to normal baseline levels, and it seems that this period of sleep was sufficient for the full return of cerebral function, despite some residual sleepiness. Other effects we noticed with the sleep-deprived subjects' behaviour, such as speech slurring, and lapses, also disappeared after this initial sleep. Like previous reports about recovery sleep (e.g. Tables 2.1 and 2.3), we found that it contained much stage 4 sleep, but only half an average night's worth of REM sleep. However, we do not know whether stage 4 sleep was the key to the return of normal behaviour and performance. By midnight the sleep-deprived subjects had returned to bed again—this time to their own beds. They were allowed to sleep for as long as they wanted. Eight out of the ten woke at their normal rising time, quite refreshed, and claimed not to be in need of further sleep until the next (Tuesday) night, when they slept quite normally again.

To restate the two key conclusions that can be drawn from my study: first, and the most important, is that if people really apply themselves then cerebral function apparently can be maintained at virtually normal levels for up to the second night of sleep deprivation, but beyond this point it seems to be affected noticeably. So, initially during sleep loss, motivation is the main cause of impaired performance. Thereafter this seems to be increasingly due to some form of cerebral impairment. Second, for a return of normal cerebral function only a portion of the lost sleep needs to be reclaimed.

For the moment, let me stay with the first point, and I will come to the second later. It could still be argued that the apparent decline in detection on the second night continues to be due to motivation rather to cerebral impairment, as my incentives were still not strong enough. We cannot threaten subjects with fear of losing life or limb, and a laboratory experiment will never resolve this problem. But surely, if sleep was solely some sort of drive behaviour for occupying the unproductive hours of the night[31,32], then I would have expected Nature to have given us an override to it, when the incentive to stay awake was very high, or in an emergency when life is threatened. Although life and limb has not been threatened in the laboratory, there are, sadly, many real-world examples which can be drawn upon, particularly from wartime. For example, shipwrecked sailors exposed to the cold sea know full well that if they fall asleep they may never wake up again, because a fall in body temperature (hypothermia) will set in much more rapidly, partly because of physical inactivity. Nevertheless, the time still comes when sleep overwhelms them and they die. A similar situation applied to Battle of Britain fighter and bomber pilots flying sortie after sortie without sleep. Falling asleep in the cockpit will be fatal one way or another, but many were killed in this manner, usually on the return home.

Although my stance is that the cerebrum does need some sleep for its repair, all I have is indirect evidence, and the argument, that I cannot see why Nature should maintain sleep in such behaviourally advanced mammals as humans only as a drive or instinctual process for occupying time, conserving energy, etc. As we have so few basic drives or instincts left in our repertoire of waking behaviour, why should the other third of our lives be governed by such mechanisms? Sleep certainly can act as a time filler for us, as well as seeming to have a restorative role for the cerebrum, and this is what I will be arguing—that sleep in advanced mammals has an essential core component for cerebral repair, etc., and a more flexible 'optional' component for occupying time. Whether or not human sleep provides any special degree of growth and repair for the rest of the body will be a matter for the debates in Chapter 4.

But I have not yet finished with the topic of cerebral function and sleep deprivation, and I want to pick up the threads of why detection, as well as such cerebrally demanding tasks as IQ tests and stimulating 'battle games' are so relatively unaffected by up to two nights of sleep loss.

2.12 Spare cerebral capacity

Even though at least some sleep seems essential to the cerebrum, I also argue that it is reasonable to expect Nature to have built in a form of reserve to cope with limited sleep deprivation. We can draw parallels here with several days of food deprivation, where various back-up systems are brought in and internal energy supplies are drawn on without any real harm occurring—so why not the same for sleep and the brain? Besides, most organs can cope well with some restrictions on their function. We can survive fairly healthily on only one kidney, or with a metre less small intestine, or with part of a lung removed, or with one ovary or testis. We know that during the first 36 hours of sleep deprivation the cerebrum has the capacity to perform normally, and this could be a sign of a back-up or reserve system. So, one reason why complex tasks such as IQ tests are not affected by up to two nights of sleep deprivation is that the cerebrum uses a spare capacity to withstand a short period of sleep loss, and that with effort and motivation we can mobilize these reserves to overcome the initial effects of sleeplessness.

The ways in which this presumed spare capacity of the cerebrum could cope with short-term sleep deprivation is a matter for speculation, but one possibility I find attractive would be analogous to the 'error correct' facility of advanced computers, whereby spare circuits are built into complex networks. If one of the usual circuits fails, then there is an automatic rerouting through the spare circuits to bypass the problem. The computer operator notices nothing wrong as the whole system functions normally. Such failures can continue to increase, still unnoticed, until the spare circuitry runs out, and only then will the operator detect a fault. At first glance this may seem minor, as it is only the last fault that is apparent, but when the machine is opened up for investigation not one fault is discovered, but many.

Something similar might happen to the cerebrum. It must develop faults in its networks during wakefulness—after all, it is one of the most complex machines in existence. These must be bypassed somehow, presumably by rerouting through other neural networks. I propose that normally these faults are largely repaired during sleep, or, to use computer terminology, 'off line'. There is no reason to assume that there are only enough spare circuits to keep us going for the 16 hours of one waking day, and there is probably provision for a reserve capacity. It seems that for the average person this capacity may be good for up to the second night of sleep deprivation, when, despite our best efforts, performance begins to fail. Increased effort by the subject to combat the initial sleepiness may be encouraging the use of the spare cerebral capacity. This, then, may be a reason why stimulating and complex tasks can withstand short-term sleep loss, whilst performance at simple and dull tasks deteriorates more quickly because the subject can summon up no effort to do well.

2.13 Performance measures are too limited

Although complex tasks used in sleep deprivation studies, such as IQ performance and decision making, need a high level of skill, they rely on techniques that are already well developed in the subject. Furthermore, IQ tests and their like are 'convergent' tasks. That is, they encourage the person to 'home in' progressively on the solution. To help with this process a selection of possible answers is given from which the correct one is selected. This makes scoring the test easier, but it does not encourage creativity, novelty or flexibility of behaviour, which are 'divergent' thinking skills. These are difficult to measure and are seldom looked at by sleep deprivation researchers. The emphasis with psychological performance measurement in sleep deprivation has been on those tests that are the most sensitive to sleepiness, are easy to score, and are not vulnerable to large practice effects that would cancel out any impairment due to sleepiness. So we are back with the dull, monotonous, and unstimulating tasks such as 10–20 minutes of simple reaction time testing, which are primarily assessing the motivation of the subject rather than the inherent capacity to perform. Also, of course, just because these tests soon show profound effects of sleep deprivation, we cannot assume that they are also tapping areas central to our understanding of sleep function. Conversely, we cannot conclude that because the interesting tasks like IQ performance are slow to be affected by deprivation, they are not so central to sleep function, as they may be drawing on spare cerebral capacity.

Tests of cerebral impairment during sleep deprivation that could be developed much further come from two sources. The first is from one of the Walter Reed rating scales—Cognitive Disorganization. Spontaneous thinking becomes progressively impaired in the ways shown in Table 2.4 and Fig. 2.2, but not noticeably until the second night of sleep loss. Unfortunately, because this scale is not very precise, it is hardly ever reported on nowadays. However, the scale range could be developed further and expanded with more detailed criteria.

The second possibility for testing material comes from another research area, neuropsychology—the psychological effects of cerebral damage due to disease, accidents, etc. Of course, these are extreme situations, and I am not suggesting that sleep deprivation causes such damage. Merely, that in a much more modest way we might gain clues from this field of research about what to look for during sleep deprivation by considering cerebral impairment. Much has been written about behaviour following cerebral damage. So to avoid dwelling too long on this topic I will concentrate on just one part of the cerebrum, the frontal lobes. These are the largest lobes of the cerebrum and seem to be concerned with intriguing aspects of behaviour that have been much neglected by sleep deprivation research, for example the more 'divergent' thinking I mentioned earlier. Below are some further aspects of divergent thinking, together with other psychological and behavioural difficulties found in patients with frontal lobe damage:

Rigidity—repeating old routines (perseveration), even if these are inappropriate. Lacking a flexible approach to new situations.
Reduced spontaneity—less activity with general behaviour and speech. Difficulty in making new plans.
Language impairment—confused and fewer words used. Bad spelling.
Poor memory—for recent events ('short-term' memory).
Difficulty in organizing body movements—e.g. copying the movement of others.
Poor spatial ability—confusion about where one is in the environment, and about planning a new route to go elsewhere, even locally.
Less inhibited about behaviour—more likely to show socially unacceptable behaviour, and become irritable, coarse, facile, and unmannered.

These are only some examples, with most not easy to measure and requiring special tests. One exception is short-term memory, which has been

assessed in several sleep deprivation studies. This usually shows a decline by
the second night of deprivation, as demonstrated by the Walter Reed experiments, and by Wilkinson in his studies. However, the type of memory tasks
they used were dull and unstimulating, and again we do not really know how
much of the memory impairment was due to a lack of the subjects' interest
and motivation in the task, rather than to any real cerebral impairment.
Nevertheless, many of the problems outlined above are often found to some
extent during sleep deprivation, particularly speech impediments, of the type
reflected in the Cognitive Disorganization Scale.

One fascinating, as yet only partly answered question, is whether sleep-
deprived subjects can overcome their speech difficulties if they are motivated
more? Whilst the answer seems to be, no, this cannot be done beyond about
two nights of sleep loss, most of the evidence we have is again anecdotes from
wartime. There are many accounts of how soldiers in prolonged combat lose
the ability to understand orders. Field commanders cannot give coherently
worded verbal instructions, and often forget what they ordered. This has
other consequences, as the commander loses control of his leadership
because communication with his men is lost one way or another. But there
are, of course, other obvious factors apart from sleep deprivation contri-
buting to the battle scene, and I cannot claim sleep loss to be the sole cause of
the problems.

Neither do we know whether sleep deprivation seriously impairs the ability
to adapt to a novel situation. We know that, given the incentive, the hospital
doctor, pilot, and army commander can keep up with their usual well-trained
complex skills for about two nights of sleep deprivation. But could they
respond appropriately to a novel situation of which they have little
experience? Or would they be inflexible in their behaviour, at a loss for ideas,
and just sticking to standard routines and skills that might well be inappropriate? Then they may become so concerned with trying to cope with this
situation that they forget to attend to new developments, and a serious crisis
may evolve through oversight. This puts pressure on already strained
emotions, which for one reason or another may become less controlled,
unmannered, and lead to quite irrational behaviour. Such a scenario happens
in real life, but is uncommon in the laboratory.

I would like to end this discussion on performance measures by relating the
points made here to those of the previous section on 'Spare Cerebral
Capacity'. We have seen how sleep deprivation initially affects motivation
rather than the inherent ability of the cerebrum to work. Although cerebral
impairment may be occurring at this time, the cerebrum probably has the
capacity to overcome this problem without a loss in its overall performance.
At least, that is, it can deal with complex 'convergent' tasks. But the
commonly used psychological tests only tap certain abilities, and, for
example, we do not know whether flexibility of behaviour or creativity are

affected at this early stage of deprivation, or whether they can also be maintained at usual levels through the use of the spare capacity. It is possible though that this spare capacity has already been used, for example, for creative thinking. If this were so, then creative ability would be impaired sooner during sleep deprivation, perhaps on the first night, or even in the last part of our normal waking day—that is as soon as spare cerebral capacity has to be used to replace faults in standard circuits.

2.14 Two types of sleepiness?

I have already introduced you to one of the key themes of this book—that human sleep has two main functions each served by a different form of sleep:

1. A sleep that repairs the effects of waking wear and tear on the cerebrum. It centres around the first few hours of sleep, particularly SWS and the 'deeper' form of stage 4 sleep. I call this *core sleep*, and some of REM sleep is also included. It is particularly evident on the first recovery night after sleep deprivation. One further point, as will be seen in the forthcoming chapters, is that I doubt whether the rest of the body requires core sleep or any other sleep for its repair—relaxed wakefulness is sufficient.
2. A sleep that fills the tedious hours of darkness until sunrise, maintaining sleep beyond the point where core sleep declines. This sleep I call *optional sleep*, and is probably under the control of a behavioural drive to sleep. It is influenced by a circadian rhythm much more than is core sleep, and, as will be seen in Chapter 6, is modifiable to some extent to suit one's circumstances. *At the onset of normal night-time sleep, both core and optional sleep are active, with core sleep subsiding after a few hours to let optional sleep continue* (see Fig. 6.1).

If these proposals hold, as I believe they do, and as I hope readers will see as they progress through this book, then we might well consider looking for two types of sleepiness. One relates to increased cerebral impairment (a reversible process) and the need for cerebral repair that becomes readily evident by the second night of deprivation. The other relates to a build-up of whatever governs optional sleep, which is present at the beginning of deprivation. Because this optional sleep drive is very much governed by a circadian rhythm, switching in at night and lifting by day under normal sleep-wake habits, it may well do this to a large extent during sleep deprivation. However, as it would not have been dissipated through sleep, it is likely that there would be some carry-over in the daytime, followed by a larger build-up the next night.

Given the various findings with incentives during the first phase of deprivation, I suggest that this drive to sleep can be countered by the subject applying more effort. But· by the second night, perhaps longer for some people, sleepiness due to cerebral impairment begins. Increasing effort fails to ward off this type of sleepiness and performance drops. Using the metaphorical car again (Section 2:8), it is like saying that in the early stages of sleep deprivation power loss in the engine is mostly due to a sticking accelerator, overcome by pushing harder on the accelerator pedal. However, after two nights of sleep deprivation the loss of power becomes increasingly associated with engine wear. It is a forlorn hope that greater effort on the accelerator at this stage will overcome engine wear—all that happens is that the engine uses up more fuel, makes more noise and smoke, but produces little extra power. By the third day of deprivation both core and optional sleepiness are very apparent.

Dividing sleep and sleepiness up in this way has a counterpart with eating. We can isolate the feeling of hunger from the actual need for food. This point has been emphasized in the classical text on starvation, *The Biology of Human Starvation*, by Dr Ancel Keys and colleagues[33]. In their massive review of the literature and detailed account of their reknown 'Minnesota Experimental Starvation Project', they emphasized the need to separate these two aspects of feeding. The feeling of hunger is seen to centre on stomach pangs, whereas a need for food involves physical weakness, tiredness, and the sufferer's awareness that more food is necessary. Put into the sleep deprivation context, hunger pangs may be equivalent to sleepiness produced by the optional sleep drive, while the physical weakness and food need are equivalent to cerebral impairment and the need for core sleep.

Of particular interest to me in their review were the repeated observations that hunger pangs usually subside after about 5 days of total starvation, but do not totally disappear. So, the subjective feeling of 'hunger' changes its meaning from predominantly hunger pangs and increasing weakness over the first few days, to one of increasing weakness alone. Sufferers still claim to be 'hungry' throughout both stages, but analysis of what they really mean shows this difference. For this reason Keys and colleagues emphasized that the observer should not simply record the extent to which the starved person feels 'hungry', but break down the meaning of this feeling into its components. Similarly, for sleep deprivation we might be able to break down the feeling of 'sleepiness' into more subtle divisions, and I have suggested two—that produced by a need for core sleep and that by a need for optional sleep.

It may just be a coincidence that both hunger and sleep deprivation have 'fifth-day turning points'. The 205-hour sleep deprivation study clearly observed this phenomenon with sleepiness, as can be seen in Fig. 2.1. If there is a sleep drive, occupying the unproductive hours of the night etc., then one could well reason that during prolonged sleep deprivation there would come a point (the fifth day) when the mechanism controlling this drive would somehow 'acknowledge' that some sort of crisis was present. So for it to continue increasing its pressure to sleep beyond this time would be pointless, particularly if there is a build-up of cerebral impairment as well. Some sort of

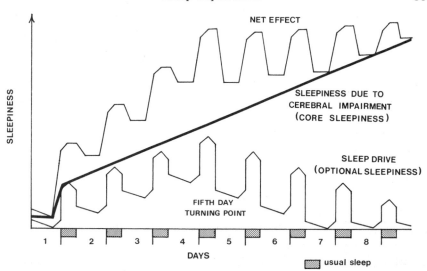

Fig. 2.4 Changes over time for the two types of sleepiness during sleep deprivation. Sleepiness due to cerebral impairment and a *need for core sleep* increases steadily from the second night (heavy line). Sleepiness from a *drive for optional sleep* (bottom line), which normally has a pronounced circadian rhythm, also increases for about the first 5 days, still with a night-time rise and daytime fall. The two types of sleepiness summate to give the overall feeling of sleepiness (top line). During the first few days when both types of sleepiness are active, the net effect distorts the circadian rhythm of summated sleepiness, owing to the steady increase in core sleepiness. Therefore, the daytime circadian fall will be reduced and the night-time rise enhanced. Around the fifth day, optional sleepiness declines, leaving core sleepiness to continue its rise, with the net effect being a levelling of the summated feeling of sleepiness.

relief from the overall increasing sleepiness, by reducing the sleep drive, might well help the individual's survival. Maybe the 'fifth-day turning point' during sleep deprivation is just such an event, with optional sleepiness lifting. After this point, sleepiness would mostly be due to an increasing need for core sleep, with the net effect of some overall improvement in sleepiness. These trends are shown in Fig. 2.4.

Changes with time for the summated effect on sleepiness can be compared with the real values obtained from the 205-hour deprivation study, given in Fig. 2.1. Although the graphs from the two figures look very similar, it is of course easy for me to be wise after the event, and to have produced a model of sleepiness having the same outcome to that of the real findings. New work will have to evaluate this idea.

Of course, there may be a much easier explanation for the fifth-day turning point in sleepiness—that subjects see the end of the experiment in sight, and become more enthusiastic about the project! So far, all I have done is to introduce you to core and optional sleep/sleepiness, and much more support

for these views will be forthcoming in this book. The discerning reader may
have realized that, so far all I have produced is a circular argument. I used the
sleep deprivation results to create the core and optional sleep hypothesis,
which led to the proposal for two types of sleepiness. Then support for this
latter idea came from the original sleep deprivation findings! But as will be
seen, especially in Chapters 5–7, breaking out of this circle is not difficult.

2.15 Short-term sleep restriction

In Sections 2.11 and 2.12, I described how core sleep might well be involved
with the repair of faulty cerebral circuits. However, there is probably spare
capacity within these circuits, as the effects of one night of total sleep
deprivation can be counteracted if we are given the incentive to put more
'effort' into whatever mental tasks are being done. The intriguing question
now arises: what is the minimum amount of sleep necessary for psychological
performance to remain normal, without incentive and compensatory effort?

One of the most systematic studies that has shed much light on this topic
was carried out by Wilkinson[34]. Although this was 20 years ago, a fairly clear
picture came out, and few other experiments have come up to his level of
thoroughness. The subjects were sailors who volunteered in groups of six,
and stayed at the laboratory for 6 weeks at a time, including extended weekends off. Every Tuesday and Wednesday night their sleep was restricted to
one of six levels—7.5, 5.0, 3.0, 2.0, 1.0, and 0 hours of sleep. They completed
all of these restrictions, at one per week, in a different order for each subject
so that in any week each man underwent a different condition from the rest of
his shipmates. During the daytime of the first Monday and Tuesday they
became familiar with the laboratory and various psychological tests, which
were: Wilkinson's Auditory Vigilance Task, a simple addition test, and a
coding test. Each lasted for 1 hour, and were given in a 3-hour session. From
7.45 a.m. to 10.40 p.m. on both Wednesday and Thursday, subjects repeated
these tests four times daily, with 1–2-hour breaks between sessions. This
seems quite an ordeal, and I must emphasize that the subjects were given little
incentive to put extra effort into the tasks—they were just told to do their
best. However, the schedule was familiar to them as it was like a 4-hour watch
system on board ship, involving the monitoring of equipment such as radar
or sonar.

I will not go into details about all of the findings, as the most interesting
outcome was from the vigilance task. Wilkinson calculated the detection
values, and these, averaged over the day, are shown in Fig. 2.5. Before going
further, I must point out that the detection scores are on a different scale
from those of Fig. 2.3, mainly because of differences in the duration of the
task. Wilkinson found that following one night of reduced sleep, detection
remained unchanged unless sleep was below 3 hours, in which case it fell

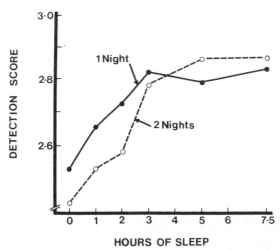

Fig. 2.5 Sleep restriction and performance—changes in detection over two nights under various sleep restrictions. Three hours of sleep is a critical minimum for the first night, rising on the second night to 5 hours. This latter effect is partly due to the increased wakefulness over the day. See text for details. (Adapted from Wilkinson's findings[34])

noticeably. However, following the second night of reduction, the fall in detection began around the 5-hour point.

Whilst Wilkinson did not measure sleep EEGs, he did make some astute comments about what was probably happening (this was 20 years ago):

The significance of these findings for those interested in sleep is, of course, that it is not until sleep is reduced below three hours that there is any substantial loss of stage 4 sleep. It is tempting to conclude from one night of partial sleep deprivation that, provided the normal amount of stage 4 sleep is obtained, there will be no loss of the capacity to perform discriminative functions, but only a reduction in motivation to do so. This conclusion, however, must be qualified by the results after two nights at which point detection* appears to fall when sleep is reduced to five hours, and was lower than normal at the three hour level. Findings (from the work of others) that partial sleep deprivation can increase stage 4 sleep on recovery nights may help to explain this. After one night of reduced sleep, there may have been a tendency for stage 4 to extend further into the night (because prior daytime wakefulness was longer—my words**), so that it was curtailed even by the modest reduction of sleep below five hours. These results argue the importance of stage 4 sleep for the maintenance of intrinsic performance capability (ref. 34, p. 41).

Around the same time, another famous pioneer in sleep research, Dr Bernie Webb, from the University of Florida, also ran an experiment restrict-

*My substitution for the technical term 'd prime'.
**In Section 5.2 I will explain in more detail how SWS, particularly stage 4 sleep, increases with lengthening wakefulness.

ing sleep to 3 hours a night, but for eight nights in succession[35]. To a large extent this study complements that of Wilkinson. It bears out Wilkinson's views on stage 4 sleep, because Webb made sleep EEG recordings on each of these nights, as well as on preliminary and recovery nights. Eight subjects volunteered, and during the evenings they underwent various psychological performance tests. None of these involved detection, though, and we do not know for how long the tests were given.

Performance did not begin to deteriorate until the seventh day, and it is tempting to claim that 3 hours sleep a night is sufficient. However, it will be remembered that Wilkinson found that on the second night of sleep restriction this minimum sleep rose to 5 hours. So it is possible that Webb's tests may not have been sensitive enough to spot smaller changes that may have occurred earlier. Also, repetition of the tests over the days may have led to an improvement (a practice effect) that could have counteracted any decline through sleep loss. But the particularly important finding by Webb, was that stage 4 sleep was spared much more than any other type of sleep. For example, whilst stage 4 sleep only fell from 92 to 85 minutes from baseline to restriction nights, REM sleep dropped from 103 to 13 minutes. Even so, 3 hours sleep was probably too short, as a stage 4 rebound increase still occurred on the ninth night of unrestricted sleep. There was a small rebound with REM sleep.

Wilkinson's experiment could also have suffered from improvement through practice. However, this was unlikely because not only were his subjects well trained beforehand, but they underwent the various reductions in different orders, and this would have evened out any residual practice effect. Wilkinson considered that beyond one night, 3 hours sleep a night seems too short.

So, what about 4 hours a night? With two colleagues, Wilkinson went on to carry out a further study looking at 4 days of 4 hours sleep per night, compared with 6 hours, and a normal 7.5 hours per night[36]. A total of 16 sailors underwent each of the three conditions (4, 6 and 7.5 hours) over 6 weeks. In a similar arrangement as before, a battery of psychological tests, including the vigilance task, was given during the daytime. Detection scores were calculated. Although it seemed that the 4-hour schedule was just about long enough to avoid any fall in detection, a small practice effect was also found (despite the experimenters' best efforts beforehand), which would have distorted these findings. So it looks as though 4 hours sleep is just under a minimum sleep requirement. If sleep reduction was to be on a longer-term basis, then maybe about 5 hours daily sleep would be the minimum.

In Section 6.3 I will be describing the extent to which we can adapt to cutting down our normal amount of sleep on a more or less permanent basis. Such 'long-term' sleep reduction is a different topic to the short-term studies lasting a few days, I have just described, as the latter incorporate sleep deprivation. 'Deprivation' implies that more sleep may be needed, but this appears not to be the case for the long-term experiments, as adaptation occurs. 'Adaptation' indicates that there is no real sleep loss, and a satisfactory but lower amount of daily sleep has been established—that is there is no increase in daytime sleepiness, and normal levels of psychological performance are present, without the subject having to apply increased effort. About 5 hours daily sleep does seem to be the comfortable limit here, although it may be possible for some people to go down a little further. But this is enough discussion on sleep reduction, as it is leading me away from the main theme of this chapter—total sleep deprivation, where there is still more to be covered.

2.16 Age and sleep deprivation

Almost all sleep deprivation experiments have used young adults, more specifically men, and usually from colleges or the Forces. Consequently, much of our knowledge is based on people who are not typical of the normal population. Webb has begun to redress this imbalance through a recent series of deprivation studies that have compared the psychological and behavioural responses of younger and older male subjects. In the first experiment[37] ten 40 to 49-year-old and six 18 to 22-year-old men were recruited. In a later study[38], twelve 50 to 60-year-old versus six 20 to 25-year-old men were used. Both studies monitored the subjects through a baseline period, two nights total sleep deprivation, and two recovery days. Subjects were given a wide range of psychological performance tests, falling into the broad categories of:

Sleepiness and mood: subjects rated themselves on scales.
Ability to persist with attention: at 20–30 minute tests such as the Wilkinson Auditory Vigilance Task (detection scores were not calculated), and an adding test made up of a long series of sums.
Precision: how accurately were the above tasks performed; were the sums correctly added?
'Cognitively demanding' tasks: of greater complexity, e.g. long and short-term memory for words, comparing the length of lines, and finding the common theme in groups of words.

The main outcome from the first study was that the older men were affected more by the deprivation. Not only was this apparent in the subjective ratings of sleepiness and in the persistence measures, but only the older men showed any impairment at the cognitively demanding tasks. Whilst Webb concluded that older subjects do not cope so well with sleep deprivation, he was cautious about the actual extent of this age effect, as another interesting outcome was that older subjects tended to do better at several of the tests during the baseline period, and therefore had a greater way to fall. This was probably because they were more motivated to do well initially, and therefore put more into the tasks. Nevertheless, during deprivation the older subjects certainly claimed to feel sleepier than their younger counterparts, suggesting that the greater fall in performance for the older subjects was real.

The second study was more detailed, and tried to clarify some of the issues that arose in the first experiment, for example the higher baseline values for older subjects. Some modifications and extensions of the tests were also made. The findings were mixed, although generally similar to those before. One complication was that from the subjective ratings of sleepiness, it was now the younger men who seemed to be more affected by the deprivation! Whilst both groups started at the same point on this rating scale, the older men showed less of an increase in sleepiness during deprivation. Nevertheless, perplexing as this may seem, the older subjects still showed a greater deterioration at the tests of persistence/attention. Whilst their precision scores were not so badly affected by sleep loss, this was partly due to their starting off at a lower level. Some of the cognitively demanding tests showed the greatest decline for those older men who did better at the beginning (i.e. they had further to fall). Neither group demonstrated any impairment to either long- or short-term memory. One clear outcome was that motivation and the amount of extra effort put into the tasks played a crucial role.

Webb tried to untangle this rather confusing picture by concluding that:

In these age ranges where a differential effect was found, the older subjects showed less decline in subjective ratings, but greater decline in tests of persistence/attention, precision and cognitive processing. Where there were exceptions, these reflected higher levels of baseline performance by the younger subjects, declining to equal performance under deprivation.

Generally, he felt that apart from the subjective ratings, this conclusion also held for his previous study, even though there were some contrasts between the two experiments, particularly for baseline levels.

To add my own comments on these studies, it seems that the older men in Webb's study may have been more prone to increased sleepiness over 2 days of deprivation, despite what is claimed on their subjective ratings—perhaps they like to think that they are as good as the younger men. Performing well on simple and monotonous tasks is a greater struggle for the older subject and needs more added effort. Interesting and stimulating tests show little difference between young and old subjects, and it is possible that the older men are applying even more compensatory effort. Overall, it seems that for the older subjects the course of events with the behavioural and psychological effects of sleep deprivation is the same as those for the younger subject, except that changes happen more rapidly. Applying my concept of two types of sleepiness to these two short studies, it seems that core sleepiness may begin earlier for the older subjects—soon after the first night of sleep loss.

2.17 Does repeated deprivation produce any immunity to sleep loss?

No, seems to be the answer. However, this intriguing and important question has only been examined twice, once by Wilkinson[39] and more recently by Webb's laboratory[40]. Wilkinson deprived 12 young men of sleep for one night, on six occasions. Each time, he measured their performance during 30 minutes of choice reaction time. He was also interested to see how changing incentives would interact with repeated sleep deprivation, and so for three of the occasions an incentive for the subjects to do well was also included. This was given through immediate feedback to the subjects on how well they were doing. For the other three sessions the incentive was omitted. Wilkinson found that rather than becoming 'immune' to sleep deprivation, performance deteriorated under both conditions, although the deterioration was cut by half using the incentive. He concluded that the monotony and decreasing novelty of both the conditions was the main cause of the fall—a line of reasoning fitting in with Kjellberg's ideas (Section 2.9).

However, Webb had a different outlook, and believed that sleep deprivation could be seen as a stress, with subjects becoming desensitized to it. He used six young men, and extended Wilkinson's experiment by increasing deprivation to two nights on five occasions, and used more tests. But he was forced to agree with Wilkinson, as performance at most tests got steadily worse—subjects were not becoming immune. As might be expected, the more challenging tasks were less affected by both deprivation itself and the repetition of deprivation. Wilkinson's viewpoint seems to be right—repeated deprivation just adds to the monotony.

2.18 Can sleep deprivation effects be sped up or slowed down?

The best way of reducing the effects of sleep loss is, of course, to take naps, and there have been many investigations into this area. This is not a line I wish to pursue just yet, though, as I want to stay with uninterrupted sleep deprivation. Whilst this leaves us with relatively little other research to go on, two types of study do come to mind where either: (a) physical, or (b) mental activity are varied during the deprivation programme. Starting with the former, it is well known that mild exercise in the form of walking temporarily reduces the feeling of sleepiness. Will heavier exercise be more beneficial, or will it make matters worse? As I mentioned in Section 2.3, several military studies of sleep deprivation have incorporated exercise, but none of them have looked at this factor systematically. Furthermore, often they also included food restriction. So, this leaves only three investigations, which all looked at high versus low physical activity on psychological performance during sleep deprivation. One was again by Webb[41], another by a group from the Naval Health Laboratory in San Diego, run by Dr Ardie Lubin and coworkers[42], and the third by Dr Robert Angus and colleagues from the Defence and Civil Institute of Environmental Medicine, Ontario[43]. In Webb's study, eight subjects were sleep deprived for two nights under each of two conditions: (1) complete bed rest, and (2) 15 minutes of strenuous work on an exercise cycle every hour. Performance at the Wilkinson Auditory Vigilance Task, at memory for words, and at numerical addition were all assessed before, during and after deprivation. The results showed no differences between the conditions for any of these measures, or for the amount and quality of the recovery sleep (which was monitored). Webb concluded that the performance decline due to sleep deprivation was the same for rest or exercise.

Webb gave his subjects an hour or so rest period between the exercise and performance testing, unlike the following study by Lubin and colleagues, who tested their subjects soon after the exercise. This may be a reason for the different outcome, as will now be seen. The San Diego experiment was a much larger enterprise, with 40 subjects, even though it only lasted for one night of deprivation and the following day. Subjects were assigned to one of three experimental groups that were given, for an hour at a time, exercise, relaxation in bed, or a nap. Every 4 hours during sleep deprivation, following an hour at one of these three activities, they were given a 2-hour battery of psychological tests (including Wilkinson's Vigilance Task). Obviously, the nap group fared the best, but it was the exercise group that generally performed the worst. It was clear that bed rest was no substitute for sleep, and that exercise did not combat sleepiness—quite the contrary in fact. However, had the exercise subjects been given a longer recovery time prior to testing, the outcome might have been different, as the findings of the previous experiment suggest. Nevertheless, both studies agree that exercise during sleep deprivation benefits performance little, and may make matters worse.

Angus and colleagues came to the same conclusion in their longer enterprise of 60 hours of sleep loss. They questioned the outcome from the other two studies, as quite reasonably they thought that bed rest did not make a good comparison for exercise—the subjects should be out of bed but fairly inactive. Two groups of subjects were used: exercise versus no exercise. Angus's study gave the highest exercise load of all three studies, whereby the subjects pedalled on an exercise cycle at 25–30 per cent of their maximum level, for 1 hour in 3—that is a total of 20 hours of exercise. An impressive battery of psychological tests and subjective rating scales was given, more substantial than those of the other two studies. But no differences were found for any test, as both conditions showed similar declines in performance and increases in sleepiness.

I have described these exercise studies at some length in order to demonstrate that taxing the body in this way does not seem to alter sleepiness, or seemingly the need for sleep. If this were so, then performance and sleepiness would have deteriorated further. Besides, there is an impressive mass of evidence that the body does not specifically need sleep to recover from the effects of exercise, only rest—a topic dealt with in more detail in Section 4.10. On the other hand, extra 'brain work' through continued sensory stimulation during sleep deprivation certainly increases sleepiness and psychological impairment.

This is something I looked at a few years ago[44-46], at a time when I was concerned about unwanted effects of keeping sleep-deprived subjects confined to the monotonous environment of a laboratory—an artificial situation where there is only limited involvement with the outside world. In particular, laboratories are visually dull. In Section 2.6 I suggested that this might be one reason why visual misperceptions occur during sleep deprivation—the brain becomes 'fed up' with looking at the same views. It should be remembered that vision is our dominant sense (e.g. one-third of all the nervous pathways entering the brain from all the senses added together—touch, smell, taste, hearing, etc., come from the eyes), and it is through this sense that most of our understanding of the environment comes.

So, in my experiment, for most of the time when the subjects were not otherwise undergoing psychological and physiological tests, I exposed them to an interesting and changing visual environment. The trouble is that it becomes progressively more difficult during sleep deprivation to keep up the subjects' interest in their surroundings. Consequently, the entertainment value of the environment becomes important, and I arranged a daytime itinary of visits to zoos, museums, botanic gardens, and beauty spots. For the nights, subjects went to the cinema to see various 'action' films. There was also a control condition, typical of most deprivation studies, where the subjects were laboratory bound.

The subjects, six young men, were deprived of sleep for 64 hours (i.e. three days and two nights) on two occasions: with the stimulation, or confined to the laboratory and its environs. Half the subjects did one condition first and the others vice versa. During the laboratory confinement they exercised to the same extent as in the other condition. A test battery was given every 6 hours, and included self-ratings of sleepiness, as well as vigilance performance (not on Wilkinson's task, as I did not know about it then), tests of visual acuity and eye focusing, and various measures of respiration and heart function. Up to the end of the first night's deprivation both conditions produced similar rises in sleepiness and falls in vigilance. But then it became increasingly obvious that the stimulation condition was causing more sleepiness and greater difficulties on the vigilance task. Problems with focusing the eyes and with double vision were also more apparent. Such differences between the conditions were greatest at 4.00 a.m. on the second night. Interestingly, there were a few reports of visual misperceptions, but these only occurred during the confinement condition, adding weight to the notion that visual monotony facilitates their appearance (Section 2.6).

Neither condition resulted in any physiological change of significance, except that the stimulation condition caused more breathing irregularities, mostly due to more frequent sighing, yawning, and changes to breathing that occur when sleep begins (i.e. these subjects were having more 'microsleeps' or 'lapses'). These were making the heart-beat more variable, but not abnormal. By the end of the deprivation in the stimulation condition the subjects were quite exhausted and felt that they could not go on for much longer, unlike the other condition where life was more tolerable. The overall findings from this study were quite clear—the signs all pointed to the stimulation condition causing a more rapid advance of the effects of sleep deprivation.

The experiment ended on the third night and the subjects slept in the laboratory that night, and for the next one. On both occasions they were allowed to sleep for as long as they wanted to. Although the recovery sleep on the first night had the typical characteristics of not only being longer, having a large rebound of stage 4 sleep and smaller rebound in REM sleep, there were certain differences between the conditions. Following the stimulation condition, subjects slept for just over 11 hours, compared with 10 hours for the other condition, and showed a 40 per cent greater rebound in stage 4 sleep. There was no difference in the rebound for REM sleep. On the second recovery night, subjects slept for only about 20 minutes longer than normal, after both conditions. Whilst the stage 4 sleep rebound on the second night had fallen, it was still greater (33 per cent) after the stimulation condition. Again, there were no differences in the REM sleep rebound.

We do not really know how or if the extra stage 4 sleep taken after the stimulation condition was related to the greater sleepiness. From my 'core/optional' sleep perspective, I would suggest that the extra stimulation produced more cerebral 'wear and tear', thus enhancing core sleepiness. I suspect that the extra stage 4 sleep (core sleep) was associated with greater cerebral recovery.

Since that experiment we have done further studies[47,48] which have looked at the effects of stimulation during wakefulness on sleepiness and sleep. As these did not involve sleep deprivation, but just covered the waking day (albeit a busy day of sightseeing, etc.), I will describe them in more detail in Section 5.5. Suffice to say, in the evenings following these days the subjects felt more sleepy—they were 'worn out'. They fell asleep rapidly and showed more stage 4 sleep, although total sleep was not longer. There were no other obvious changes to sleep.

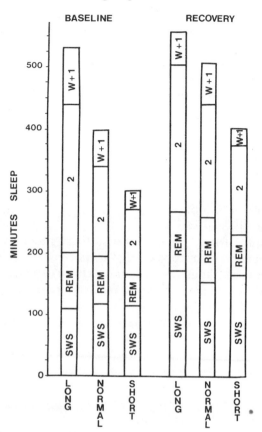

Fig. 2.6 Sleep stage amounts for natural long, normal, and short sleepers, before (baseline) and after 36 hours of sleep loss (recovery).

Usual sleep (baseline) contains similar amounts of SWS for all three groups. The differences lie with the other stages, particularly stage 2 sleep. On recovery, all subjects show large increases (around 40 percent) in SWS, and smaller increases (around 20 percent) in REM sleep, leading to more total sleep in the short and normal sleepers. Long sleepers seem to 'absorb' this, and show only a small lengthening of sleep (see text). (From Benoit et al.[49])

2.19 Do long and short sleepers differ in their recovery sleep?

As far as it is known, there is little difference between natural long and short sleepers (within any age group) in their ability to cope with sleep deprivation. On the other hand, there are interesting differences in their recovery sleep. Enough sleep deprivation studies have told us that only a portion of lost sleep needs to be regained. However, one question that has remained unanswered until recently is whether natural long sleepers need more recovery sleep than short sleepers. An experiment has now been carried out, albeit for only one night of sleep loss, by Drs Odile Benoit, Jean Foret, and colleagues[49], from the Laboratoire d'Etude du Sommeil in Paris. Following a questionnaire survey amongst medical students, the investigators selected out five short sleepers (averaging 5 hours of sleep a day), five long sleepers (averaging 9 hours), and nine normal sleepers (averaging 7 hours). All were healthy, good sleepers, and had been sleeping for several years at their respective sleep lengths. So, for example, the short sleepers were not insomniacs. All subjects first had their sleep monitored in the laboratory and were allowed to sleep as usual. Their baseline sleep stage characteristics can be seen in Fig. 2.6.

The main differences between the long and short sleepers in their baseline sleep were, for the long sleepers, 2 more hours of stage 2 sleep and another three-quarters of an hour of REM sleep (for normal sleepers these values lay roughly around the half-way point). SWS (i.e. stages 3 plus 4 sleep) was remarkably similar for all three groups, differing by only a few minutes. Stage 4 sleep alone was not reported on. I do not want to dwell on these baseline sleep differences, though, as the more central issue is sleep deprivation. Besides, I shall be looking at the normal sleep patterns of long and short sleepers in more detail in Section 6.2.

On two separate occasions, all the subjects underwent one night's sleep deprivation, ending either the following morning or the following night—that is sleep deprivation was for 24 or 36 hours. There was a problem following the shorter sleep loss, as this meant sleeping during the daytime, which happened to be more difficult for the longer sleepers. So to avoid complications, I shall concentrate on the results for sleeping at night after the 36 hours of sleep loss. Whereas the normal and short sleepers increased their usual sleep lengths by about 25 per cent and 33 per cent respectively, the long sleepers showed only a notional rise of 5 per cent. SWS rose by about 40 per cent in all three groups. But REM sleep showed varying rises (3–32 per cent), with the lowest for the long sleepers. Stage 2 sleep seemed to act more as the 'filler', making up the remaining sleep to varying extents according to the type of sleeper.

My interpretation of these findings is that long sleepers usually have 'excess' sleep, which to some extent can absorb an increase in SWS. Hence, they do not require extra sleep after a limited period of sleep deprivation. On the other hand, short sleepers may be near to a minimum sleep length, and any extra SWS and REM sleep that is required has to be added on. Normal sleepers fall between the two extremes. Such findings not only reflect the importance of SWS, and to some extent REM sleep, but also give further weight to my core and optional sleep proposals. Long, normal, and short sleepers have similar amounts of core sleep. Whereas the sleep length of short sleepers is almost down to core sleep, for long sleepers there is much optional sleep following on. This optional sleep can be partially sacrificed for the extra needs of core sleep. I will come back to this outlook on long and short sleepers in Section 6.2.

2.20 Epilepsy

During both the 264- and 205-hour deprivation studies, described earlier, neurologists were brought in to make careful examinations of the subjects. In both cases these specialists reported only minor neurological problems, apart from the problems with cerebral functioning I have already mentioned. Nevertheless, as only a total of five subjects were covered in these investigations, and as the great majority of other deprivation studies have not carried out neurological assessments, it is still possible that more substantial changes do occur in some people. Only general practitioners, rather than neurologists, are usually present during these other studies, as detailed neurological assessments have usually been considered unnecessary because nothing much seems to be happening. Whenever EEGs have been carried out during sleep deprivation, the only finding is that the EEG is typical of extreme sleepiness. One interesting finding, though, is that there is ever increasing evidence that sleep deprivation may promote epilepsy in those people who have some history of this disorder. For those without such a history, the outcome is unclear, except that the occurrence is unlikely.

Before discussing these eventualities, I will give a brief overview of some relevant aspects of epilepsy. Although epilepsy is an abnormal phenomenon, mainly of the cerebrum, it is not necessarily an unusual state of the brain, as everyone has the potential to have an epileptic episode given the appropriate circumstances. Normally, this potential is kept in check by inhibitory processes within the brain. In those people with epilepsy where there is no obvious cause (such as minor brain damage) it can be brought on simply by a lack of this inhibition, so that the brain is more easily triggered into having an attack. Epilepsy comes in a variety of forms, some minor and unnoticeable, and others more obvious, especially the 'grand mal' type of generalized seizure, where there is collapse, loss of consciousness, followed by rigidity and convulsions. The EEG shows that the whole of the cerebrum is affected, and displays a characteristic 'spike and wave' activity, of small spikes accompanied by very large delta waves.

However, as grand mal is an exceedingly rare occurrence during sleep deprivation experiments, I will concentrate on two other, more subtle types of epilepsy that may be more relevant—'petit mal', and a variety of 'partial' epilepsy (as only part of the cerebrum is involved), known as 'psychomotor' epilepsy. Both types last only about half a minute, and can go unnoticed. The cerebrum shows the 'spike' discharge, but only in petit mal are spikes accompanied by delta waves. If the spikes occur alone, as in psychomotor epilepsy, then they are difficult to detect unless the EEG electrodes happen to be sited over the affected part of the cerebrum. In psychomotor attacks there is usually no loss of consciousness, although whilst the attack is happening the sufferer may experience strange sensations, such as tingling in the skin, a peculiar smell, taste or sound, visual illusions/hallucinations, and emotional changes. A stereotyped motor activity usually develops ('automatisms'), such as licking, chewing or fumbling with the hands—hence the term 'psychomotor' (affecting the senses and muscles) for this type of epilepsy. In petit mal epilepsy, consciousness is lost, although there is no collapse and posture is maintained. A vacant look appears on the face, and the eyelids may flutter. Often there are repetitive movements of the head or upper body, such as head turning, arm bending, and twitching. The sufferer has no recollection of the event afterwards; hence petit mal epilepsies are also known as 'absences'.

People who have had some form of epilepsy are normally excluded from sleep deprivation studies, as usually the experimenters give a preliminary medical screening to all prospective subjects, and those with other than minor medical disorders are not taken on. Usually, epilepsy is not looked for specifically in this screening and is simply one of a collection of disorders listed for excluding a subject. Until recently, strong evidence linking sleep deprivation with epilepsy has been scant. But this is now coming from several reports from hospital EEG clinics, and a recent substantive review[50] of these has concluded that sleep deprivation is a very useful tool in helping diagnosis in those people where epilepsy may be suspected. Typically, patients are deprived of sleep for a single night, and EEGs are performed the next morning. Then usually over 25 per cent of people suffering from epilepsy of one sort or another will show clear EEG abnormalities.

The reason why sleep deprivation has this effect is not really known, although it could well be due to a reduction in the inhibitory mechanisms I have mentioned. We do know that, outside sleep deprivation, psychomotor epilepsy is more likely to occur during drowsiness and sleep than during wakefulness, as apparently the inhibitory mechanism lifts somewhat at sleep onset. In fact, it is believed that a high proportion of sufferers never know that they have the disorder as it is normally confined only to their sleep. As there is much drowsiness during sleep deprivation, this may increase the chances of a psychomotor episode being noticed. Consequently, volunteers for sleep deprivation studies who normally have psychomotor epilepsy only in their sleep could slip through the medical screening and end up as acceptable subjects.

For the great majority of people who have no history of epilepsy, sleep deprivation is most unlikely to cause obvious attacks, particularly for the first 1–2 nights of sleep loss. At least this seems to be the picture at the moment. But there is the problem that if a psychomotor attack happened to subjects during sleep deprivation, would they realize that this is what they were having, or would they simply put it down to a bizarre event of sleep deprivation? For example, they may see it as some sort of intrusion of dreaming into wakefulness, or even as a misperception or hallucination, as I described in Section 2.6. Of course, most misperceptions are unlikely to be psychomotor attacks. In the case of petit mal, the 'absence' it produces means that the sufferer would have little recollection of the event anyway, and it is not likely that they would report such behaviour to an experimenter.

Because both psychomotor and petit mal attacks last for such a short time and are relatively infrequent, it is unlikely that an experimenter would happen to be looking at the subject at the time the attack occurred. Even fellow subjects might be too sleepy to notice. This is why the monitoring of the EEG throughout sleep deprivation is now seen to be important. To avoid restricting the subject, 'ambulatory' monitoring can be performed. However, this is a new innovation for sleep deprivation research, and few findings have been reported so far. For this technique, EEG electrodes are connected to a battery-powered miniature recorder, similar in size and shape to a 'personal stereo recorder' and carried on a belt at the waist. In this manner, up to 24 hours of EEG can be accumulated at a time. But there is one problem with such ambulatory monitoring, as physical movement produces artefacts on the recording which can overwhelm the EEG trace. Good recordings can only be obtained with the subject sitting or lying quietly. The problem may not be serious, though, as drowsiness is less likely during physical activity, and so the likelihood of an epileptic event is reduced. There-fore, little of interest may be hidden by the artefact, anyway.

The degree to which the sleep-deprived subject is otherwise stressed is another factor which must be considered within the context of epilepsy. Anxiety, particularly that leading to increased cortisol output, enhances the likelihood of epileptic attacks in those people with a history of epilepsy. So it is interesting to note that, outside the hospital studies of patients, most of the accounts of epileptic phenomena occurring during sleep deprivation all come from military-type experiments, especially when sleep loss exceeds two nights[51,52] with prolonged flying or battlefield simulation.

Clearly, the putative link between sleep deprivation and epilepsy is another area requiring more investigation and clarification, not only from the practical viewpoint, but because it may shed more light on the topic of sleep deprivation and cerebral impairment.

2.21 Other effects on the human EEG

For the majority of sleep-deprived subjects the EEG just indicates extreme sleepiness. Whilst this suggests that nothing unusual is happening within the brain at this time, it should be remembered that the EEG, as normally recorded (Section 1.3), only reflects activity in the surface layers of the cerebrum (i.e. the cerebral cortex). This is reasonably satisfactory for looking at alpha activity and the spikes of epilepsy, which are found in these upper layers, but such methods tell us little about what else may be going on electrically, deep within the cerebrum. To investigate this, electrodes would have to be placed inside the brain, which is of course impossible. Deep recordings have been taken from sleep-deprived rats, but these have not been closely examined for abnormalities.

To avoid various artefacts occurring in the EEG, subjects have to lie or sit quietly, and then they are liable to fall asleep. Whilst this may be useful from the perspective of epilepsy, it is not so good if one is trying to measure the normal waking EEG. With progressive sleep deprivation all that may be measured is an increasing propensity to fall asleep. So, EEG measurement of the recumbent sleep-deprived subject has to be brief, before drowsiness sets in, and this requires a skilful recording procedure. One of the most notable studies in this respect was, again, the 205-hour sleep deprivation experiment (Section 2.7). Dr Paul Naitoh, a leading figure in sleep deprivation research, now working at the Naval Health Research Center in San Diego, was responsible for EEG assessment during that study. With colleagues, he carefully measured and analysed the EEGs of the subjects before, during and after sleep loss[22]. Nothing clinically abnormal was noticed. They looked in detail at the delta, theta, alpha, and beta frequency ranges (see Section 1.3), and it was alpha activity that showed the most obvious change. Alpha activity normally appears during relaxed but alert wakefulness, when there is little external stimulation, and particularly no visual stimulation.

Little happened at first, until about the third night of sleep loss, then alpha activity began to disappear markedly up to 120 hours (the fifth-day turning point), and then levelled off. This trend reflected the changes found in the subjects' own ratings of sleepiness, and in their psychological performance measures (Fig. 2.1). There was also a clear circadian rhythm in the appearance of alpha activity, where low levels occurred not only in the small hours of the morning, but also in the early afternoon. High points appeared in the later morning and early evening. This circadian effect persisted up to the end of the deprivation. Two recovery nights were needed to bring alpha activity back to normal. However, it should be remembered that sleep on these nights was restricted. Whilst the most obvious explanation for the changes in alpha activity is 'sleepiness', this sign of the inability of the cerebrum to maintain itself in relaxed readiness may belie more subtle effects of sleep loss on the brain.

EEG technology for humans is improving, and we now have more than just the 'spontaneous' EEG, where the experimenter usually does little to the subject whilst the EEG is monitored for several minutes. A newer method is to give a series of very short stimuli to one of the senses, for example light flashes to the eyes, 'clicks' to the ears, or pricks to the skin. EEG electrodes are placed on the scalp over the brain area dealing with the sensory process concerned—that is at the back of the head for vision (occipital area), side of the head for hearing (temporal area), and top of the head for touch (frontal-parietal area). The minute response evoked in the EEG is recorded for about 0.5 seconds following each stimulus, and is stored in a computer. About 50 or more of these are averaged together to produce a clearer signal, called the 'averaged evoked response' (AER). Because many stimuli can be given fairly rapidly the whole process takes no more than a minute or so. Sometimes the EEG response to a signal is recorded for a longer duration, around 10 seconds, and about 10 of these periods are averaged. This variant of the AER is called the 'contingent negative variation' (CNV), and is largely a measure of one's ability to maintain an attitude of 'alert and ready to respond'. Both the AER and CNV are made up of a series of complex waves which have standard identifications.

In effect, this process of averaging helps us to see more subtle electrical events within the cerebrum, and enhances small signals coming from the lower brain areas that are normally obscured by the electrical activity of the upper layers. AERs to sound stimuli have been obtained from sleeping subjects, and give further clues about what is happening to the cerebrum during the various sleep stages, and I will come to this topic in Section 5.10. However, within the context of sleep deprivation there have been very few investigations using AER or CNV techniques. One of the most notable was again by Naitoh and colleagues[53], concentrating on the CNV. Following one night of total sleep loss the CNV declined significantly, indicating a pronounced deterioration in the ability to hold oneself in immediate readiness to respond. According to Naitoh, the sleep-deprived brain 'lives from moment to moment, without pre-planned preparation'. Although subjects can quickly respond to stimuli when these arrive, subjects seem to react to each stimulus as a sudden surprise, rather than treat it as an expected event.

A more recent investigation[54] lasted for 2 days of sleep deprivation, and found rather puzzling AER and CNV changes which the authors attributed to a 'decrease in (cerebral) efficiency' (p. 354). To date, we have no information on what might happen to AERs over longer deprivation periods, particularly when sleep loss goes well into what I have called 'core sleepiness', beyond the second night (Section 2.14). Hopefully, these intriguing titbits of findings with AERs and CNVs will encourage others to go in to this much neglected approach to sleep loss.

References

1. Kleitman, N. (1963). *Sleep and Wakefulness* (second edition). University of Chicago Press, Chicago.

2. Licklider, J.C.R. and Bunch, M.E. (1946). Effects of enforced wakefulness upon the growth and the maze-learning performance of white rats. *Journal of Comparative Psychology*, **39**, 339–350.

3. Selye, H. (1976). *The Stress of Life* (second edition). McGraw Hill, New York.

4. Rechtschaffen, A., Gilliland, M.A., Bergman, B.M. and Winterer, J.B. (1983). Physiological correlates of prolonged sleep deprivation in rats. *Science*, **221**, 182–184.

5. Everson, C., Bergmann, B., Fang, V.S., Leitch, C.A., Obermeyer, W., Refetoff, S., Schoeller, D.A. and Rechtschaffen, A. (1986). Physiological and biochemical effects of total sleep deprivation in the rat. *Sleep Research*, **15**, 216.

6. Bergmann, B., Fang, V.S., Kushida, C., Everson, C. and Rechtschaffen, A. (1986). Hypothalamic-adrenal variables in paradoxical and total sleep deprivation of rats. *Sleep Research*, **15**, 212.

7. Kushida, C., Bergmann, B., Fang, V.S., Leitch, C.A., Obermeyer, W., Refetoff, S., Scholler, D.A. and Rechtschaffen, A. (1986). Physiological and biochemical effects of paradoxical sleep deprivation in the rat. *Sleep Research*, **15**, 219.

8. Gilliland, M.A., Bergmann, B. and Rechtschaffen, A. (1986). High EEG amplitude NREM sleep deprivation in the rat. *Sleep Research*, **15**, 218.

9. Gulevich, G., Dement, W. and Johnson, L. (1966). Psychiatric and EEG observations on a case of prolonged (264 hours) wakefulness. *Archives of General Psychiatry*, **15**, 29–35.

10. Naitoh, P., Pasnau, R.O. and Kollar, E.J. (1971). Psychophysiological changes after prolonged deprivation of sleep. *Biological Psychiatry*, **3**, 309–320.

11. Pasnau, R.O., Naitoh, P., Stier, S. and Kollar, E.J. (1968). The psychological effect of 205 hours of sleep deprivation. *Archives of General Psychiatry*, **18**, 496–505.

12. Opstad, P.K. and Aakvaag, A. (1983). The effect of sleep deprivation on the plasma levels of hormones during prolonged strain and calorie deficiency. *European Journal of Applied Physiology*, **51**, 97–107.

13. Patrick, G.T. and Gilbert, J.A. (1896). On the effects of loss of sleep. *Psychological Review*, **3**, 469–483.

14. Wilkinson, R.T. (1965). Sleep deprivation. In: Edholm, O.G. and Bacharach, A.L. (ed.) *Physiology of Survival*. Academic Press, London. pp. 399–430.

15. Naitoh, P. (1976). Sleep deprivation. *Waking and Sleeping*, **1**, 53–60.

16. Ross, J.J. (1965). Neurological findings after prolonged sleep deprivation. *Archives of Neurology*, **12**, 399–403.

17. Johnson, L.C., Slye, E.S. and Dement, W. (1965). Electroencephalographic and autonomic activity during and after prolonged sleep deprivation. *Psychosomatic Medicine*, **27**, 415–423.

18. Morris, G.O., Williams, H.L. and Lubin, A. (1960). Misperception and disorientation during sleep deprivation. *Archives of General Psychiatry*, **2**, 247–254.

19. Gillin, J.C. (1983). The sleep therapies of depression. *Progress in Neuropsychopharmacology and Biological Psychiatry*, **7**, 351–354.

20. Vogel, G.W. (1983). Evidence for REM sleep deprivation as the mechanism of

action of antidepressant drugs. *Progress in Neuropsychopharmacology and Biological Psychiatry*, **7**, 343–349.

21. Rubin, R..T., Kollar, E.J., Slater, G.G. and Clark, B.R. (1969). Excretion of 17-hydroxycorticosteroid and vanillymandelic acid excretion during 205 hours sleep deprivation in man. *Psychosomatic Medicine*, **31**, 68–75.

22. Naitoh, P., Kales, A., Kollar, E.J., Smith, J.C. and Jacobson, A. (1969). Electroencephalographic activity after prolonged sleep loss. *Electroencephalography and Clinical Neurophysiology*, **27**, 2–11.

23. Kales, A., Tan, T-L, Kollar, E.J., Naitoh, P., Preston, T.A. and Malmstrom, E.J. (1970). Sleep patterns following 205 hours of sleep deprivation. *Psychosomatic Medicine*, **32**, 189–200.

24. Williams, H.L., Lubin, A. and Goodnow, J.J. (1959). Impaired performance with acute sleep loss. *Psychological Monographs*, **73**, part 14, 1–26.

25. Williams, H.L., Gieseking, C.F. and Lubin, A. (1966). Some effects of sleep loss on memory. *Perceptual and Motor Skills*, **23**, 1287–1293.

26. Broadbent, D.E. (1955). Variations in performance arising from continuous work. In: *Conference on Individual Efficiency in Industry*, Medical Research Council, Cambridge. pp. 1–5.

27. Kjellberg, A. (1977). Sleep deprivation and some aspects of performance. III Motivation, comments and conclusions. *Waking and Sleeping*, **1**, 149–153.

28. Wilkinson, R.T. (1964). Effects of up to 60 hours sleep deprivation on different types of work. *Ergonomics*, **7**, 175–186.

29. Green, D.M. and Swets, J.A. (1966). *Signal Detection Theory and Psychophysics*. Wiley, New York.

30. Horne, J.A. and Pettitt, A.N. (1985). High incentive effects on vigilance performance during 72 hours of total sleep deprivation. *Acta Psychologica*, **58**, 123–139.

31. Webb, W.B. (1975). *Sleep the Gentle Tyrant*. Prentice Hall, New Jersey.

32. Meddis, R. (1977). *The Sleep Instinct*. Routledge & Kegan Paul, London.

33. Keys, A., Brozek, J., Henschel, A., Mickelsen, O. and Taylor, H.L. (1950). *The Biology of Human Starvation*. University of Minnesota Press, Minneapolis.

34. Wilkinson, R.T. (1968). Sleep deprivation: Performance tests for partial and selective sleep deprivation. In: Abt, L.A. and Reiss, B.F. (ed.), *Progress in Clinical Psychology—Vol. 3*, Grune and Stratton, London. pp. 28–43.

35. Webb, W.B. and Agnew, H.W. (1966). Sleep: effects of a restricted regime. *Science*, **150**, 1745–1747.

36. Hamilton, P., Wilkinson, R.T. and Edwards, R.S. (1972). A study of four days partial sleep deprivation. In: Colquhoun, W.P. (ed.) *Aspects of Human Efficiency*. The English Universities Press, London. pp. 101–112.

37. Webb, W.B. and Levy, C.M. (1982). Age, sleep deprivation and performance. *Psychophysiology*, **19**, 272–276.

38. Webb, W.B. (1985). A further analysis of age and sleep deprivation effects. *Psychophysiology*, **22**, 156–161.

39. Wilkinson, R.T. (1961). Interaction of lack of sleep with knowledge of results, repeated testing, and individual differences. *Journal of Experimental Psychology*, **62**, 263–271.

40. Webb, W.B. and Levy, C.M. (1984). Effects of spaced and repeated total sleep

deprivation. *Ergonomics*, **27**, 45–58.
41. Webb, W.B. and Agnew, H.W. (1973). Effects on performance of high and low energy expenditure during sleep deprivation. *Perceptual and Motor Skills*, **37**, 511–514.
42. Lubin, A., Hord, D.J., Tracy, M.L. and Johnson, L.C. (1976). Effects of exercise, bedrest and napping on performance decrement during 40 hours. *Psychophysiology*, **13**, 334–339.
43. Angus, R.G., Heslegrave, R.J. and Myles, W.S. (1985). Effects of prolonged sleep deprivation, with and without chronic physical exercise, on mood and performance. *Psychophysiology*, **22**, 276–282.
44. Horne, J.A. (1975). Binocular convergence in man during total sleep deprivation. *Biological Psychology*, **3**, 309–319.
45. Horne, J.A. (1976). Recovery sleep following different visual conditions during total sleep deprivation in man. *Biological Psychology*, **4**, 107–118.
46. Horne, J.A. (1978). The effects of sleep deprivation upon variations in heart rate and respiration rate. *Experientia*, **33**, 1175–1176.
47. Horne, J.A. and Walmsley, B. (1976). Daytime visual load and the effects upon human sleep. *Psychophysiology*, **13**, 115–120.
48. Horne, J.A. and Minard, A. (1985). Sleep and sleepiness following a behaviourally 'active' day. *Ergonomics*, **28**, 567–575.
49. Benoit, O., Foret, J., Bouard, G., Merle, B., Landau, J. and Marc, M.E. (1980). Habitual sleep length and patterns of recovery sleep after 24 hour and 36 hour sleep deprivation. *Electroencephalography and Clinical Neurophysiology*, **50**, 477–485.
50. Ellingson, R.J., Wilken, K. and Bennett, D.R. (1984). Efficacy of sleep deprivation as an activation procedure in epilepsy patients. *Journal of Clinical Neurophysiology*, **1**, 83–101.
51. Bennett, D.R., Mattson, R.H., Ziter, F.A., Calverly, J.R., Liske, E.A. and Pratt, K.L. (1964). Sleep deprivation: neurological and EEG effects. *Aerospace Medicine*, **35**, 888–890.
52. Gunderson, G.H., Dunne, P.B. and Feyer, T. (1973). Sleep deprivation seizures. *Neurology*, **23**, 678–686.
53. Naitoh, P., Johnson, L.C. and Lubin, A. (1973). The effects of selective and total sleep loss on the CNV and its psychological and physiological correlates. *Electroencephalography and Clinical Neurophysiology*, Suppl. **33**, 213–218.
54. Gauthier, P. and Gottesmann, C. (1983). Influence of total sleep deprivation on event-related potentials in man. *Psychophysiology*, **20**, 351–355.

3. Physiological effects of sleep deprivation

So far, I have mainly concerned myself with the effects of sleep deprivation on the brain, as it is here where the problems seem really to lie, with the rest of the body relatively unaffected. This latter claim has been based on the absence of any findings of physiological significance from the 264- and 205-hour studies. But now I want to examine the claim more thoroughly, particularly as it may be remembered that in Section 2.3 I pointed out that most of the sleep deprivation studies using measures of general body physiology were directed towards presumed stress effects, rather than towards possible functions sleep might have for the body. Over the last decade, measures have become more sophisticated, and whilst still generally stress oriented they have given more depth to the earlier findings, even though the outcome still points to an absence of any harmful effect of sleep deprivation on the body, beyond the brain.

But before describing the recent findings, I would like to set the scene by looking briefly at some of these earlier results, as there are several important investigations in addition to the two very long deprivation studies I have already described. One final note—I will be concerned with physiological changes in parts of the body other than the brain, and rather than refer continually to the 'body except the brain' I will just use the term 'body', being distinct from the brain. This is not a modern version of dualism that sees the brain as a completely separate entity, but a simplification of writing style.

3.1 The first major physiological study—Kleitman (1923)

After his work on dogs (Section 2.1), Kleitman carried out pioneering sleep deprivation experiments on humans. These physiological studies were the first of their kind and complement those of Patrick and Gilbert, who concentrated on human behaviour and psychological performance. Like all good investigators he tried out the methods on himself, as well as on others, and wrote[1], 'Most of the work that involved long periods of normal control testing was done on the writer, who went through more than a dozen sleepless periods himself. The other subjects were used to check the results obtained on him'. Sadly, many latter-day researchers criticize Kleitman's work as he

79

spent too much time looking at himself, and used too few other subjects. The problem is of course, that he could have (unwittingly) introduced his own biases into the findings, which makes poor science. However, in his defence, he was a methodical experimenter who separated out the data on himself from those of the other subjects. His own experiences of sleep deprivation give considerable depth and insight into his clear and lucid accounts, found for example in his book *Sleep and Wakefulness*[2]. His work must be highly regarded, not only for this insight, but also because he is one of the few sleep researchers who has taken a broad perspective on our understanding of sleep, and who really strode to discover why we sleep.

His main experiments with humans used a total of six young men, excluding himself, who were sleep deprived for 40–115 hours. Regular measurements were made of heart rate, temperature, respiration rate, blood-pressure, and metabolism at rest (oxygen consumption). Blood samples were taken daily for red and white blood cell counts, and for measurements of haemoglobin level, blood sugar, and certain electrolytes. All urine was collected, and assessed for certain aspects of kidney function (e.g. excretion of chlorides), and to see how the body was utilizing food (i.e. nitrogen, phosphates, and creatinine). These latter measures were of particular interest to Kleitman, as he was puzzled by Patrick and Gilbert's reported increases of body weight.

But Kleitman had to remain perplexed about those increases, as none of his subjects put on weight, and there were no notable changes to metabolism or any of the blood or urine measures. Also absent were any changes to the pulse and blood pressure. Although respiration became irregular, this was probably due to sighing, yawning, etc. Kleitman was a physiologist, but he soon realized that the greatest effects of sleep deprivation were on the brain, and he began to concentrate more on neurology and behaviour.

At the time of his experiments there were several current and perhaps bizarre theories about the causes of sleep (see Section 1.1), for example that waking progressively impairs the heart and circulation, leading to insufficient blood for the brain. Another theory hypothesized that sleep is due to a build-up of toxic substances in the blood. His sleep deprivation findings caused him to reject these, and instead go for theories centring more on neural activity. Kleitman was sceptical about the vogue then for a Pavlovian approach, that sleep is an 'inhibitory reflex', and argued instead for sleep being caused by 'increased synaptic resistance'. This was based more on the earlier views of the famous neurologist, John Hughlings Jackson, who in 1898[3] argued that, 'sleep was for the highest levels of the nervous system, which are modifiable and more susceptible to fatigue'—a view that I very much support, and is central to my proposals for core sleep.

3.2 The next 50 years

In 1978 I wrote a review of the published experiments dealing with the physiological and biochemical effects of sleep deprivation since the days of Kleitman[4]. Over 50 experiments had been carried out during this 50-year period, and, excluding the 264- and 205-hour studies already mentioned, most fell in the range of 2–5 nights without sleep. Many were stress oriented, and several had problems with their methodology, of the sort I outlined in Section 2.3. In this chapter I want to concentrate more on the recent research since my review, and so I will only briefly summarize those early studies, before proceeding to the new findings.

Of the 11 deprivation experiments in this 50-year period that monitored the output of the stress hormone cortisol, all but three reported no change, and by far the weight of evidence suggests that there was no significant alarm response. Two of the three studies that did find such a response were military-type experiments[5,6] that included additional psychological strain beyond the sleep deprivation itself. The third study[7] gave no information about how the subjects were kept awake, apart from what the authors described as 'psychic and physical stimulation', which could well have been stressful in itself. Several of the 11 experiments also looked for other effects of stress, particularly with respect to blood sedimentation rate, and 'packed cell volume'—an index of the density of blood cells. These two indices are influenced by cortisol output, and are also fairly sensitive to any developing illness. Only one of these studies[7], the one giving the psychic and physical stimulation, found anything significant. There are ten reports where adrenaline and related substances were measured (see Section 2.3), but only two found any noticeable rise, with one of these studies being the military experiment[5] just mentioned. Many investigations monitored heart rate and blood-pressure, but the overall outcome favours no clear change to either, as, for example, three reports found a rise in heart rate, five a decrease, and nine no change. Systolic blood pressure fell in three studies and remained the same in nine.

Despite the lack of evidence showing any harmful effects of sleep deprivation on general body functioning, there has been a prevailing belief that sleep is a state of heightened body tissue repair following the apparent 'wear and tear' of wakefulness. But if this was really so, then surely sleep deprivation would produce more serious effects on the body? However, one could counter that as most of the measures used in these studies were directed largely towards stress, they may not have picked up subtle impairments due to lack of body tissue repair. Whilst this riposte is reasonable, any such tissue malfunction would itself have caused an alarm response in cortisol levels, and affected some of the blood measures such as white cell count and sedimentation rate. As far as we can tell from these earlier experiments, this was not the case.

3.3 Body 'restitution' and sleep

Very few of these earlier studies had taken measurements that shed any clear light on the topic of body restitution and sleep, and whether this might be failing during sleep deprivation. However, before I go on to describe what few measurements have been made, let me give a quick account of what I mean by tissue restitution and repair. Tissues are largely made of proteins. But proteins are unstable and, to varying extents, they are in a continuous state of *breakdown* and *synthesis*. Together, these two processes are part of *protein turnover*. The building blocks of protein are amino acids, which can be likened to the bricks of a wall, with the wall itself being a protein molecule. The bricks are always falling out (i.e. protein breakdown), and having to be replaced (synthesis). Some of the bricks that fall out remain intact, and these can be placed back into the wall. Others are damaged and have to be disposed of.

Transportation of new amino acids to the cell is via the blood, which also removes those that are 'damaged'. These latter amino acids are *oxidized* in the liver to form urea, which is disposed of by the kidneys in the urine. Plenty of new amino acids enter the bloodstream from the gut following the digestion of proteins (into amino acids) in the diet. Most of us in the Western world are well fed, and eat far more protein than is required for tissue rebuilding, and so any excess amino acids from the gut are also oxidized into urea and excreted. A more detailed account of these processes is given in Section 4.1 and illustrated in Fig. 4.1.

In order to understand what is happening to protein turnover, its three phases (synthesis, breakdown, and oxidation) have to be measured at the same time. So returning to the brick wall analogy, when bricks are replaced at a higher rate than those falling out, then a condition of restitution and/or growth prevails. On the other hand, if more bricks fall out than can be replaced then disrepair predominates. Those who support the body restitution viewpoint for sleep consider that wakefulness is a condition of overall wear and tear—that is tissue disrepair. In other words, 'catabolism' prevails during wakefulness, and 'anabolism' during sleep. If this were the case, then sleep deprivation would presumably extend the disrepair. Unfortunately, no sleep deprivation study has looked at the three phases of protein turnover simultaneously to test this theory. The only phase that has been monitored in this respect is urea output, which tells us little on its own. Proponents of the body restitution role for sleep would expect more protein to be broken down and oxidized than synthesized during sleep deprivation, through continued tissue wear and tear—leading to a greater urea output.

Over the 50-year period of sleep deprivation research only three studies have measured urea output. Although none found any significant changes, only one regulated food intake and measured the protein content of the food eaten by their subjects[8]. It is necessary to know this intake, of course, otherwise any increase in urea production might simply be due to the subjects eating more—which is a common tendency during sleep deprivation. So, the intake of protein from food has to be subtracted from the total urea output. Remember, urea comes from the oxidation of old amino acids and new ones from recent food intake. In that study[8], sleep deprivation lasted for two nights, and the urea output of each subject was assessed daily. On the first day this increased by a nominal 6 per cent, and on the second it went down by the same amount. These small changes could, for example, be due to a small 'carry-over' of urea in the liver and bloodstream from one 24-hour period into the next. However, the key point is that the sum effect over the 2 days was for no change in urea output, and there is little support here for the restitution theory. But I must emphasize, again, that urea output concerns only one aspect of protein turnover, and is no more than a very crude guide to the total process involved in protein turnover.

The body's use of its energy supplies is also relevant to the restitutive theory of sleep. However, the underlying rationale is somewhat complex and I will describe this in more detail in Section 4.6, dealing with the concept of 'cell energy charge'. Suffice it to say that the body's energy supply mainly centres on compounds called the 'adenylates'—adenosine tri-, di-, and monophosphates (ATP, ADP, and AMP). These can be viewed as an energy 'currency' or 'cash'. The body's carbohydrate and fat reserves can be likened to savings bonds that can only be converted to 'ready cash' by a series of transactions (that I will not go into). The real 'cash' for spending energy is ATP, and the subsequent 'empty purse' needing to be topped up by the conversion of more savings bonds is represented by ADP and AMP.

The reason why I raise this topic of energy now is that in the early 1960s two deprivation studies[9,10], by the same group of researchers, claimed that sleep deprivation resulted in 'emergency responses' in adenylate levels. At face value these findings suggest that lack of sleep does, after all, have a serious effect on the body—evidence which could be used in support of the body restitution theory for sleep.

The first experiment[9] was carried out in 1960, on a 27-year-old male unemployed ex-local radio disc jockey who wanted to run a marathon record show. The investigators described him as an anxious individual, with some psychiatric problems when young, but otherwise healthy. His motive for doing the study was to raise money for charities, and to seek fame so that he could get a job at another radio station. For most of the marathon he sat at a disc jockey console in front of bright lights, in a Detroit store window in full public view. Until the 100-hour point he coped quite well, but then became 'expansive, hyperactive and grandiose . . . hostile towards women' up to about 160 hours, when he become subdued but very irascible. Nevertheless, he managed to keep going for 220 hours non-stop, and then collapsed.

Despite the bizarreness of the occasion, it was an irresistable opportunity for sleep deprivation researchers. But because of the circumstances, quite unlike the more sanguine set-up for Randy Gardner (Section 2.5), the findings should be viewed cautiously. This is why I did not include it amongst my earlier account of the longest studies. Blood samples were taken once before sleep deprivation and only twice during the deprivation, on the fourth and seventh days of the marathon. ATP activity rose significantly on the fourth day, but returned to baseline levels on the seventh day. However, the authors interpreted this latter change in a strange way, seeing it only in terms of a substantial fall. They declared that it 'could well represent a failure of the mechanisms responsible for the increased synthesis of ATP' (p. 190). I cannot agree with such an interpretation, and would simply describe it as a return to normality.

The second study[10] was conventional and was run with 12 subjects in a laboratory, with sleep deprivation lasting for 5 days. Once more, blood samples were only taken twice during deprivation, on days two and four. These were compared with a baseline measurement. Again, ATP activity rose on the first occasion and returned to baseline levels on the second. In the same way as before, the authors described this fall as a 'precipitous drop' (p. 75).

Although these findings have never been followed up, they have had quite an impact on sleep deprivation research that is still evident today. Nevertheless, both experiments had problems with their methods, particularly as the adenylates were measured only in blood samples. This gives little indication of what is going on inside the cells of other body tissues, especially as red blood cells are peculiar in their use of adenylates.

A real fall in ATP levels within cells represents a crisis that cannot be endured for more than a few minutes. Typically, it occurs during very heavy (anaerobic) exercise. Under these circumstances there is a safety mechanism for temporarily speeding up the manufacture of ATP, resulting in a by-product called 'creatine' being produced. This is converted to creatinine in the kidneys and excreted in the urine. So, measurement of urinary creatinine gives an indication of any true emergency responses with the ATP supply to cells. Creatinine is very easy to assess, and it has been monitored by six sleep deprivation experiments over the last 50 years since it was first measured by Kleitman[1]. But the only finding of any increase in creatinine came from the study on the disc jockey. Here, urine was collected and sampled daily and, although several of the days had statistically significant rises in creatinine output, these were still small, with all but one being within a 'healthy' range and not of clinical interest.

This prompts me to end this short account of the earlier sleep deprivation studies with a note of caution about the concepts of 'statistical' and 'clinical' significance—often mistakenly seen to be the same. A change of statistical significance may well be of little clinical relevance if it still falls within the range for healthy individuals. So it is prudent to be aware of the normal ranges for any biochemical or physiological measure. To take an extreme example as an illustration, if as a result of some stimulus a group of 20 subjects all showed an increase of 2–5 millimetres of mercury in their systolic blood pressure, then statistically this would be highly significant. On the other hand, the clinician would dismiss this as trivial. Of course, clinically significant changes are usually also highly statistically significant.

3.4 Effects on exercise

In Section 2.18 I described experiments investigating whether sleepiness is offset or made worse by exercise. Little effect was found, with perhaps some worsening. Other sleep deprivation studies have been interested in exercise from a different perspective—is one's inherent physiological ability to do exercise impaired? It is the field that I now want to concentrate on. It is particularly interesting to me as it is of some relevance to the issue of body restitution and sleep, although the investigations themselves were not really concerned with this theme. Their objective was to find out whether and how exercise might be affected by sleep loss.

If sleep deprivation impairs tissue repair or ATP production, especially in muscle, then one might reason that the ability of muscles to work would deteriorate as sleep loss progresses. However, there are also psychological factors to contend with, as sleepy subjects are often less motivated to persevere at exercise, and rest up sooner than normal. For similar reasons, sleep-deprived subjects are more likely to view the same exercise load to be heavier than usual. If certain physiological measurements are made, which I will be coming to, then it is possible to see whether the reduced endurance of the sleep-deprived subject is due to physiological or psychological factors.

Ideally it would be best to look inside muscle, but this can be a painful procedure. One deprivation experiment has done this, though, by removing minute samples of muscle via a needle (i.e. a biopsy)[11]. Subjects were sleep deprived for 5 days and a biopsy was taken from leg muscle on the last day and compared with a pre-deprivation sample. Changes were found in several enzymes associated with certain metabolic process, some of which related to ATP use. But it is difficult to say whether these changes were of clinical significance, particularly as there was no control group of subjects sleeping normally. There was no indication of how the subjects were kept awake, and especially whether this involved any exercise. All of these factors could have affected the outcome of the biopsies. Certainly the authors pointed out from blood tests, which were also taken, that the subjects showed physiological signs of stress. What we do not know is the real cause of this stress—was it sleep deprivation, or apprehension about other aspects of the study such as the biopsies? Unfortunately, no further experiment has followed up these findings, and we have to wait for confirmation. Other, more indirect measures of muscle function that I am now going to cover indicate that there is little obvious impairment during sleep deprivation.

These other studies have used less specific ways of assessing muscle activity, including general athletic performance. One of the most carefully conducted experiments of this type gave 12 subjects three nights sleep deprivation, and measured a variety of abilities such as grip strength, running speed over a 40-metre dash, jump height, and leg strength[12]. Although none of these indices deteriorated during the deprivation, there are strong psychological factors again, as it could be argued that there may have been some physiological deterioration that was compensated for by increased psychological effort. One way or another, how subjects view such studies is of critical importance to the outcome. Highly motivated people can show great feats of physical endurance during sleep deprivation. For example, there are reports of 92 hours of almost-continuous five-a-side football matches, producing no physical ill-effects[13]. Similarly unaffected was an athlete exercising nearly continuously for 100 hours[14].

The mechanical efficiency of the body in its use of energy gives another index of the ability of muscle to work. This is not so affected by psychological factors, and reduces the problem of motivation. It is assessed by measuring (via a mouthpiece) the amounts of oxygen consumed per minute ($\dot{V}O_2$) and carbon dioxide ($\dot{V}CO_2$) produced by a subject exercising at a fixed workload—usually cycling on a stationary cycle 'ergometer'. The speed has to be constant and at an 'aerobic' level (i.e. at a speed well below the subject's maximum—e.g. at 60 per cent of the maximum), otherwise there is the complication of anaerobic exercise and 'oxygen debt' (which I will not go into). From this information the amount of energy used up during the exercise can be calculated and, when it is compared with the actual physical workload set on the ergometer, we can estimate the individual's mechanical efficiency, or in a loose sense 'miles per gallon' and see whether this deteriorates during sleep deprivation.

Another aspect of the ability to do work is 'physical fitness'. One method again uses oxygen uptake, and assesses the maximum possible exercise output within the 'aerobic' range. This is referred to in shortened form as '$\dot{V}O_{2max}$'. The fitter the subject, the greater is the $\dot{V}O_{2max}$. Both $\dot{V}O_{2max}$ and mechanical efficiency not only relate to the working of the muscles but also give a guide to the ability of the lungs and blood to absorb oxygen from the air and to transport it to the muscle. If ATP turnover were becoming impaired, or muscle cells were weakening in some way because of a lack of repair during sleep deprivation, then mechanical efficiency and $\dot{V}O_{2max}$ would fall, since more oxygen would be used for a given workload.

Mechanical efficiency and $\dot{V}O_{2max}$ also relate to the uptake of oxygen by the lungs and blood, and the distribution of oxygen around the body by the cardiovascular system. So these indices can be further refined, and used for example as a guide to heart function by calculating the oxygen uptake at a certain heart rate, say at 150 beats per minute. There are other aspects to the physiology of work, especially endurance, but this is affected by psychological factors that are a particular problem for sleep deprivation. Another relates to the physiological recovery processes after the exercise has finished—how many minutes does it take for these to return the body to pre-exercise levels? As one might expect all of the indices I have described are interrelated, and endurance, for example, increases with fitness and recovery is quicker. The recent studies that have looked at the effects of sleep deprivation in relation to physical exercise have used permutations of the various measures I have just described.

The majority of the recent experiments in this field come from Dr Bruce Martin at the Indiana University School of Medicine[15]. Several carefully conducted studies have been run by his group since the beginning of the 1980s. Initially, these were only for one night's deprivation, and none found any reduction in $\dot{V}O_{2max}$ or changes in various cardiovascular measures, such as blood-pressure. The only outcome of note was that subjects (mistakenly) perceived that their exercise loads were greater during deprivation. Also, their endurance (the time it took for them to feel exhausted by the exercise and give up) fell by about 10 per cent. However, this could not be substantiated by the physiological measures, and Martin reasonably presumed that the underlying cause was psychological.

Another of his exercise studies, of one-night sleep deprivation, concentrated in more detail on stress and these apparent psychological factors. Here, he measured the blood levels of adrenaline, noradrenaline, the related substance dopamine, as well as cortisol, and, of particular interest, beta endorphin. This has many actions, and to some extent relates to the individual's control of stress. Although all these substances were affected by the exercise, none was additionally influenced by the sleep loss. In this study, the subjects' perception of their workload remained unchanged. Unfortunately, the time to exhaustion could not be measured here.

Lastly, a further, longer two-night deprivation study by Martin also found no effect on $\dot{V}O_2$ values, or for that matter any changes with blood levels of adrenaline, noradrenaline, and related substances. Now, the time to exhaustion fell, by 20%, for no apparent physiological reason. Overall, it seems that one night of sleep loss may or may not change the psychological aspects of exhaustion, but two nights is more likely to do so.

What about the findings from other laboratories? After all, Martin's experiments were only up to 2 days deprivation, and it is possible that this is too short for detrimental effects to appear in the usual physiological measurements of exercise. Prior to Martin's work, the major study in this field was in 1969, carried out by Dr V. Brodan and colleagues at the Institute of Nutrition in Prague[16]. Although it was not so long ago, those were the days when sophisticated devices for measuring oxygen uptake were not readily available, and the popular method for assessing physical fitness depended on the heart-rate response to exercise. Heart rate is mostly concerned with the function and efficiency of the circulation, and is strongly correlated with $\dot{V}O_2$ levels over a fairly wide range of exercise loads.

Brodan and colleagues used the 'Harvard Step Test', which is based on stepping up and down on a 45 cm (18'') bench once every 4 seconds for several minutes. Heart rate is monitored for the first 8 minutes of rest immediately after the stepping stops. This recovery can be compared with norms for physical fitness—the fitter the subject, the quicker is the recovery. In this experiment, 26 subjects were sleep deprived for 3–5 days, and the Harvard Step Test was carried out every 24 hours. No loss of performance was found, and levels remained relatively stable for the first 4 days. Interestingly, on the last day there was a slight improvement. However, no control group was used to monitor for any training effect, and it is quite possible that the subjects, who were not particularly fit to start with, were getting fitter because of this regular physical activity. Such an effect could have counteracted any small detriment due to sleep deprivation.

I became very interested in the effects of sleep deprivation on the physiological responses to exercise, and we ran our own experiment[17]. Seven subjects were sleep deprived for three nights and days following a baseline day. Twice a day, in the morning and afternoon, they exercised on a cycle ergometer at three different workloads (light, moderate, and heavy) on each occasion. Levels of $\dot{V}O_2$ uptake and $\dot{V}CO_2$ output were measured, together with heart rates. Since our subjects were only of average fitness, there was the likelihood that this frequent exercising might make them fitter, and we would have the problem I have just outlined for Brodan's study. Therefore we used a second group of people of similar initial fitness who also went through the same procedures, but slept normally. On each measurement occasion we calculated the subjects' mechanical efficiency, $\dot{V}O_2$, and $\dot{V}O_2$ at a heart rate of 150 beats per minute. None of these showed any difference between the two groups. The only outcome of interest was that both groups of subjects indeed became slightly fitter with successive exercising, and to similar extents. We used very sensitive statistical techniques to try and tease out what may have been very small effects of sleep deprivation, but again nothing was found.

3.5 The control of body temperature (thermoregulation)

In the experiments on rats at the Chicago Sleep Laboratory (Section 2.2), the main finding seemed to be a failure in the animals' ability to retain body heat.

Seemingly, this heat loss could not be counteracted by the increased food intake, and the animals had to draw on their own energy reserves. This apparent problem with thermoregulation leads to the obvious question of what happens in the case of humans? Before I go on to answer this, it should be remembered that rats have a relatively large body surface area in proportion to their body size, and it is likely that any problem with thermoregulation will be of greater consequence to them than to a mammal our size.

Few investigators have looked carefully to see whether human thermoregulation is affected by sleep deprivation, partly because attention has only very recently been drawn to this area. Nevertheless, there are some interesting changes, but nothing pointing to any loss of thermoregulation. Let me begin with a common finding with a simple measure—body temperature. But I must emphasize that this is not a measure of thermoregulation, only a product of thermoregulation, as it is the net result of the balance between heat produced and heat lost. Most sleep deprivation studies from the days of Patrick and Gilbert have found a small fall in body temperature in their subjects. Its circadian rhythm is maintained, and the whole rhythm just gets shifted downwards. This can be seen in Fig. 3.1, from our own study, described in Section 2.11. Sleep deprivation ran for 72 hours over a weekend following a Friday baseline day. It will be recalled that there

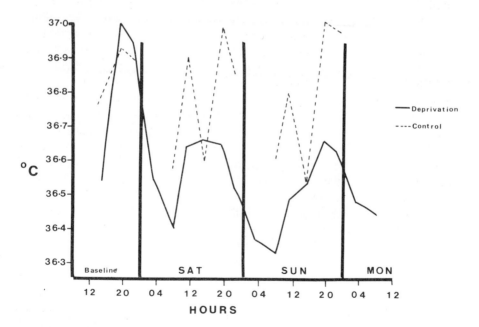

Fig. 3.1 Body temperature during sleep loss—oral temperature changes over 72 hours in sleep-deprived and normally sleeping control subjects. The fall begins on the first night, although the circadian rhythm remains.

were two sleep-deprived groups; however, as they showed similar trends in body temperature the results have been combined here. Compared with subjects in the control group sleeping normally, the sleep-deprived subjects showed an average fall in temperature of about 0.3–0.4°C, starting during the first night of deprivation. Similar temperature changes can be seen in Fig. 2.1 for the 205-hour study.

It is a common finding that sleepless subjects feel colder and put on more clothes, or turn up the heating. Unfortunately, this possibly important behaviour has been overlooked in sleep deprivation research, and no study has kept a record of it. I have to confess that this criticism also applies to my own experiments. Increased clothing cuts body heat loss down, of course, but during sleep deprivation we do not know if or how this would affect body temperature.

Whereas humans show a fall in body temperature as soon as sleep deprivation begins, this was not apparent in the rats from the Chicago Sleep Laboratory study until they had been without sleep for at least a week. Nevertheless, the animals seemed to show an immediate rise in metabolic rate, reflected in voracious eating and weight loss. Humans also usually want to eat a lot during sleep deprivation, at least during the first few days, but for reasons that are not clear. This increased appetite could partly have a psychological basis related to the loss of REM sleep (see Section 8.6). Despite the rise in food intake, human body weight seems to show little change, although it should be noted that few studies have kept very detailed records of weight. As far as it is known, the subjects of the 264- and 205-hour studies did not show any obvious changes in body weight.

Maybe we humans also need more food to fuel a rise in metabolic rate during sleep deprivation, to overcome an increase in body heat loss rather like the rats? Only one human sleep deprivation experiment has measured metabolic rate to the level of thoroughness required to answer this question. Certain precautions need to be taken before such measurements can be collected. The thermal environment has to be carefully controlled, and the subjects fasted for at least 6 hours (to exclude the metabolic cost of digestion, which can be very large). The usual method is to monitor the rates of $\dot{V}O_2$ uptake and $\dot{V}CO_2$ production in a similar way to that of the exercise studies (Section 3.4), but this time with the subject resting and relaxed. This is what was done by Dr Vincent Fiorica and colleagues[18], at the Federal Aviation Administration Physiology Laboratory in Oklahoma. Six subjects were sleep deprived for 4 days, and six control subjects slept normally. Each morning all had their resting metabolic rate measured for half an hour, in the nude, and in a neutral environmental temperature of 27°C. No effects on metabolism from sleep loss were found. There was no rise, and both groups showed almost exactly the same results. Unfortunately, no record was kept of the food eaten by the subjects, although, according to the investigators, it 'was approximately similar between the two groups'. Daily weighings were made, but no changes were reported.

Additionally, Fiorica and colleagues did something particularly interesting, by putting their subjects' thermoregulation under a strain. Each afternoon subjects were monitored for a further hour while in the cold, at 10°C. They wore only shorts. As well as having their resting $\dot{V}O_2$ and rectal temperature measured, skin temperatures at several sites over the body were also recorded. When weighted together these latter temperatures give a guide to heat loss. For example, a drop in skin temperature in a cold environment usually indicates less heat loss from the body, as blood flow to the skin is being restricted (peripheral vasoconstriction), and skin temperature falls to approach that of the environment.

Fig. 3.2 shows the outcome for both the control and sleep-deprived subjects over the baseline day and the three deprivation days. The results for $\dot{V}O_2$ and mean weighted skin temperature are plotted at 5-minute intervals for the hour's exposure to the cold, following an initial 10-minute period at normal room temperature. Although skin temperature showed a slightly greater fall (of around 1.0°C) in the sleep-deprived group, the reduction in body heat loss was very small. From the rising $\dot{V}O_2$ levels it can be seen that both groups increased their metabolic rate and internal heat production by similar amounts. Rectal temperature was lower during sleep deprivation, as one might expect, but it showed no greater fall during the cold exposure.

Using all these findings, Fiorica and colleagues were further able to make various other calculations, particularly body heat storage. This dropped from the beginning to the end of each cold exposure. The fall was expressed as Calories per kilogram of body weight over the hour. For the sleep deprived group, from days one to four, these values were 1.9, 2.3, 2.3, and 1.9 respectively—remarkably similar to the comparable levels of 1.9, 2.2, 2.2, and 2.0 for the control subjects.

From these findings it seems that we have little reason for suspecting that sleep loss impairs thermoregulation in humans, despite the original suspicions based on the animal findings. Before leaving Fiorica's experiment, it is worth noting that there were no signs of any subject being particularly stressed by the cold exposure, or for that matter by the deprivation. Although cortisol was not monitored, urine samples were assessed for total levels of adrenaline, noradrenaline, and dopamine. Adrenaline usually responds to most types of stress (although not to the same extent as cortisol), but it remained unchanged during sleep deprivation.

A little more insight into thermoregulation in humans during sleep deprivation comes from two studies that were mainly exercise based. In the first, from Martin's laboratory, subjects ran regularly on a treadmill, in an environmental temperature of 0°C, during 2 days of sleep deprivation[19]. The usual measures, of rate of $\dot{V}O_2$ uptake, heart rate, etc., were taken, as well as

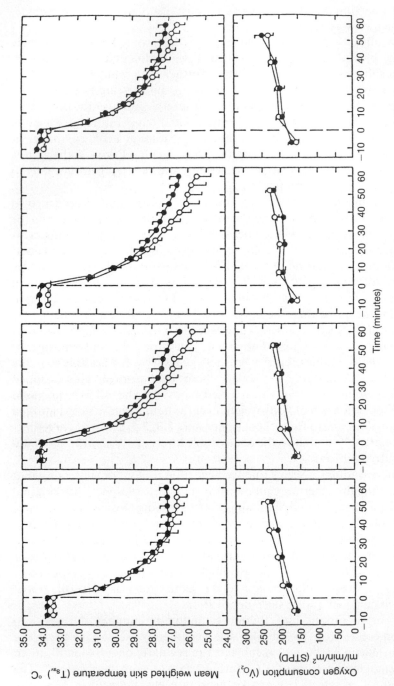

Fig. 3.2 Heat loss and heat production measured daily over 82 hours of sleep loss, in sleep-deprived (open circles), and control subjects (filled circles)—as determined by (upper) skin temperature weighted from several sites, and (lower) metabolic rate (oxygen consumption). All subjects were exposed to a cold (10 °C) environment for 1 hour, following an initial 10 minutes in a neutral environment. Some small differences can be seen between the groups in the rate of fall of skin temperature, but this is minor. Overall, sleep deprivation had no effect on thermoregulation. (From Fiorica et al.[18]. Reproduced by permission of the American Physiological Society)

rectal temperature. As usual, this latter measure was lower for the sleepless subjects before the exercise began, but during the exercise it rose to a level similar to that of the control subjects. From this and other findings, Martin's conclusion was that the sleep-deprived subjects produced as much heat as normal, but conserved more of it by losing less.

The second experiment had a greater emphasis on thermoregulation, although at a normal environmental temperature and humidity. Its conclusions were similar to those of the last experiment. Dr Michael Sawka and colleagues at the Yale School of Medicine, showed that after one night of sleep loss there was an interesting change in thermoregulation[20]. Five fit men pedalled on a cycle ergometer for 40 minutes at half their maximum rate. Apart from monitoring rectal temperature and $\dot{V}O_2$, the investigators also measured sweat rate (i.e. 'evaporative' heat loss from the body) as a guide to body heat loss. Compared with baseline measurements, sweat rate fell by about 25 per cent during deprivation—that is evaporative heat loss dropped. Rectal temperature changes were similar to those just reported—lower than normal before the exercise, and rising to the expected level by the end of exercise period. Again then, sleep deprivation led to a greater 'storage' of body heat during exercise. Sawka and colleagues believed that the cause lay in mechanisms within the brain regulating sweating and blood flow to the skin. But why this change should happen during sleep deprivation remains a mystery.

To conclude, all these findings fail to show that humans experience any serious problem with thermoregulation during sleep deprivation. However, there is a small fall in body temperature, or, to put it differently, body temperature seems to be reset and regulated at a slightly lower level. This may be associated with the greater feeling of being cold. Less heat may be lost from the body, and these two findings combined—a drop in body temperature and a reduced heat loss—suggest that the resting metabolic rate should fall a little, but there is little evidence of this so far. Rodents appear to respond quite differently to sleep deprivation, as the signs are that metabolic rate and body heat loss both rise as soon as the deprivation begins, but deep body temperature remains unchanged, at least for the first week or so of sleep loss. Whilst none of these few experiments on humans has gone beyond 4 days of sleep loss, it still seems that we fare considerably better than rodents within this period—perhaps because of less stress or our greater body size.

3.6 Other aspects of homeostasis

Let us see what can be gleaned about the regulation of other physiological systems during human sleep deprivation. There is something of interest with respiration. Firstly, it should be remembered that when the oxygen level of the blood falls (hypoxia), or the carbon dioxide level rises (hypercapnia), sensors within the control centres for respiration in the base of the brain lead to the rate and depth of breathing being increased until normal blood levels of these gases are re-established. Three recent studies[21-23], all of one night's sleep deprivation, have looked at the response of respiration to hypoxia or hypercapnia. All found that sleep deprivation reduced these responses by about 20 per cent. However, the extent to which this could be regarded as an impairment rather than as a relatively harmless 'dampening', or a resetting of the response at a lower level, in the same way that body temperature seems to be reduced, is difficult to say. Other aspects of respiration are clearly affected by sleepiness, with yawning and sighing being prime examples. These seem to be under a behavioural rather than physiological influence, but may be responsible for the irregular heartbeat that is also found during sleep deprivation (Section 2.18).

Overall then, for humans, sleep deprivation may be having apparently harmless effects on control mechanisms within the brain that regulate certain physiological events (i.e. homeostasis) like respiration and heat balance. Homeostasis certainly undergoes some fascinating changes during sleep itself, particularly in REM sleep. But this is another story, and will be left for Chapter 8.

3.7 Update on hormone changes

Over the last few years our knowledge about the hormonal effects of sleep deprivation has been broadened, mostly through work at the Laboratory for Clinical Stress Research in Stockholm, where a leading investigator in this field is Dr Torbjörn Åkerstedt. He and his colleagues have published many detailed accounts covering a variety of hormones[24-26]. In one of their major studies 12 young men were deprived of sleep for three nights. Blood and urine samples were taken regularly, and various aspects of behaviour were monitored. Blood was assessed for: cortisol, adrenaline, noradrenaline, several sex hormones including luteinizing hormone (LH), follicle-stimulating hormone (FSH), variants of testosterone and progesterone, and the thyroid hormones. Additionally, levels of the rather mysterious hormone melatonin were measured in the urine. Melatonin is released by the pineal gland during the night-time, and is suppressed by daylight—therefore it has a pronounced circadian rhythm. Whilst its function in humans is not understood, in lower mammals it regulates reproduction and the seasonal sexual cycles. This hormone is discussed more fully in Section 4.8.

Åkerstedt and coworkers found that none of the adrenal or sex hormones showed any rise in output during deprivation; in fact several showed a fall. This latter change was interpreted by these investigators as simply another sign of sleepiness and a drop in physiological activation, certainly not an indication of any emergency or stress reaction. Although thyroid activity rose, this seemed to be a natural effect of the need for more energy through being continuously awake. The circadian rhythmicity of melatonin was particularly fascinating, as it rose and fell over the day with almost exactly the same pattern as did body temperature and the subjects' self-ratings of their sleepiness. Heightened melatonin output and the most 'sleepy' time of the day both coincided with the temperature trough, at 5 a.m., with all of these reversing in the early evening. Superimposed on this rhythmicity was an overall rise in melatonin output over the sleep deprivation days, coupled with increased sleepiness. However, it was not clear if and to what extent the melatonin rhythm caused the sleepiness rhythm.

Circadian rhythms in all of these and other physiological variables during sleep deprivation have been a subject of considerable research by Åkerstedt, and he has produced an excellent review on the topic[26]. Whilst some variables show a remarkably persistent circadian rhythm during deprivation, for example adrenaline release, body temperature, sleepiness, and melatonin output, others such as heart rate, systolic blood-pressure, and noradrenaline lose almost all their rhythmicity. It seems that either directly or indirectly the circadian rhythms of these latter measures are heavily dependent on the presence of sleep and wakefulness, usually with sleep reducing their levels. One obvious underlying factor here is physical activity. This certainly has a profound influence on the noradrenaline rhythm, for example, where the circadian change of this hormone is almost entirely dependent (positively correlated) on the level of physical activity. Increases in such activity at night during sleep deprivation prevent the usual night-time fall of noradrenaline.

3.8 The immune system

Many people believe that 'lack' of sleep makes us more vulnerable to infections, and that late nights lead to colds and influenza, etc. This may well be true, but the cause is not necessarily lack of sleep itself, but stress, due to overwork for example. Sleep loss and increased susceptibility to infection may both be the result of the overwork. One prominent mechanism behind all this is probably the increased cortisol output resulting from the stress, and cortisol depresses several aspects of the immune system. We know that sleep deprivation studies have seldom reported any rise in cortisol, but only two such studies have looked at the immune response. Both were run by Dr Jan Palmblad and colleagues, also from the Laboratory for Clinical Stress Research[5,27]. However, before turning to these studies, let me give a perhaps too simple guide to this highly complex biological system. I should add that some of this will also be relevant to Section 5.12.

The immune response centres on white blood cells, for example granulocytes, killer cells, macrophages (monocytes), and, above all, lymphocytes—which have a dominant role in orchestrating the immune response. Lymphocytes are divided into two types, the T and B cells. The former, together with most of the other white cells, destroy invading bacteria, viruses and other foreign bodies (i.e. antigens) by surrounding and consuming them in a process known as phagocytosis. T lymphocytes also produce various substances, the 'lymphokines', that stimulate phagocytosis. Interferon is a good example of a lymphokine. More recently discovered stimulatory substances (from monocytes) are interleukin-1 (IL-1) and interleukin-2, which also produce fever (i.e. they are pyrogens). They are currently creating great interest from the perspective of sleep substances, and I shall be dealing with this in Section 5.12.

All these immune responses come under the major category of 'cell-mediated immunity'. The other category is 'humoral immunity', centring around the B lymphocytes. This concerns the production of antibodies, the immunoglobulins—substances that become attached to the surface of antigens to render them harmless either directly, or indirectly, by identifying and targeting the invader for phagocytosis by other white cells. There are several types of immunoglobulin.

I must emphasize that the immune response is a highly intricate process involving many interacting mechanisms. Trying to measure the total immune response is impossible, and all the immunologist can do is to look at small aspects of it. Not only are there many technical limitations, but to do a comprehensive series of tests would require months of work and large samples of blood. So, to return to the experiments by Palmblad and colleagues, it must be appreciated that both their investigations covered only a small portion of the immune system. In fact, in both studies humoral immunity was not able to be investigated at all, and only limited aspects of cell-mediated immunity could be assessed.

Their first report[5], of three nights of sleep deprivation in eight women, incorporated some simulated battle stress, referred to by the authors as 'stressor exposure'. It may well have been the cause of the small rises in cortisol and catecholamine output that were found. The main immunological measure adopted was the rate at which a virus was consumed by phagocytosis, which turned out to be depressed a little during the deprivation. Interferon production was also measured, and this increased during the deprivation period, continuing to do so on the first day after recovery sleep. Nevertheless, as the investigators pointed out, neither this rise nor the decreased phagocytosis were of clinical significance, as both changes were small.

Their second report[27] used the 12 subjects monitored by Åkerstedt and others which I described in the previous section. It was 'pure' sleep deprivation without any battle stress, and for our purposes is a more important study, even though the blood sample for measures of the immune response was taken on the second day and not on the last day of deprivation. This time the immunological measures centred around the rate of proliferation of lymphocytes and granulocytes in response to an antigen. Proliferation fell, but it was still within normal limits—as the investigations pointed out, the effect was not clinically significant even though it was statistically significant. So the subjects could not be considered to be ailing in any way. Five days later, the subjects returned to the laboratory, and the proliferation rate was almost back to baseline values.

Given the limited measurements, neither investigation found anything really remarkable, and there was nothing to suggest that sleep deprivation had any great impact on the immune system. If stress is to have a hand in immune suppression, then it has to rise to a greater level than that found here, even for the 'military type' study, which in this case was still not very stressful. We are still very much in the dark in our understanding of the immune system's response to sleep deprivation, as sadly no more work has been done. It is a key area for sleep deprivation research, especially as recent findings with 'sleep substances' (see Section 5.12) suggest that sleep, particularly SWS, is associated with some boosting of the immune system. But we do not know if such an effect is really beneficial. This boost may just be counteracting some undesirable effect of sleep and be due, for example, to the fall in body temperature bringing an increased risk of infection. After all, a lack of this boosting, which presumably happens during sleep deprivation, seems not to impair immune function. This last point is based not only on the results of Palmblad and his group, but also on the findings from the sleep-deprived rats in the studies by the Chicago Sleep Laboratory (see Section 2.2).

3.9 Conclusions about sleep deprivation in humans

With the exception of the brain, specifically the cerebral cortex, sleep deprivation is surprisingly uneventful for the rest of the body. But there are still gaps in our knowledge, especially in relation to the immune system. Nevertheless, there are no reports of physical illness, and no signs of any alarm response; there is simply a general physiological slowing up. In humans, minor changes or resettings occur in the regulation of certain physiological processes, particularly with thermoregulation. For small mammals, though, such changes seem to be more serious.

This nil outcome with respect to body functioning, from over 50 sleep deprivation experiments on humans, is not what one might expect from any viewpoint that sleep is a condition of heightened tissue growth and repair ('restitution'), overcoming the wear and tear of wakefulness. Apparently, for humans at least, this restitution is carried out effectively during the wakefulness of sleep deprivation. On the other hand, the obvious effects of sleep deprivation on behaviour and psychological performance could well support this restitutive hypothesis for the brain, or at least for the cerebrum. In summary, for humans:

Sleep seems to be essential for the brain, but not for the rest of the body.

My conclusion is not new, and is no more than an update on Kleitman's views, for example. Over 20 years ago he wrote in his magnum opus[2]:

The failure to find specific predictable changes in the visceral activities points to an absence of effect on these activities from lack of sleep. Mental and muscular performance in various tests can be maintained at normal levels if the tests are of short duration, but sustained effort is impossible. The increased sensitivity to pain, impairment of the disposition, tendency to hallucinations, and other signs of this character are the outstanding and significant findings in all studies on lack of sleep. They suggest a fatigue of the higher levels of the cerebral cortex—the levels that are responsible for the critical analysis of incoming impulses and the elaboration of adequate responses in the light of one's previous experience. (p. 229)

In the next section I will be providing more evidence showing that, excluding the cerebrum, body restitution in humans mostly occurs during wakefulness. It will be seen that the key stimulus to body restitution is the absorption of amino acids from the gut after feeding. For most of us, sleep is a fasting state, as the last meal of the day is consumed several hours before sleep. In fact, tissue dissolution is the more likely event during sleep than is tissue restitution. But there is something else that is desirable before body restitution can proceed without hindrance during wakefulness, and that is physical rest, for example sitting. Most people spend much of wakefulness resting in this way. However, because small mammals have much greater energy needs owing to their higher metabolism, they have to spend most of their wakefulness very actively foraging. The remaining waking time is spent in other essential physical activities such as grooming, nest building, infant rearing, etc. Besides, as will be seen, sitting down and doing 'nothing' is an advanced form of behaviour. To do this, an animal needs the ability to, for want of a better word, 'contemplate'. Rodents do not have a sufficiently advanced brain to allow them to rest and do nothing for more than a minute or two. For them, sleep is the only way they can be immobilized for any appreciable length of time. Because body restitution is dampened down by physical activity, the physical rest of sleep may allow this restitution to proceed unhindered. My key point is that it is not sleep which facilitates this restitution for these animals, but the physical rest accompanying it.

For most human organs, whatever goes on during sleep also occurs during wakefulness. A good example relates to skeletal or voluntary muscles—the muscles we have conscious control over. This is the commonest tissue found in the body. If one lies down and relaxes on a comfortable bed in a quiet room and shuts one's eyes without falling asleep, then the tonus of nearly all the voluntary muscles (excluding the neck) falls to a level similar to that found during sleep. In fact metabolic rate, which is a good guide to the level of relaxation, only drops about another 9 per cent in sleep (including REM sleep) compared with the level found during relaxed wakefulness[28]. This small increase in relaxation will not, as far as it is known, lead to any further rise in body tissue restitution, given the same state of food absorption from the gut. Even sitting rather than lying down is sufficient for body restitution to proceed unhindered.

Excluding the brain, certain changes occur in the activities of various organs during sleep that are only to be found during sleep. However, none of these changes has yet been shown to be necessary for survival. Several are simply due to peculiarities in the brain's control of these mechanisms, for example penile erection and the loss of neck muscle tone in REM sleep (see Chapter 8). There is little sign that such events are essential to our well-being, and they are often called 'epiphenomena'. For example, they cannot be taken as indicators of enhanced body restitution occurring during sleep.

However, within many parts of the brain, particularly the cerebrum, there are numerous alterations in activity that are not found outside sleep. Some of these are reflected as EEG changes, and form the criteria for determining the sleep stages. We know that the effect of sleep loss on the brain is life threatening, for one reason or another. At one level, sleepiness is hazardous, at another I have been conjecturing that neuronal networks within the higher centres increasingly fail without the necessary repair processes of sleep. But I cannot yet prove this latter point, and must admit that the cerebral events of sleep could be just part of a process to keep us occupied during the unproductive hours of darkness. In other words, all of our sleep may be under the control of some behavioural drive to sleep.

But if this were the case, then why is there no cut-out mechanism for the whole of sleepiness in emergencies? Certainly I think it is likely that part of our sleep—optional sleep—is under such a drive, which may lift at around the 'fifth-day turning point' of sleep deprivation. But I also believe that some of sleep—core sleep—is critical for one organ in particular—the cerebrum, or more likely the cerebral cortex. I shall be developing these arguments for core and optional sleep in Chapters 5 to 7, but meanwhile consider the following.

Unlike voluntary muscles, the cerebrum cannot really slow up and relax during wakefulness, even when we are lying relaxed in tranquillity with the mind 'cleared'. The EEG (predominantly alpha activity—see Section 1.3) shows that the cerebrum remains in a state of quiet readiness, fully aware of what is going on around. This vigilance still needs a high rate of cerebral activity, which is near to its maximum. Even when we get very excited and mentally very active, the cerebrum's own metabolic rate seldom increases by more than another 15 per cent. In this respect the waking cerebrum is like a computer, where the power consumption is near to its peak whether it is idling on stand-by, awaiting instructions, or is involved with programs and taking in information.

The cerebrum is a highly complex electrochemical engine and like all engines it must need adjustment and repair. The question is, can this be done with the engine still running almost at top speed, or in other words during wakefulness? Even if this were possible, it is likely that repairs would be done more effectively with a slower running speed. Obviously the brain cannot be entirely switched off like a computer and other engines, otherwise we would die. The point that I want to make is that, unlike other body organs, the cerebrum cannot 'relax' to any appreciable extent during wakefulness. If cerebral restitution is enhanced through reduced brain activity, then such reduced activity is only provided during sleep. The type of sleep where this activity is the lowest is SWS, particularly in stage 4 sleep.

Evidence supporting sleep's release of the cerebrum from the quiet readiness of wakefulness has come from a remarkable study of the electrical activity in the cerebral cortex of cats[29]. During non-REM sleep the deeper layers were shown to shutdown partially and become isolated. Such happenings did not occur during wakefulness, or for that matter in REM sleep. Although the authors would not commit themselves on the meaning of this isolation, some sort of recovery process was suspected. Of course, because of ethical and technological limitations we cannot get inside the human brain during sleep to see what happens to nerve growth, repair, and other events that would indicate cerebral restitution. But there is circumstantial evidence, and this is covered in more detail in Chapter 5.

I must emphasize that there are other parts of the brain, the more 'basic' areas of the midbrain and hindbrain controlling vital body functions, that have to continue their activities throughout wakefulness and sleep, and can therefore never relax. Any restitution here must be done 'on line' with the engine still fully running, so to speak. But here, types of response are both limited and fixed. There is little potential for adaptability, or changes in connections with other neurones (e.g. learning) that typically seems to occur in the cerebrum in response to the day's events. Adaptability presumably creates more neuronal wear and tear compared with the stereotyped events within the basic areas of the brain. In Sections 2.11 and 2.12 I described how this adaptability seems to fail during sleep deprivation.

To summarize the key points about human sleep deprivation, covered in the last two chapters:

1. *Of all organs, it is the brain, and specifically the cerebrum (i.e. the cerebral cortex), that shows the greatest effects of sleep deprivation.*
2. *However, the cerebrum has the capacity to cope with at least one night's sleep loss.*
3. *The rest of the body seems relatively unaffected by sleep deprivation.*

4. *Only about one-third of lost sleep is made up. This recovery sleep contains much of the missing stage 4 sleep and about half of the missing REM sleep.*

From these findings, it is proposed that:

1. *Human sleep particularly restores cerebral function.*
2. *The rest of the body seems not to need sleep in this respect; food and relaxation are probably sufficient.*
3. *Only a portion of sleep (core sleep) is necessary for the cerebrum, and seems to be typified by the first part of a normal night's sleep, especially stage 4 sleep.*
4. *The latter part of a night's sleep is influenced by some form of behavioural drive to sleep (optional sleep).*
5. *The feeling of sleepiness may have two components—owing to a loss of core sleep and a loss of optional sleep.*

Finally, here is a note of caution. Sleep deprivation has been carried out only on fully grown adults, and we do not know what would happen in the case of children. To the extent that sleep deprivation gives clues to the functions of sleep, these only really apply to the adult, and, for example, do not help us to understand whether sleep is necessary for physical growth. Unfortunately, most of the findings outside the area of sleep deprivation that are relevant to the issue of body restitution and sleep also come from adult mammals. So we can only infer about what might be happening in the young.

References

1. Kleitman, N. (1923). The effects of prolonged sleeplessness on man. *American Journal of Physiology*, **66**, 67–92.
2. Kleitman, N. (1963). *Sleep and Wakefulness* (second edition). University of Chicago Press, Chicago.
3. Jackson, J.H. (1958). Evolution and dissolution of the nervous system. *In*: Taylor, J. (ed.), *Selected Writings of John Hughlings Jackson*. Staples Press, London. pp. 45–75.
4. Horne, J.A. (1978). A review of the biological effects of total sleep deprivation in man. *Biological Psychology*, **7**, 55–102.
5. Palmblad, J., Kantell, K., Strander, H., Froberg, J., Karlsson, C.-G., Levi, L., Grantstrom, M. and Unger, P. (1976). Stressor exposure and immunological response in man: interferon-producing capacity and phagocytosis. *Journal of Psychosomatic Research*, **20**, 193–199.
6. Francescioni, R.P., Stokes, J.W., Banderet, L.E. and Kowal, D.M. (1978). Sustained operations and sleep deprivation: effects on indices of stress. *Aviation, Space and Environmental Medicine*, **49**, 1271–1274.
7. Kuhn, E., Brodan, V., Brodanova, M. and Rysanek, K. (1969). Metabolic reflections of sleep deprivation. *Activitas Nervosa Superior*, **11**, 165–174.

8. Scrimshaw, N.S., Habicht, J.P., Pellet, P., Piche, M.L. and Cholakos, B. (1966). Effects of sleep deprivation and reversal of diurnal activity on protein metabolism of young men. *American Journal of Clinical Nutrition*, **19**, 313–319.

9. Luby, E.D., Frohman, C.E., Grisell, J.L., Lenzo, J.E. and Gotlieb, J.S. (1960). Sleep deprivation: effects upon behaviour, thinking, motor performance and biological energy transfer systems. *Psychosomatic Medicine*, **22**, 182–192.

10. Luby, E.D., Grisell, J.L., Frohman, C.E., Lees H., Cohen, B.D. and Gotlieb, J.S. (1960). Biochemical, psychological and behavioural responses to sleep deprivation. *Annals of the New York Academy of Sciences*, **96**, 71–79.

11. Vondura, K., Brodan, N., Bass, A., Kuhn, E., Teisinger, J., Andel, M. and Veselkova, A. (1981). Effects of sleep deprivation on the activity of selected metabolic enzymes in skeletal muscle. *European Journal of Applied Physiology*, **47**, 41–46.

12. Takeuchi, L., Davis, G.M., Plyley, M., Goode, R. and Shephard, R.J. (1985). Sleep deprivation, chronic exercise and muscular performance. *Ergonomics*, **28**, 591–601.

13. Reilly, T. and Walsh, T.J. (1981). Physiological, psychological and performance measures during an endurance record for 5-a-side soccer play. *British Journal of Sports Medicine*, **15**, 122–128.

14. Thomas, V. and Reilly, T. (1975). Circulatory, psychological and performance variables during 100 hours of paced continuous exercise under conditions of controlled energy intake and work output. *Journal of Human Movement Studies*, **1**, 149–155.

15. Martin, B.J. (1986). Sleep deprivation and exercise. *Exercise and Sports Science Reviews*, in press.

16. Brodan, V.J., Vojtechovsky, J., Kuhn, E. and Cepelak, J. (1969). Changes in mental and physical performance in sleep deprived healthy volunteers. *Activitas Nervosa Superior*, Supplement **11**, 175–181.

17. Horne, J.A. and Pettitt, A.N. (1984). Sleep deprivation and the physiological response to exercise under steady-state conditions in untrained subjects. *Sleep*, **7**, 168–179.

18. Fiorica, V., Higgins, E.A., Iampietro, P.F., Lategola, M.T. and Davis, A.W. (1968). Physiological responses of men during sleep deprivation. *Journal of Applied Physiology*, **24**, 167–176.

19. Kolka, M.A., Martin, B.J. and Elzondo, R.S. (1984). Exercise in a cold environment after sleep deprivation. *European Journal of Applied Physiology*, **53**, 282–285.

20. Sawka, M.N., Gonzalez, R.R. and Pandolf, K.B. (1984). Effects of sleep deprivation on thermoregulation during exercise. *American Journal of Physiology*, **246**, R72–R77.

21. Cooper, K.R. and Phillips, B.A. (1982). Effect of short-term sleep loss on breathing. *Journal of Applied Physiology*, **53**, 855–858.

22. Schiffman, P.L., Trontell, M.C., Mazar, M.F. and Edelman, N.H. (1983). Sleep deprivation decreases ventilatory response to CO_2 but not load compensation. *Chest*, **84**, 695–698.

23. White, D.P., Douglas, N.J., Picket, C.K., Zwillich, C.W. and Weil, J.V. (1983). Sleep deprivation and the control of ventilation. *American Journal of Respiratory Disorders*, **128**, 984–986.

24. Åkerstedt, T., Froberg, J.E., Friberg, Y. and Wetterberg, L. (1979). Melatonin excretion, body temperature and subjective arousal during 64 hours of sleep deprivation. *Psychoneuroendocrinology*, **4**, 215–225.
25. Åkerstedt, T., Palmblad, J., de la Torre, B., Marana, R. and Gillberg, M. (1980). Adrenocortical and gonadal steroids during sleep deprivation. *Sleep*, **3**, 23–30.
26. Åkerstedt, T. (1980). Altered sleep-wake patterns and circadian rhythms. *Acta Physiologica Scandinavica*, Supplement 469 (whole).
27. Palmblad, J., Petrini, B., Wasserman, J. and Åkerstedt, T. (1979). Lymphocyte and granulocyte reactions during sleep deprivation. *Psychosomatic Medicine*, **41**, 273–278.
28. Shapiro, C.M., Goll, C.C., Cohen, G.R. and Oswald, I. (1984). Heat production during sleep. *Journal of Applied Physiology*, **56**, 671–677.
29. Livingstone, M.S. and Hubel, D.H. (1981). Effect of sleep and arousal on the processing of visual information in the cat. *Nature*, **291**, 554–561.

4. Body restitution and sleep

The findings from sleep deprivation research indicate that, apart from the cerebrum, the remainder of the body continues to function fairly normally. So I concluded in the last chapter that if one had to argue that sleep has a restitutive role which is confined to sleep, whereby tissues are somehow repaired following the wear and tear of wakefulness, then the only organ where this seems to apply is the cerebrum. The rest of the body appears able to restore itself during wakefulness. Nevertheless, many sleep researchers believe that not only does sleep provide restitution for most of the body, as well as for the cerebrum, but that this restitution is almost wholly confined to sleep, and is largely absent during wakefulness. In summary, there are two issues at stake:

1. Is sleep a generalized condition of heightened tissue restitution for the body as a whole?
2. Can this restitution also occur in wakefulness?

Whereas a commonly held opinion, at least for humans is, 'yes', on the first account, and 'only to a limited extent' on the second, I propose the opposite: that for humans (but excluding the cerebrum) the respective answers are 'no—it is proceeding more slowly', and 'yes—most of it occurs during wakefulness'. For other mammals, my answers vary, because the crux of this debate as I see it, does not centre so much on sleep itself, but on two other factors:

1. *Whether or not sleep is a fasting state.* Tissue restitution requires an adequate supply of nutrients to cells, but fasting prevents this.
2. *The extent to which relaxation occurs in wakefulness.* Is sleep the only way of allowing prolonged periods of physical inactivity? Near constant physical activity will depress tissue restitution, and delay it until a period of rest. If sleep is the only occasion for rest, then restitution will predominantly occur at this time—not because sleep itself stimulates this restitution, but simply because sleep is the only provider of rest.

For humans, sleep generally involves a fast, and adequate relaxation usually occurs during wakefulness—two reasons why I shall be arguing that body restitution happens mostly in wakefulness. For the rodent, the other mammal most studied in these respects, the reverse situation holds for both these answers—restitution may be mostly confined to sleep, but by default.

Why then, despite the seemingly minor effects of total sleep deprivation on body functioning in humans, is there such strong support for the idea that human sleep is a state of heightened body tissue restitution? It is because there seems to be other evidence pointing to this conclusion, coming from several sources, for example:

1. *Increases in rates of cell division during sleep.*
2. *The sleep-related release of growth hormone in humans.*
3. *Rises in SWS following daytime exercise.*

As will be seen, these and other findings apparently make a plausible argument favouring the body restitutive theory for human sleep. That is, until they are scrutinized more closely. Then it becomes clear that the evidence is circumstantial. The problem has been that such findings have usually been interpreted with the theory firmly in mind to start with, rather than with an open mind letting the theory develop from the facts. In this chapter I will take you through this evidence in more detail, and show how it is so misleading, starting with humans and then going on to the rodent. First though, let me give a little more background on what is meant by tissue restitution—cell growth and repair.

4.1 Tissue restitution: protein turnover and cell division

Tissues are made up of cells, which in most cases can divide (mitosis), and hence multiply. In the fully grown adult, mitosis normally only balances out the cell death rate, and so there is no net gain in cells to produce any physical growth. In children, of course, the rates of cell division exceed those of cell death, resulting in physical growth. In some tissues, like the lining of the gut, the lifespan of a cell is only days, whilst in others, such as most blood cells, the lifespan is a few months. However, for neurones and most types of muscle cell, mitosis ceases soon after birth, and usually their life is as long as that of the person. For these and all other cells there is another aspect to growth, in addition to an increase in cell numbers, as they can also increase or decrease in size. This involves protein turnover, a topic I introduced in Section 3.3.

Cells are made of proteins, which in turn are constructed of amino acids. Earlier, I used the analogy of a brick wall for the protein, and the bricks, as the amino acids. All proteins are to varying extents unstable, and are in a continuous state of *turnover*: breaking down into their constitutent amino acids (*breakdown*), that can *either*:

1. Be destroyed to provide fuel for the energy needs of the body by conversion into urea (*oxidation*) for excretion in urine,
or

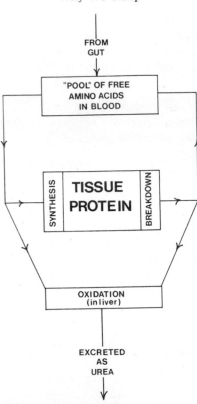

Fig. 4.1 Tissue protein and the fate of amino acids. Protein is in continuous turnover, breaking down and being synthesized. Amino acids for synthesis come from a 'pool' found mostly in the blood, made up of old amino acids from previous protein breakdown and new ones from a recent meal. The alternative fate for amino acids, new and old, that are surplus to the needs of protein synthesis is oxidization in the liver to provide energy for the body. The by-product, urea, is excreted.

2. Be re-used for the synthesis of new protein (*synthesis*), together with fresh amino acids in the diet. These processes are shown in Fig. 4.1.

Tissue repair (restitution) occurs when the rate of protein synthesis exceeds that of breakdown, leading to an increase in the amount of protein within the cell. If this condition continues then the size of the cell will increase. Another term for this state of affairs is 'anabolism', whereas 'catabolism' reflects the opposite condition, of tissue dissolution, which prevails when protein beakdown exceeds synthesis. However, simply measuring synthesis rates alone provides little guide to whether the cell is in a state of restitution or dissolution. In order to know this the protein breakdown rates must also be measured. An analogy here is that we cannot tell whether the population of a country (cell protein content) is changing simply by looking at the birth rate—the death rate is also needed. Although the birth rate may be going up, the death rate may be rising faster, causing a population decline. On the other hand, a falling birth rate might accompany a rise in the total population if the death rate was even lower.

The measurement of protein synthesis is an easier process than is that of protein breakdown, and few experiments have looked at both. Unfortunately, most of the animal studies that are cited in support of the hypothesis that sleep is for body restitution only have findings for protein synthesis rates. Although increased protein synthesis does not necessarily mean increased cell growth, to be fair, growth is generally the case.

Protein turnover and mitosis are the key aspects in the life of a cell that are of most interest to us within the context of restitution and sleep. However, in those cells able to divide there are other phases which complete its life cycle, and together these make up what is called the 'cell cycle', culminating in mitosis. But I shall not dwell on these, except to mention that cells can be held up in the cycle by various inhibitors such as exercise and rises in adrenaline and corticosteroid output (see next section).

The instructions or recipe for the manufacture of protein from amino acids come from DNA via a series of different forms of RNA. Just before protein synthesis begins these RNAs increase in activity. So one method of monitoring the rate of protein synthesis is to assess the amount of RNA in a tissue. There have been many studies on rodents, measuring circadian rhythms in RNA activity, protein synthesis, and mitosis. Together, these can give some picture of the cell cycle, particularly in relation to an animal's sleep and wakefulness. What is now very clear in rodents is that the circadian peaks in these activities are largely confined to the sleep period, and the lowest daily rates to the waking period. This has been shown in an excellent summary of the literature by Dr Kirstine Adam and Professor Ian Oswald from the Department of Psychiatry at Edinburgh University[1]. Such findings have been the mainstay to their proposal that sleep is a state of heightened tissue restitution for humans and rodents alike. There is little doubt that for the rodent this is true. However, what I am arguing is that for this animal, sleep is not the real cause, but the physical inactivity of sleep, coupled with its feeding patterns.

4.2 Factors influencing protein turnover and the cell cycle

There is a variety of mechanisms which speed up and slow down protein turnover and mitosis. Some mechanisms are more powerful than others, although at any one time of the day several may be at work in a co-ordinated way. Generally, whatever influences protein turnover will have a knock-on effect to slow or speed up other phases of the cell cycle, especially mitosis.

The most powerful stimulus to an increase in the protein content of a cell (i.e. restitution, or anabolism) is *an increase in the availability of amino acids to the cell* (beginning an hour or so after eating).

Several hormones, particularly growth hormone and insulin, encourage increased protein synthesis, mitosis, etc. I must stress that feeding will stimulate anabolism, whereas growth hormone only facilitates it. There is a subtle difference in these words, as 'stimulation' indicates an order whereas 'facilitation' only offers the increased opportunity. Such facilitation is of little help if the amino acid availability to the cell is limited. In these circumstances, for example during a fast, growth hormone has an alternative effect on tissue protein turnover. It protects the protein content of tissue by slowing down both protein breakdown and the oxidation of amino acids (i.e. it slows down catabolism). This alternative role could well be happening during sleep, and may be a reason for the large output of growth hormone during human sleep—a topic I shall be returning to in Section 4.7.

In the case of humans, when considering the action of sleep in relation to body restitution, it must be remembered that for most of us night-time sleep is a fasting state. There is little or no eating for about 12 hours, from about 7 p.m. to 7 a.m.. Digestion, absorption, and oxidation of amino acids from the gut is usually completed within about 5 hours of eating, depending, of course, on what and how much is eaten. Assuming that protein has been eaten in the meal, then the supply of amino acids to the cells from the blood (the amino acid 'pool') will be plentiful during these postprandial hours, but by around 2 a.m. the pool will have become depleted. So, how could tissue restitution still be high at this point in time—where would the amino acid building blocks for the tissue protein come from? In fact, tissue restitution would have occurred earlier in the evening, and in the afternoon following lunch.

Whereas we usually eat our food in relatively large quantities as meals, the laboratory rodent, on the other hand, has a different feeding routine. It is a 'nibbler' taking numerous small quantities of food throughout the 24 hours. Whilst it consumes most (around 75 per cent) of its daily food during the normal waking period, it will still wake up frequently during sleep to nibble at the everlasting supply of food provided by the laboratory staff and available within a few inches of its nest. This is a crucial point, as almost all of the animal research on protein synthesis and mitosis, referred to in the debate on body restitution and sleep, is based on the laboratory rodent. These differences in feeding style between humans and rodents is the first of several reasons why we cannot draw simple comparisons between these two species when discussing the subject of sleep and tissue restitution.

The second major influence on tissue restitution is exercise. This clearly depresses mitosis[2] and increases protein breakdown and oxidation, even in humans[3,4]. It may also decrease protein synthesis, depending on the intensity and duration of the exercise. There are several reasons why this happens, for example:

1. Exercise can elevate the output of adrenaline and cortisol—both of which increase protein breakdown and inhibit mitosis.
2. Exercise can lead to a diversion of blood from the gut to muscle, reducing digestion and the absorption of amino acids and other foodstuffs through the gut wall.
3. Protein synthesis consumes much energy in the form of ATP (see Section 3.3), and probably accounts for 20 per cent or more of our resting metabolic rate. If the exercise is energy demanding, then less energy is available for protein synthesis and the rate of synthesis will fall.

Exercise is not such a critical factor as is food intake to protein synthesis. In order for exercise to depress tissue restitution substantially, it has to occupy much of the day and be at the level of at least a slow jog[3]. As most of us spend much of the waking day relatively inactive, sitting or standing, this situation

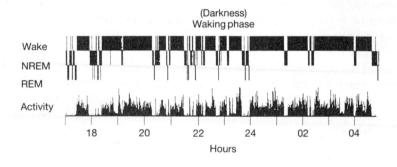

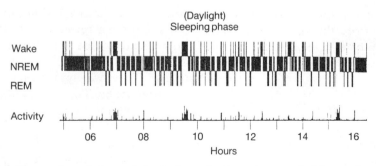

Fig. 4.2 Sleep is the only form of physical rest for the rodent—wakefulness, sleep (REM and non-REM sleep), and physical activity in the laboratory rat over 24 hours, under a 12-hour daylight, 12-hour darkness schedule. Wakefulness is a time of much activity but little rest for these animals. Periods of more than a few minutes of rest only come with sleep. See text for details. (Adapted from data kindly supplied by Alex Borbély)

seldom applies. Even when we exercise, it is usually for less than an hour a day, and any resultant depression of protein synthesis, etc. will be caught up on in the ensuing relaxed wakefulness[3].

Whilst humans can sit and relax for much of wakefulness, thus allowing protein synthesis, mitosis, etc. to proceed unhindered, most small mammals cannot do this. Rodents and insectivores are good examples—they are almost continually physically active throughout wakefulness, and in the absence of sleep they cannot sit still for more than a minute or so. Wakefulness is filled with movement of one sort or another: exploring, foraging, grooming, feeding, drinking, infant rearing. Relaxed wakefulness requires a highly developed cerebrum, which they do not have. Sitting still is not an absence of behaviour, but a sophisticated behaviour associated with contemplation, daydreaming, manipulative skills, etc. only demonstrated by advanced mammals. The relentless physical activity of wakefulness in laboratory rodents is quite apparent in Fig. 4.2, which shows changes in physical activity over 24 hours (measured by movement sensors in the cage) plotted against sleep and wakefulness determined by the EEG. Wakefulness is accompanied by considerable activity and little rest. Prolonged periods of inactivity are only to be found during sleep. These detailed and impressive findings are from the work of Professor Alex Borbély, a leading European sleep researcher, from the Institute of Pharmacology, at the University of Zurich[5]. Some of his other work will be discussed in Section 5.3.

Physical activity in the rodent will slow down tissue restitution[4], and, as will be seen, especially mitosis[2]. Consequently, in these animals much of restitution may be delayed until the inactivity of sleep. Here, sleep is only the vehicle for restitution, not its cause.

4.3 Feeding and protein turnover

The central role of feeding (or to be more precise, the absorption of amino acids from the gut following digestion) for protein turnover was clearly shown by a leading research group in this field that used to be based at the Clinical Nutrition and Metabolism Unit, St Pancras Hospital, London, at the time headed by Professor John Waterlow. Their widely acclaimed text, *Protein Turnover in Mammalian Tissues and in the Whole Body*[6] heavily emphasizes this key point. They have also pioneered the measurement of circadian rhythms in human protein turnover. In fact, to date, they have been the only group to have measured protein turnover during human sleep, which is why their findings shed so much light on body restitution and sleep.

In one of their major studies, run by Drs Graham Clugston and Peter Garlick[7], ten obese and five lean subjects rested throughout daytime wakefulness and slept at night. From 8 a.m. to 7 p.m. the subjects ate at every hour one-twelfth of their daily food ration. From 8 p.m. until the following morning at 8 a.m., they ate nothing, as was their usual habit. Dividing the normal three meals of the day into 12 hourly portions is unusual, but was necessary in order to establish stability of measurement. However, this does not really affect the outcome from my viewpoint, as I am interested in what happens during the night-time fast. Whole-body protein turnover was measured continuously in these subjects for 24 hours, using a method involving the slow intravenous infusion of a radioactively labelled amino acid (leucine). It enters the amino acid pool (see Fig. 4.1) just like any other amino acid from recent food absorption or cell protein breakdown, and undergoes the same fates. But because it is labelled its course can be tracked to see how much ends up incorporated into tissue protein, or being oxidized.

The outcome for both the lean and obese subjects was the same, and to avoid replication I shall just give the findings for the obese subjects. Table 4.1 summarizes the amounts of protein involved in each of the three phases of protein turnover, for the two 12-hour periods. The feeding period led to 129 g of protein being synthesized and 101 g being broken down, so the net effect was a 28 g increase in the protein content of tissue during the daytime (suggesting anabolism and enhanced restitution). Oxidation was also relatively high, indicating that the amino acid pool contained excess amino acids that were being disposed of. The 12-hour night-time fast led to a fall in synthesis, to 87 g of protein, that was exceeded by the 107 g of breakdown, giving a loss of 20 g protein from tissue—a finding against anabolism and tissue restitution, but for catabolism and dissolution. Oxidation also fell, to less than half the daytime amount, indicating that the amino acid pool was getting low, and that amino acids were being spared from oxidation.

More detailed hour-by-hour information over the 24 hours was also reported on. Protein synthesis began to increase about an hour after the start of morning feeding, and reached a plateau within 5 hours. Oxidation lagged about 2 hours behind in its rise and plateau times. However, of greater importance to us was the fairly rapid fall in both synthesis and oxidation after the last meal at 7 p.m. By midnight, around the beginning of sleep, both synthesis and oxidation had almost bottomed out. Refeeding in the morning,

Table 4.1 Human sleep is a state of tissue dissolution, not restitution: body protein turnover during daytime feeding and night-time fasting in human subjects. During the day synthesis exceeded breakdown, indicating tissue restitution. At night the reverse occurred, suggesting tissue dissolution. (From Clugston and Garlick[7])

	Synthesis	Breakdown	Oxidation
	(grams of protein per 12 hours)		
Daytime fed	129	101	50
Night fast	87	107	19

not wakefulness, led to the re-establishment of daytime protein turnover levels. Such findings clearly indicated that sleep had not stimulated any increase in tissue restitution—it was the feeding.

The investigators were looking at protein turnover in the whole subject, and these findings were general trends for all tissues combined. But before we also conclude that these findings fail to support a brain restitution role for sleep, it must be noted that the investigators pointed out how it is possible for a minority of tissues, for example the brain, to have shown opposite trends during sleep, with protein synthesis rising and breakdown falling. Nevertheless, for the bulk of our tissues it certainly looks as though sleep is a state of degradation, although as I have already suggested the growth hormone release during sleep may be slowing up the catabolism.

This research group have carried out other studies relevant to restitution and sleep, which again point to the key role of feeding for protein turnover. In one study[8] subjects were fed a liquid diet *continuously* over 24 hours via a tube through the nose into the stomach. The technique is not so bad as it sounds and people soon get used to it. As before, the three phases of protein turnover were measured, and it was found that all three stayed constant throughout the 24 hours, irrespective of sleep and wakefulness. That is, sleep and wakefulness made no difference—it was the feeding that mattered.

Another of their investigations[9] demonstrated that the type of food influencing body protein turnover was, indeed, the protein content of the food itself. As in the first study, subjects ate hourly in the daytime and fasted at night, with protein turnover monitored in the same way. Their daily protein intake was 70 g, which is about average. Again, as can be seen in Table 4.2, this fasting caused falls in synthesis and oxidation at night, and a rise in breakdown. Then the subjects spent 3 weeks on a zero protein diet, still given in the daytime, with fasting at night. Protein turnover was once more monitored over 24 hours. Now, the difference in protein turnover between

Table 4.2 The influence of the protein content of food on whole-body tissue protein turnover: whole-body protein turnover during daytime feeding and night-time fasting in humans, on normal, and protein-free diets. Note that day-night differences in protein turnover depend on the protein content of food, not whether subjects were asleep or awake. (From Clugston and Garlick[8])

	Synthesis	Breakdown	Oxidation
	(grams of protein per 12 hours)		
Normal diet			
Daytime fed	121	77	41
Night fast	92	112	20
Protein-free diet			
Daytime fed	72	79	7
Night fast	70	77	6

day and night found previously was abolished. This was, of course, because there was insufficient protein in the second diet to stimulate anabolism. As might be expected, protein synthesis and oxidation were low during the daytime feeding, and sleep had no effect.

Unfortunately, we know little about protein turnover during sleep and wakefulness in the rodent, although many studies have looked at protein synthesis alone. As I have mentioned, this generally shows its daily peak during the animal's sleep period, and a low point during its waking period—findings contrasting with those for humans. A rise in protein synthesis during sleep could indicate an increase in the protein content of its tissues (i.e. body restitution), or on the other hand it is possible that the breakdown rate could be running faster, resulting in a net protein loss from tissues. However, let us accept that the protein synthesis peak during the sleep period does reflect a time of increased tissue restitution. My contentions are, of course, that in rodents such peaks are not due to sleep itself, but are: (1) postponed until sleep, owing to the physical activity of wakefulness, and (2) partly due to eating during the sleep period.

I have little experimental proof for the first point, as the necessary experiments have not yet been done on protein turnover in animals. But there is strong evidence for the inhibitory effect of physical activity on another aspect of the cell cycle, mitosis, and I shall be dealing with this in the next section. With regard to feeding style, as I have already pointed out, rodents are nibblers, and will periodically wake up to eat during their sleep period. Feeding will stimulate tissue restitution, and as these events are also within the sleep period, the enhanced restitution will coincide with sleep. Because food intake is crucial to the issue of restitution and sleep, differences in feeding behaviour between rodents and humans, together with their contrasting abilities to display relaxed wakefulness, will grossly distort any comparison between them in relation to sleep function.

4.4 Mitosis, sleep, and physical activity

The signs from the protein turnover findings in humans are, at least for those of us who lead fairly sedentary lives, that heightened tissue restitution occurs in wakefulness following a meal. Larger meals containing more protein are likely to have longer-lasting effects on body tissue protein turnover, although this is a poorly investigated area. For most people the largest meal is in the evening, and, as we usually remain relaxed and awake for several hours afterwards, protein turnover can proceed at full speed. In those cells with the ability to divide, this can lead on to increased mitosis, which coincidentally happens to be in the early part of sleep. However, I must stress that feeding may only facilitate mitosis, as little is known about whether or not, in humans, feeding can stimulate mitosis. What is certain is that there is a

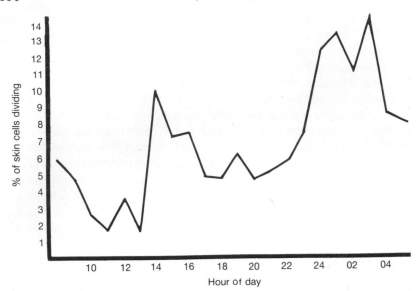

Fig. 4.3 Circadian changes of mitosis in the human skin (epidermis)—note the early after-noon and early morning peaks. Sleep is not necessary for these to occur. (From Scheving[10]. Reproduced by permission of Alan R. Liss Inc.)

circadian rhythm of mitosis, of which the night-time peak is a part.

One of the best examples of the circadian changes in mitosis in humans is shown in Fig. 4.3, coming from a meticulous study of human skin (epidermal cells), carried out by Dr Lawrence Scheving from Arkansas Medical School[10]. There are two clear peaks, one at about 2.30 p.m. and a larger one between 1 and 3 a.m. Prior to the early morning measurements, most subjects remained awake, and so the circadian rise at night could not be due to sleep—the typical early morning peak in mitosis just coincides with sleep. Even Scheving concluded that 'in man it is not the onset of sleep that is responsible for increased epidermal (mitotic) activity, because the majority of night volunteers had not slept prior to presenting themselves for biopsy during the peak of activity' (p. 13).

In the rodent, the circadian rhythm in the rate of epidermal mitosis looks very similar to that of the human, and this can be seen in Fig. 4.4, coming from animals under a daily 12-hour dark/light cycle[11]. However, such studies have not been oriented towards sleep and wakefulness *per se*, but simply towards circadian rhythms, and understandably none has carried out any sleep EEG recordings. But we know, from the work of Borbély for example (Fig. 4.2), that during darkness these animals spend most of their time awake, and most of the daylight hours asleep.

In mammals, including rodents and humans, mitosis is depressed by rises

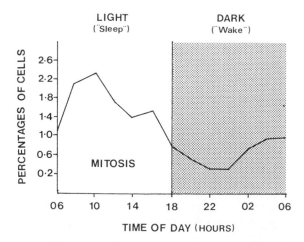

Fig. 4.4 Circadian changes of mitosis in the epidermis of the laboratory mouse. Animals were under a 12-hour light/12-hour darkness schedule (see text). The circadian trends are very similar to those of humans (Fig. 4.3). (From Clausen *et al.*[11]. Reproduced by permission of Blackwell Scientific Publications Ltd)

in the output of cortisol, adrenaline, and probably noradrenaline. These hormones show clear circadian rhythms, and in humans all have their daily troughs around late evening to early morning. Cortisol peaks at about 6–8 a.m., and adrenaline peaks in the afternoon. Because the noradrenaline rhythm is almost entirely dependent on the level of physical activity[12], it falls during sleep, owing to the physical rest sleep brings. Whereas this rhythm has indirect links with sleep, the rhythms of the other two hormones are largely *independent of sleep and wakefulness* although, in humans at least, sleep does depress the trough in cortisol a little further (see Section 4.8). The most convincing evidence from humans of the independence of the cortisol and adrenaline rhythms from sleep comes from the sleep deprivation findings (Section 3.7), where *both rhythms remain.*

I must emphasize that none of these three circadian rhythms (cortisol, adrenaline, and noradrenaline) is large enough to have a profound effect on mitosis alone[13]. Nevertheless, the early morning circadian troughs of all three will facilitate mitosis, and the peaks dampen it somewhat. My point is that this facilitation is not due to the sleep itself, but only coincides with sleep. But, as will be seen, probably the greatest inhibitor of mitosis is moderate to heavy physical activity, with a major underlying cause being the exercise-induced rises in cortisol, adrenaline, and to some extent noradrenaline.

Mild exercise, such as slow walking, has little effect on adrenaline and cortisol levels, but noradrenaline will begin to rise[12]. Exercising at about 40 per cent of one's maximum capacity (e.g. jogging) will double adrenaline output and increase noradrenaline by about 75 per cent[12]. Cortisol will rise, but to varying amounts. Such increases in these hormones, particularly in adrenaline, seem to be large enough to have powerful depressing effects on mitosis in both humans and rodents. Unfortunately though, there are only a few human studies relating to this point, but many more for rodents.

One of the most notable studies on the effects of physical activity on mitosis in humans was by Dr L.B. Fisher, at the time working at the Institute of Dermatology in London[14]. Volunteers had small skin biopsies taken at 2-hour intervals throughout the day, from 8 a.m. to 11 p.m., and measurements were made of mitotic rates. Little information is available about food intake, except that he supplied sandwiches between 1 and 2 p.m. and water was constantly available.

Having established the normal daily trends in mitosis in a no-exercise control group of subjects, Fisher required another group to play badminton from 9 a.m. to 5 p.m., with 15 minutes rest after each hour of playing. For them, this exercise load was of a moderate level, and although their energy output was not measured, we know from other work that the dashing and resting of badminton averages out to be roughly equivalent to a slow jog[15]. Fisher found that mitosis was not just 'dampened', but reduced to almost zero throughout the day from the beginning of the exercise until 10 p.m. in the evening. Nothing is known about what happened after that. Although blood levels of adrenaline and cortisol were not measured, Fisher believed that the continued depression of mitosis in the evening was due to rises in the output of these hormones, resulting from the exercise.

Fisher's exercise was not light, but neither was it heavy, and it certainly suppressed mitosis. I mention this as this exercise load was rather like that found for the rodent during wakefulness—'on the go' most of the time, with the animal having brief periods of running interspaced with walking, foraging, etc. So, we go on to the rodent. Some of the most meticulous and thorough investigations on the effect of physical activity on mitosis in these animals were carried out over a period of 20 years starting in the late 1940s, by Professor W.S. Bullough from Birkbeck College, London. He, often together with a colleague, Dr Edna Laurence, conducted a series of experiments looking at mitosis in a variety of tissues from the mouse, particularly the skin and the lining of the gut.

In one of his earlier studies[16], barbiturates were used to induce 3 hours of sleep in his animals at the beginning of the dark phase when their activity and wakefulness would normally be high, with mitosis entering its circadian low point. Compared with a non-drugged group which was awake at this time, mitosis in the drugged animals rose (but not quite up to the usual peak), only falling when the animals recovered consciousness and became active. Bullough concluded that inactivity encouraged mitosis. I should add that food was always available to both groups of animals.

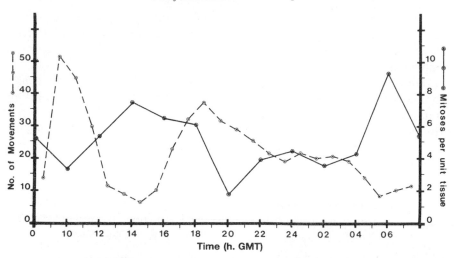

Fig. 4.5 The inverse relationship between physical activity and rate of skin mitosis in mice. The greater the activity, the lower is mitosis. (From Bullough[1]. Reproduced by permission of The Royal Society)

Another finding of his helped establish that activity-inactivity, rather than sleep and wakefulness, seemed to be the key, as an inverse relationship between levels of physical activity and rates of mitosis was found[1]. Animals were placed in a two-roomed box with food on one side and water on the other, and were allowed to move between the two sides through a hole containing a movement sensor that recorded physical activity. Epidermal mitosis was measured frequently and as can be seen in Fig. 4.5, showing rates of mitosis plotted against levels of activity, one is a clear mirror image of the other. The greater the activity, the lesser was the mitosis.

Bullough was one of the first investigators to propose that potent mechanisms for depressing mitosis in the mouse seemed to be rises in the output of the hormones cortisol, adrenaline, and perhaps noradrenaline. In later studies he concentrated on adrenaline, and showed clearly that it interferes with mitosis in two ways[17]: (1) it prevents cells from entering mitosis, and (2) for those cells already in mitosis it speeds it up from the usual 2.8 hours from the start to finish of mitosis to 1 hour. So within an hour of an adrenaline increase, few cells are in mitosis or are entering it.

More evidence for Bullough favouring this crucial role of adrenaline came from the effects of adrenalectomy—the removal of the adrenal glands, and therefore loss of just about all adrenaline release and much of noradrenaline output[18]. Following adrenalectomy, he discovered that the circadian rhythm in epidermal mitosis almost disappeared, giving way to a large rise in mitotic rates. Of even greater interest was that when these animals were exercised moderately for 4 hours in a slowly rotating box mitosis did not fall, which, as expected, was the case for a control group of similarly exercised animals with their adrenals intact. When the adrenalectomized animals were given adrenaline by injection then mitotic rates fell.

However, Bullough emphasized that, at least for rodents, adrenaline does not control mitosis, but only influences it, because the main inhibitors of mitosis seem to be the 'chalones'—natural substances found within tissues. By themselves chalones are not very active, but when bound to adrenaline molecules arriving from the blood the adrenaline-chalone complex makes a powerful inhibitor of mitosis. Adrenaline alone, like chalones alone, has little effect on mitosis. According to Bullough[19]:

the circadian mitotic cycle is evidently the outcome of fluctuations in the adrenaline content of the blood; with reduced adrenaline secretion in sleeping mice the adrenaline–chalone complex breaks down and the epidermal mitotic rate rises (p. 193).

Where does cortisol come into this picture? The effects of this hormone were also examined in more detail by Bullough[20]. He discovered that it too has little anti-mitotic activity by itself, but when present with the adrenaline–chalone complex it acts to prolong the suppression of mitosis by reducing the rate of adrenaline loss from the complex.

We can be fairly certain that, for humans, sleep is not the cause of the circadian rhythm of mitosis. But, to be truthful, we do not know for certain whether this conclusion really applies to rodents, as the appropriate experiments can never be conducted. The procedures by which these animals can be deprived of sleep are stressful in several respects (Section 2.1). Humans can be sleep deprived whilst sitting quietly, but to keep the animal awake, it has to be kept physically active, and this will increase adrenaline release, etc. It is hardly surprising that sleep deprivation even 'by gentle handling' leads to a depression of mitosis, as has been found in a very recent study[21].

Another apparently impossible experiment with rodents addresses the question of whether it is really physical immobility rather than sleep that allows their rates of mitosis to rise? Ideally the animals would be immobilized but prevented from sleeping to see if mitosis rises. But physical restraint would be pointless, as the animal's struggling would still result in heightened physical activity. And there would be the stress of the situation, which would certainly raise adrenaline and cortisol output. An alternative would be a drug-induced waking paralysis, but this would also cause fear and stress. So would the converse, that is somehow artificially producing physical activity in sleep. This would simply wake the animal unless the sleep was drug induced. It is because of these problems that the human findings with mitosis and protein turnover during sleep and wakefulness are so valuable, even though they are limited in other ways. In humans, where relaxed wakefulness exists naturally and can be examined without the problems of stress etc., the evidence points to relaxation, feeding, and circadian rhythms, but not sleep, being the stimuli or facilitators of body restitution.

To recap on the key points I have described in relation to physical activity and body restitution for laboratory rodents:

1. *Periods of relaxed wakefulness are at best only momentary.*
2. *The relatively high physical activity levels in these animals during wakefulness slow down body restitutive processes such as mitosis.*
3. *Adrenaline, cortisol, and perhaps noradrenaline may be the mediators here. Sleep is the only real immobilizer, with the rise in body restitution coming through this immobility, not through sleep itself.*

4.5 Metabolism during sleep and the energy cost of restitution

Protein synthesis needs energy, although the energy cost of this synthesis is not known exactly. In relation to the resting metabolic rate, (i.e. metabolism with the subject lying relaxed on a bed and awake), it is estimated that protein synthesis makes up at least 20 per cent of this level, and may be much greater, perhaps over 40 per cent[6]. When we sleep, metabolism falls by about 9 per cent below that of lying relaxed but awake at night, and in the same state of fasting[22]. This drop is mostly due to sleep, and is in addition to the roughly 15 per cent fall in the circadian rhythm of resting metabolism from average daytime values that occurs at night whether the person is awake or asleep. Overall, during sleep at night the metabolic rate goes down by about 25 per cent from a typical daytime resting level.

What I am coming round to saying is that if human sleep was a state of elevated body restitution then, because of the relatively high metabolic cost of protein synthesis, there would have to be an accompanying increase in metabolism, which is clearly not the case. It could be contested perhaps that muscles become more relaxed during sleep and use less energy. Such 'spare' energy could then be diverted, so to speak, in order to provide the extra energy required for restitution, with the net effect of leaving overall metabolism relatively unchanged from waking to sleep. But the problem with this argument is that the voluntary muscles (except those in the neck, which lose their tone during REM sleep) in fact show little or no reduction in tone from lying awake and relaxed to sleep. So there is little energy saving here. The reason for the fall in metabolism during sleep is, of course, simply the slowing up of most body processes, including body restitution, and especially protein synthesis due to the associated fast.

4.6 'Cell energy charge' and sleep

In order to try and explain what seems to be the impossible, how metabolism could remain low during sleep in the face of heightened body restitution and an increased need for energy, the concept of 'cell energy charge' has been invoked[1,23]. But in my opinion this is a false trail, and is quite misleading to the understanding of sleep function. The concept of cell energy charge is, however, useful to those people studying protein turnover outside the context of sleep and wakefulness.

Originally, the concept hypothesized[24] that anabolism is positively related to the cell energy charge (CEC)—the amount of ATP inside the cell, or to be more precise, the ratio of ATP (plus a portion of ADP) to the total adenylates in the cell (see Section 3.3). The higher the CEC, the greater is the anabolism. During sleep in both rodents and humans, CEC is supposed to rise, favouring more anabolism. But we have already seen that the protein content of tissue cannot increase without more amino acids being supplied to the cell, which is not the case for the fasting state of human sleep. Therefore, even if CEC was higher during human sleep, anabolism could not rise—one cannot build a new house without bricks, even if plenty of bricklayers (ATP) are around. More doubt about the usefulness of the CEC concept to human sleep comes from the difficulty that no one has ever measured CEC during human sleep, and so we have no proof that for us CEC increases here. All the evidence comes from findings with rodents that, as will be seen, cannot be generalized to humans.

Physical activity can depress CEC; however, for humans this has to be at an exercise level close to exhaustion before the effect on CEC is noticeable[25]. There is no evidence that mild exercise (for example jogging) causes any decline in CEC. Besides, as I have already emphasized, most of us spend much of the waking day in a sedentary way, and so there would be little reason for CEC to fall anyway. Another factor is that the life of an ATP molecule is very short, only a minute or two, before its energy is used and it is reduced to ADP or AMP. These products are then quickly 'recharged' and converted back to ATP, with any loss in ATP levels being made up rapidly. Because of the fleeting lifespan of an ATP molecule, it is continually having to be remade, with this cycle repeated hundreds of times over the day. When the total manufacture of ATP is added up, the figure comes to about 60 kilograms of ATP per day for an average-sized man—one body weight's worth[26]. Obviously, any fall in CEC will not last for long, and if this were to influence anabolism then the effect would also only be transitory.

A few experiments using rodents have looked at CEC changes during waking and sleep, or to be more correct during the animals' daily dark and light phases. However, none has actually measured protein synthesis or any other direct aspect of anabolism. Two studies[27,28] reported small CEC rises from waking to sleep in the brain, but one[28] then found that when the animals had adapted more fully to the laboratory environment this sleep–wake difference disappeared. A notable increase in CEC from waking to sleep in the rodent has only been reported once[29], for both brain and muscle. But close inspection of these findings shows that the CEC levels in sleep are the same as those found by other laboratories for wakefulness[30]. It seems that in this particular study it is not that CEC rose during sleep, but that for some unexplained reason the waking values were abnormally low.

Given that there is no reliable evidence that, in either rodents or humans, CEC shows any noticeable rise from waking to sleep, I could rest my case. However, before doing so I want finally to look at the extent of the relationship between CEC and anabolism, as it is apparent that under almost all normal physical activity levels, including moderate to heavy exercise, the small changes that could conceivably happen to CEC would probably have little effect on anabolism anyway. CEC changes will not affect anabolism until physiological extremes are reached—quite beyond usual everyday events for either the rodent or human. Nevertheless, these findings, implying that even small changes in CEC will noticeably affect anabolism, have been applied to the topic of restitution and sleep. Examples that have been used to demonstrate depressions of anabolism by a fall in CEC are near-death situations such as 5 minutes without oxygen[31], and total starvation of glucose[32]. It is hardly surprising that both CEC and protein synthesis fall dramatically under these circumstances, but this is no guide to what might happen in the natural state of sleep, or to the concept of body restitution and sleep.

4.7 Human growth hormone release during sleep

In both the child and the adult the first 3 hours of sleep is accompanied by a very large output of human growth hormone (hGH). It is by far the greatest natural release of this hormone over the 24 hours, and, for example, is similar in extent to that produced by a large drop in blood glucose levels during wakefulness. But I hasten to add that such a fall in blood glucose is not the cause of the sleep-related hGH surge. This surge was discovered about 20 years ago by more than one group of researchers, with perhaps the most notable being led by Dr Yasuro Takahashi, then working at the Washington University School of Medicine[33]. An example of the findings from one of their subjects can be seen in Fig. 4.6, showing a large hGH surge that is typically associated with the main period of SWS, at the beginning of sleep. The figure also shows another, small peak about 3 hours later, coinciding with a minor return of stage 3 sleep.

It is now virtually certain that the hGH surge in sleep is due to sleep, and not simply a time-of-day phenomenon. For example, it is absent during sleep deprivation. Not only is this hGH release closely associated with SWS, but SWS probably acts as its trigger. Such an output is not due to some aberration in the regulation of the hormone's release, as there is a feedback mechanism involved[34]. So, it seems to have a purpose. What this is though, no one really knows. Nevertheless, this fascinating discovery has been used as

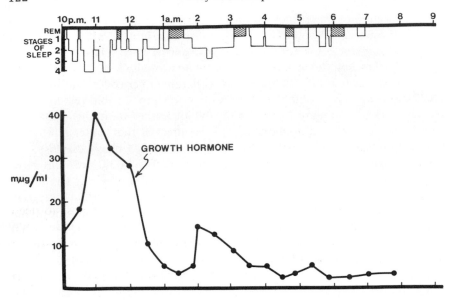

Fig. 4.6 The sleep-related growth hormone release in humans—in a young female adult subject. Note the large surge associated with stages 3 and 4 sleep at the beginning of the night, and a smaller peak around 1 a.m., coinciding with a small return of stage 3 sleep. (From Takahashi et al.[33]. Reproduced by permission of Rockefellar University Press)

a cornerstone in the evidence supporting the hypothesis that sleep is a state of heightened body restitution.

Because the hormone had been called 'growth' hormone, long before an association with sleep was known, many people have quite reasonably assumed that during sleep hGH must be promoting aspects of growth, for example mitosis and protein synthesis. However, we have already seen that the peak of mitosis probably just coincides with the hGH surge, as such a peak is clearly evident in the absence of sleep. Also, I have shown from the work of Waterlow's group (Section 4.3) that the protein content of cells falls, not rises, during sleep. Human growth hormone has many functions, and whilst it can speed up protein synthesis there must be a good supply of amino acids available to the cell at the time—which is not the case during the night-time fast. An additional hormone, insulin, usually has to be present in some quantity in the blood if protein synthesis is to increase, as it encourages cells to take up amino acids[35]. But there is no sleep-related increase in insulin. Besides, because of the night-time fast this would be quite an inappropriate response, as another effect of insulin is to reduce blood glucose levels by converting glucose into glycogen for storage. During the sleep fast, blood glucose may already be on the low side, and further reductions due to the effect of insulin could be dangerous. In fact, owing to the likely fall in blood glucose during this fast, other energy sources may have to be called in.

Several such sources are available. Apart from glycogen there are the body fat deposits, and of course amino acids from the amino acid pool (Section 4.2) which can be oxidized for energy. Whilst this pool is low during the night-time fast, it could be supplemented by an increase in protein break-down from cells. This would be a waste of valuable amino acids, and instead the body ought to be encouraged to use its fat stores. This is exactly what one of the functions of hGH is—to spare protein as a source of energy and to stimulate the use of fat instead. Here may be one possible role for the sleep-related hGH release—not the encouragment of body restitution and protein synthesis, but the sparing of protein from the risk of breakdown due to the night-time fast.

There are some obstacles to this idea. For example, a meal close to sleep onset would prevent the usual sleep fast, but we know that under such circumstances the sleep-hGH release is relatively unchanged. Also, artificial increases of blood glucose levels at the beginning of sleep, via an infusion into a vein have little effect on the hGH release unless the glucose level is abnormally high[36] (when this is done during wakefulness hGH levels fall much more readily). On the other hand, if fatty acids (a product of fat breakdown) are infused at the beginning of sleep, then the sleep-related hGH output falls[36], but still not up to the level of response obtained during wake-fulness. The greater resilience of the sleep-related hGH output to these infusions suggests that different mechanisms are controlling its output during sleep, compared with those of wakefulness. Maybe this is because hGH changes its function during sleep? This is speculation of course, but so is the more traditional interpretation for the sleep-related hGH output—of enhancing body restitution.

To continue my line of thinking for a little longer, some effects of hGH are slow acting, and it should also be noted that hGH itself is not very active. Before it produces its effects, it has to be converted by the liver into more specific products called 'somatomedins'. In fact, it is these that really influence protein synthesis and breakdown, and the mobilization of body fat for energy. But little is known about what happens to somatomedins during sleep, and whether they also show large surges during sleep[37]. Because of the time delay in the conversion of hGH to somatomedins, the sleep-related hGH output might be anticipating events later on during sleep. This could explain why hGH is not very responsive to changes in blood glucose levels, etc. earlier on in the night. The sleep fast of around 12 hours (i.e. from dinner until breakfast), common among humans, is relatively long, and the hGH output might be preparatory for the later hours of sleep when the fast heightens. Bear this last point in mind, as the surprising finding about growth hormone (GH) output during the sleep of other mammals may well shed more light on the human condition.

The surprise is that only a few mammals show any sleep-related enhancement of GH release. For example, there is little sign of it in the cat or dog (unless there is prior sleep deprivation), and, until recently, reports on the adult rat have also been negative. However, new findings[38] with immature rats have shown a positive relationship between levels of GH in the blood and the amount of sleep taken in the 10-minute period prior to the blood sampling. For the adult animal the picture is not so clear[39], as only about 70 per cent of animals showed this effect, and further clarification is necessary. Two primates other than humans, the baboon and rhesus monkey, have also been examined for a sleep-related GH output. Whilst the baboon does seem to have this[40], only two animals were studied. A more substantive investigation on the rhesus monkey found no such output[41]. Other aspects of the release of GH in this monkey are quite similar to those of humans.

Because so few species of mammal have been investigated for a sleep-related GH release, the picture is far from complete. But nevertheless it is clear that this phenomenon is not universal amongst mammals, and presents a confusing state of affairs for the hypothesis that sleep is a condition of heightened body restitution, as the sleep-related GH release is a keystone to the theory. Does this mean that only those mammals with this release show body restitution during sleep? Or that all mammals have this restitution irrespective of the sleep-related GH output? What is more likely, I suspect, is that this output has other roles unrelated to body restitution and sleep. One could be the slowing down of protein breakdown and oxidation in those mammals where sleep typically develops into a fast.

The dog and cat, who have no sleep-related GH release, are carnivores, of course, eating large quantities of protein. This is their primary food and it is the major source of energy in their diet. These animals are not 'nibblers' like the rat, or 'meal feeders' like us, but 'gorgers', usually eating one large protein-rich meal per day. Such a lot of protein will take a long time to digest, even though amino acids from this digested protein will begin to start passing into the bloodstream within an hour or so of the feed. Consequently, because of this 'protein gorge', sleep is unlikely to be a fast, and there would seem to be less need to protect these animals' own tissue protein from breakdown and oxidation. So I would argue that if the purpose of the sleep-related GH surge is to anticipate a fast, and to spare an animal's own tissue protein, then this is unnecessary in carnivorous gorgers as their amino acid pool is well topped up throughout sleep.

For the rodent, or at least the laboratory rodent, sleep is not one long continuous episode, as food nibbling still occurs during short but relatively frequent awakings. However, because of its small size it has a large requirement to feed its high metabolic rate, and needs relatively much more food than does the dog or cat. Also, being an omnivore, the protein content of the diet (particularly the laboratory rats' food pellets) is much lower than that of the carnivore, and more like that of humans. Probably then, in terms of the degree to which sleep develops into a fast, the laboratory rat lies between humans and the dog and cat—and so does the degree to which it exhibits a sleep-related GH release. My argument is tenuous, but no more so than the idea that this release stimulates body tissue restitution.

It would be prudent for further studies of GH release in the sleep of mammals to assess feeding patterns carefully, not only during the days when measurements are performed, but during the animals' rearing, when feeding and sleeping patterns are established. Laboratories differ in the type of food given, its availability over the day, and how often it is replenished. Rodents can be very particular in the food they eat, and, for example, are more partial to recently provided food than to old.

Heed should also be taken when interpreting findings concerning humans and their hGH that are outside the field of sleep, which are generalized to the role of hGH during sleep[1]. I have described this problem more fully elsewhere[42]. For example, during wakefulness, hGH given by injection leads to less urea production. A debatable assumption has been made that protein synthesis is increasing, which is then assumed to be what must also be happening during the sleep-related hGH release. But, as I pointed out in Section 4.2, the state of protein synthesis cannot be assumed simply from the urea content of urine. An increase in protein sparing by hGH is an equally tenable argument. Also, the influences of other hormones on protein synthesis are often overlooked in comparisons of daytime and sleep releases of hGH. Cortisol has a strong influence on protein turnover, and changes in output over the day, particularly during the sleep period.

However, I also have a criticism of myself, as this discussion has concerned itself only with the sleep-related hGH release in the adult, and there is the possibility that its role may differ in the sleep of the growing child, especially as most of a child's daily hGH output is confined to sleep. Undoubtedly, this hormone is central to child growth, and this is how the hormone originally obtained its name, but it is not the only hormone promoting growth. Whether this means that the child exclusively grows in sleep is another matter which is still very much of a mystery. Remember that night-time sleep in children still develops into a fast, and because they sleep for longer the fast may be greater.

There is some evidence[43] suggesting that children may indeed grow in their sleep, and this has been used in support of the body restitution hypothesis for sleep. But again the findings can be misperceived, not by the authors themselves I must add. Over a period of 3 weeks, and for most days at seven times of the day between 8 a.m. and 6 p.m., 11 boys (averaging 11.5 years of age) had the length of their ulnar bone (that runs the length of the forearm) measured very accurately. The findings can be seen in Fig. 4.7. At night, from 6 p.m. to 8 a.m. bone length seemed to increase, and some believe that sleep was responsible for this. But a more careful look at the findings needs to be

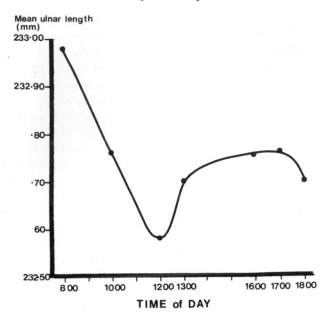

Fig. 4.7 Changes in the length of the ulnar (forearm) bone over the day in boys—average length measured at seven times of the day in 11 boys. Note the shortening in the morning. See text for details. (Taken from Valk and Van Den Bosch[43]. Reproduced by permission of the Growth Publishing Co. Inc.)

taken. It could equally be argued that what is happening is not so much growth at night, but a shortening of the bone during wakefulness, especially between 8 a.m. and midday. Physical activity will contribute to this, causing bone compression, as well as a loss of water from the cartilage cells at either end of the ulnar. No indications were given about how active these boys were in the morning, but, boys being boys, they were no doubt fairly active. At night, bone decompression takes place and the ulnar will lengthen. We do not know how much of the increase in bone length occurred between the last measurement of the day and bedtime, especially in the few hours following dinner, which is usually a physically restful period. Nevertheless, it is quite likely bone mitosis would have peaked during the sleep period, if skin mitotic rates are anything to go by (Section 4.4)—not due to sleep though, but to a circadian rhythm.

I would like to end this discussion by mentioning an additional possible role for the sleep-related hGH release, which I shall be taking up again in Section 5.12. A little-understood effect of GH in animals is to give the immune system a boost (immunoenhancement), but not much is known about this for humans. Very recent work by Dr Harvey Moldofsky and colleagues at Toronto Western Hospital[44] has shown that the onset of SWS is accompanied by increases in certain immune activities, such as the lymphocyte responses to antigens and natural killer cell activity (see Section 3.8). However, it is not known if or how the sleep-related hGH output is related to these signs of immunoenhancement, or to what extent other factors are involved, for example the fall in cortisol output that also accompanies the beginning of sleep (see below).

4.8 Other hormonal changes during human sleep

Apart from hGH, few other human hormones show any clear sleep-related release (i.e. directly caused by sleep). The most notable is prolactin. In both sexes, its levels rise rapidly at sleep onset, reaching a peak around 3 hours into sleep. This release is certainly triggered by sleep, and is blocked by sleep deprivation, but it is not as closely connected with SWS as is hGH. Prolactin is an intriguing hormone, even though little is known about it. Its chemical structure is very similar to that of hGH, with, as far as it is known, some common properties. It is more prominent in females as it encourages milk production (GH also does this to a small extent), but it has other functions that have attracted less interest. For example, it reduces water loss from the kidney, helps other hormones in the control of the body's electrolyte levels, and may have something to do with the regulation of blood levels of glucose and fatty acids. But for the time being, I am afraid that the significance of the sleep-related prolactin release for our understanding of sleep's function must remain a mystery.

Certain of the sex hormones show varying degrees of dependency on sleep, but again we know little about why this is so. Luteinizing hormone, one of the hormones regulating the production and maintenance of ova and sperm, begins to be influenced by sleep around the age of puberty, although in boys this association with sleep soon declines with approaching adulthood. In adult women, there is some inhibition of luteinizing hormone output in the first few hours of sleep. Follicle-stimulating hormone also shows some dependency on sleep, but only during puberty. In males during puberty and adulthood, testosterone output occurs mostly during wakefulness, but does show some peaking during the latter part of sleep. However, this dependency on sleep is minor compared with that of hGH and prolactin. It may be remembered from Section 3.7 that Åkerstedt and colleagues[45] found that the output of testosterone and other sex hormones were suppressed during sleep deprivation. But the investigators were unsure whether this was due to a lack of a sleep-induced secretion of these hormones, or to unknown factors.

In Section 4.4 I briefly described the circadian rhythms of cortisol, adrenaline, and noradrenaline. I would like to elaborate on these a little further. Low outputs of all three occur at night, and in all cases commence before sleep begins—that is, the circadian declines are not due to sleep. There are two caveats to this last remark. Firstly, in the case of noradrenaline, its rhythm is dependent on the level of physical activity[12]. Therefore, to the extent that sleep brings physical inactivity, sleep will influence the noradrenaline rhythm. Secondly, whilst the circadian rhythm of cortisol continues during sleep deprivation[45,46], the first few hours of sleep do depress the cortisol output a little further[47]. This makes sense given the large hGH release at the time, as in certain important respects cortisol works in opposition to hGH by stepping up both protein breakdown and amino acid oxidation.

Melatonin is an intriguing hormone that I first mentioned in Section 3.7, in the context of sleep deprivation. Although the level of melatonin is positively correlated with feelings of sleepiness[48] it is not directly linked to sleep, but somehow tied up with it. Daylight inhibits the hormone's release, and at night-time its levels rise dramatically. In fact, the circadian rhythm of this hormone is mostly dependent on daylight and darkness, regardless of sleep and wakefulness. Melatonin comes from the pineal gland within the brain, and is sensitive to light via pathways from the eyes. Indoor lighting at night is usually much dimmer than daylight, and not strong enough to suppress melatonin output[49]. Whilst melatonin may play some role in the timing of sleep and wakefulness, its role in humans is still a puzzle[49], especially as a night-time increase in melatonin is still found in nocturnal mammals[50]. In mammals other than humans, it inhibits reproduction, and is probably the controller of their breeding seasons. Melatonin is very important to the infant mammal as it can also influence growth, again on a seasonal basis, by speeding up growth when food is plentiful and slowing it down in the winter[49]. Melatonin is also involved in regulating water and electrolyte balance.

Some of the other postulated roles for the pineal gland and melatonin are tantalizing. For example, the pineal seems to have a very close association with the thymus gland[50], which also changes its activity with daylight and darkness. In the infant, the thymus has a key role in the development and function of the immune system (see Section 3.8) and, as I mentioned in the last section, there may be some role for sleep with regard to the immune response.

4.9 Thyroid activity and sleep—body versus brain restitution

This discussion on melatonin has caused me to waver a little off the topic of body restitution and sleep. However, a look now at the thyroid's hormones brings us back to this underlying theme. One of the major roles of the thyroid is the regulation of the body's metabolic rate. Bearing in mind that sleep is a resting condition during which energy is conserved, particularly for smaller mammals, it is not surprising that sleep seems to inhibit the release of thyroid-stimulating hormone (TSH), which is produced by the pituitary to regulate the release of the thyroid's own hormones. TSH has a circadian rhythm that is also influenced by sleep. It has an evening rise that declines with sleep onset. If sleep is delayed then the rise continues on into the night, declining with sleep or the hormone's normal circadian fall. However, somewhat puzzlingly, the release of thyroid hormones does not always show the same circadian pattern as TSH.

People suffering from thyroid overactivity (hyperthyroidism) are behaviourally restless and irritable, lack concentration, have a high heart rate, show raised body temperature and metabolism, warm skin, increased appetite and gut activity, but a falling body weight. Underactivity (hypothyroidism) leads to largely the opposite effects, especially apathy and sluggishness. Both conditions influence the characteristics of sleep in a way that it is of particular interest to the body restitution and sleep debate, as it is SWS that is affected[51-53].

Hyperthyroidism produces a large increase in SWS, although there is only one study to go by[51]. Here, hyperthyroid patients, aged 50–61 years, had their sleep monitored over a period of treatment aimed to bring thyroid activity down to normal. We would normally expect about 35 minutes of SWS a night for this age group—however, the patients averaged 135 minutes. Total sleep lengths were normal, and this huge amount of SWS was taken at the expense of REM and stage 2 sleep. Whilst treatment (using the drug carbimazole) brought thyroid activity down to near-normal levels within 6 months, SWS was very slow to respond, and a year later was only down to an average of 84 minutes a night. No details were given about the behaviour of these patients before, during or after the treatment.

Adult patients with hypothyroidism show little or no SWS[52,53]. Patients usually respond well to treatment with replacement thyroid hormone (thyroxine), and SWS is the sleep characteristic showing the most noticeable change, rising to normal levels. This SWS increase seems to be responsible for further delaying the first episode of REM sleep after sleep onset (i.e. a delayed 'REM sleep latency'). It is interesting to note that these changes to sleep happen sooner than in the case of treatment for hyperthyroidism.

It will be remembered that from the viewpoint of the sleep-is-for-increased-body-restitution hypothesis, SWS is thought to be particularly associated with this restitution. On such a basis, if tissue wear and tear is increased during wakefulness, then more tissue repair and SWS would be expected in the subsequent sleep. These thyroid disorders have supplied this hypothesis with ammunition which I believe turns out to be blanks. For hyperthyroidism, the hypothesis argues that the raised body metabolism during wakefulness will increase body tissue wear and tear, leading to a need for more recovery and restitution during sleep—thus apparently explaining the increased SWS during hyperthyroidism. For hypothyroidism the case runs the opposite way. But there is another explanation for these SWS changes.

Until recently it was thought that thyroid hormones are blocked from entering the brain by the blood–brain barrier—the mechanism for controlling the brain's uptake of substances from the blood. However, from the so readily evident different behaviours shown by patients—the excitability of hyperthyroidism and the sluggishness of hypothyroidism, it is clear that either directly or indirectly (e.g. via changes in brain temperature, leading to rises in cerebral metabolism), thyroid activity does affect the brain. Also, there is ever-strengthening evidence[52] that thyroid hormones do cross the blood-brain barrier to modify the release of neurotransmitters and influence nerve growth factor (a neuropeptide promoting nerve growth). Given that thyroid hormones do have direct or indirect effects on the brain, and that SWS is produced in the cerebral cortex, then it is clear that explanations of SWS changes during hyper- or hypothyroidism should centre on the cerebrum, and not in terms of what is happening elsewhere in the body (as the body restitution hypothesis seems to be keen on). Exactly why SWS is affected is a matter for debate, but I suspect that changes to the brain's waking metabolism may be a key, and this is an area that I shall be covering in the next chapter. Meanwhile, one important point that I have stressed in this Section is that SWS is not a measure of general body restitution, and this is a theme that very much applies to the next topic.

4.10 The effects of exercise on sleep—background

If sleep were a condition of enhanced body restitution overcoming the wear and tear of wakefulness, then presumably physical exercise would increase this wear and lead to more restitution during sleep? Body restitutionalists have predicted that the amounts of SWS would therefore increase, given that this is the type of sleep they associate with restitution, owing to the association between SWS, hGH output, peaks in mitosis, etc. So the actual findings of night-time SWS increases following daytime exercise fit in nicely with the restitution hypothesis, and are taken as more evidence in its support. I have already shown how, after scrutinizing various studies on protein synthesis, mitosis, cell energy charge, and hGH output, support for the hypothesis from this quarter seems to collapse—and so will the body restitution interpretation for the SWS increases after exercise.

My argument behind this last claim began with a review I carried out in 1981 of all the research on sleep following daytime exercise[54]. Some experiments used very fit subjects, and others subjects of 'average fitness', better described as 'unfit'. One of my first conclusions was to confirm the developing view of other researchers in this field, such as Dr John Trinder and colleagues from the Department of Psychology at the University of

Tasmania[55], that SWS only increases after exercise in very fit subjects, with little or no evidence pointing to such an increase in unfit people. But the reason why this difference should happen turned out to be a more complex matter for me. Was it something to do with a difference in exercise loads?

Unfortunately, the amounts of exercise performed by the subjects in many of the experiments were often vaguely described. In most cases the exercise was either running or pedalling on an exercise cycle, with only a few reports giving full details of the exercise load, while others just stated, for example, 'running for an hour' or 'pedalling at a speed of 15 miles an hour for half an hour'. However, there are tables that can be used to make rough calculations of how much energy is used up per minute for different types of activity. The characteristics I concentrated on were: (1) The *intensity* at which the exercise is performed, usually expressed as oxygen consumed per minute ($\dot{V}O_2$—see Section 3.4), and (2) the *total* energy expended, as many of the reports mentioned for how long the exercise was maintained.

At the time of most of these studies, physical fitness was not known to be of central importance, although for purposes of experimental control individual experiments used subjects of equal fitness. In some studies the subjects happened to be fit, whilst unfit in others. Therefore, direct comparisons between types of fitness could, in the most part, only be done between studies, with exercise loads varying from study to study.

Irrespective of whether the subject was fit or unfit, it soon became clear from my survey that the total amount of energy expended is largely irrelevant to whether SWS increases or not, as there were examples of unfit individuals using up large amounts of energy by walking or cycling the equivalent of many miles over many hours, but showing no SWS change. Whereas there were fit subjects who used up a quarter of that total energy in a half-hour run, and then showed a significant SWS rise. This, of course, creates a problem for the body restitution hypothesis of SWS. For someone not used to physical effort, many hours of exercise should cause as much if not more body 'wear and tear' than in the physically fit regular exerciser doing half an hour of exercise. More difficulties arise for the hypothesis when we look at the effects of prolonged bed rest in normal healthy individuals, where one might argue that wear and tear is much reduced—does SWS fall? The only experiment in this area kept healthy people in bed for 6 weeks, but found no fall in SWS[56]. A more extreme example of immobility comes from a report on the sleep of paraplegics and quadraplegics paralysed through spinal injury[57]. Although the investigators reported low amounts of SWS, these turned out to be normal for the patients' ages.

The body restitution hypothesis for SWS has no feasible explanation for such findings. As I have already stressed, SWS is produced by the brain, and is not by itself a measure of body restitution. What is more, none of these exercise and sleep studies have measured any aspect of body restitution (e.g.

protein turnover) to demonstrate that rises in SWS might conceivably reflect increased body restitution. This, together with the findings that sleep is normally a state of tissue dissolution (Section 4.3), compromise any enhanced body restitution interpretation for the SWS rise after exercise in fit people. There is one further point. Whilst certain aspects of restitution, such as mitosis, are depressed by exercise (Section 4.4), the subsequent sleep itself is not necessary for any rebound in mitosis, only rest.

So why is it only fit subjects who show any SWS increase after exercise? The answer has nothing to do with a body restitution hypothesis, but obviously centres on the brain. But first, there is another tale to unfurl. A crucial outcome from my review[54] was that the critical factor as to whether SWS would increase after exercise was the intensity of the exercise. That is, SWS usually increases after high intensity exercise—with the limitation that such exercise has to last for around half an hour or more. Now, one fundamental difference between fit and unfit people is that the former can maintain a relatively high rate of exercise for a longer time. For example, if both types of subject were asked to run as hard as they could for as long as possible, the unfit subjects would give up after a few minutes, well short of the half hour. As my estimates showed, the fit people in the exercise and sleep studies happened to be doing just this, exercising at high rate for a much longer time. However, this was only half way to what seemed to be the eventual answer to the SWS response to exercise.

Of all the physiological changes caused by exercise, the one that drew my greatest interest was body heating. The higher the intensity of exercise the greater is the heat produced by muscle. A brisk walk in a cool and dry environment normally causes little or no rise in body temperature, as excess heat production can be overcome through further heat loss via sweating, etc. As the exercise load increases, or as the heat loss from the skin falls due to a hotter, damper environment or to too much clothing, the greater is the rise in body temperature. Both fit and unfit subjects exercising at the same percentage of their $\dot{V}O_{2max}$ (see Section 3.4), under constant climatic conditions, have similar body temperature rises[58]. But because fit subjects can and will exercise for much longer, they will heat up for longer, and incur a greater total heat load. Even if unfit subjects decide to run very hard, say at 80 per cent of their $\dot{V}O_{2max}$, they become exhausted within a few minutes and do not have time to get very hot. On the other hand, the fit subject can run for up to an hour at this rate, and will be hot for most of the time.

It is also interesting to note that most of the reports of very large SWS rises in fit subjects after exercise tend to come from hot climates, even taking into consideration any differences in exercise load. A hot and/or humid environment will reduce body heat loss, and body temperature will rise further—there may even be a risk of heat exhaustion. Body heating produces many effects such as dehydration, hormonal changes, and perhaps psychological stress, and through this further physiological effects.

To summarize so far in a sentence, the SWS increases that follow exercise occur in fit people only—an effect that has something to do with their greater propensity for becoming hotter for longer. What happens to night-time sleep if someone is simply just heated up for an hour or so during the day, not by exercise but passively, for example, by a sauna, or warm bath? Until recently there was very little to go on, only two reports. One was just a very brief account on the effects of a 40-minute sauna given to subjects of average fitness, and the other, a Russian study[59], concerned weightlifters following a Turkish bath. An increase in SWS was the main finding on both occasions, and this stimulated me into doing some experiments of my own.

4.11 Is body heating the key?

To try and explore the role of body heating further we ran an experiment on a group of eight physically fit people, averaging 25 years of age[60]. There were three experimental conditions, given on separate occasions, always between 2 and 5 p.m., and in a different order for each subject. The first was high intensity (H) exercise, which consisted of running on a treadmill at 80 per cent of their $\dot{V}O_{2max}$ for a total of 80 minutes, with a 30-minute rest half way. Rectal body temperature was recorded throughout the run. We had previously found out that we could simulate exactly the exercise-induced rectal temperature rise of the H condition by sitting subjects in a bath of warm water at 39–40°C (which is still a comfortable temperature), again for 80 minutes, also with a 30-minute interim break. We called this 'passive heating' (P).

The third condition had the same total exercise load of H, but this time we wanted to minimize the rectal temperature rise. So the subjects ran on the treadmill at a low intensity (L) exercise level, at half the speed of H (i.e. 40 per cent of $\dot{V}O_{2max}$) but for twice the time, that is for 160 minutes with a break half way. This exercise load raised rectal temperature a little, by about 0.8°C, but much less than for the H and P conditions, where the rise was about 2.0°C. We could have reduced the temperature rise in L almost to nothing by running the subjects at a quarter of the speed of H, but with breaks this would have lasted for about 6 hours, which was too long and created problems with meals, etc. Besides, a preliminary pilot study had shown that the L condition was good enough for what we wanted. Before and after each condition, subjects were accurately weighed so that we could gauge their sweat loss. This turned out to be very similar for all three conditions, averaging around 3 pints per subject. This loss was made up over the following 2–3 hours by each subject drinking the equivalent amount of water, to ensure that they were rehydrated well before sleep.

Our subjects went to bed at their usual bedtimes, and their sleep EEGs were recorded, not only after each condition but also following baseline rest days. We evaluated all of the sleep EEG records on a 'blind' basis, not knowing beforehand from which experimental condition the record was taken. Also, two people assessed the records without each knowning the other's results, and an independent third person acted as referee—our sleep stage scoring was unbiased. The outcome was that virtually nothing happened with the L condition, except that, unlike the H and P conditions, the subjects not only felt sleepier at bed time, but fell asleep faster and slept for about 20 minutes longer. On the other hand, the major finding for condition H was not an increase in sleep length, but a 20 per cent rise in SWS. This was very close to the 25 per cent rise in SWS following condition P!

Indeed then, body heating seems to be crucial for the SWS increase following intense exercise. It is important to remember that following all three conditions the subjects were allowed to cool down naturally, and *within half an hour of finishing the run or heating, body temperature was back down to normal, and remained so until sleep began.* Then, on the nights following H and P when SWS increased, body temperature during sleep fell more than usual, which did not happen after L. It is quite likely that the rise in SWS was responsible for these temperature falls. Some sleep researchers have suggested that SWS might also be a type of torpor, allowing body temperature to drop—the longer the SWS the greater is this fall. I will describe this further in Section 7.5.

If body heating were the key to the SWS increase following H, then we could make a few more testable predictions. For example, if a subject was cooled during high intensity running to keep the body temperature increase down, then presumably SWS would not rise? This was the basis for our next experiment[61]. In a preliminary pilot study we found that the rectal temperature rise during H could be minimised by letting the subject run lightly clothed in a stream of air from several electric fans, with the skin damped down frequently by a water spray. This resulted in a halving of the rectal temperature increase, rising by only 1.0°C—close to that of the L condition.

A new group of young fit adults was used for the main study. This time, apart from baseline rest days, there were two high intensity running conditions, and the volunteers underwent both, about a week apart. Again, there was an 80-minute run with an interim break. One was exactly the same as before, with the subjects allowed to heat up by about 2.0°C, and the other incorporated the extra cooling. Following the hot run, SWS increased by about 25 per cent, similar to that of condition H before. But after the cool run SWS was unchanged.

From our findings I would predict that hard jogging outdoors into a cool breeeze will probably have little effect on SWS, as it is unlikely that rectal temperature would rise beyond 1.0°C. Whereas a similar run on a hot and still day, would lead to an increase in SWS. The former state of affairs seems to apply to a recent Swedish study of marathon runners[62] running outdoors at a cold time of the year. No SWS changes occurred. On the other hand, another recent study of a marathon run in the heat, in South Africa, reported large SWS increases afterwards[63]. Substantial sweat losses and body temperature rises occurred during the run.

In our cool running condition we paid particular attention to the subject's face, with one fan blowing specifically at this area. It is now known[64] that such cooling, given when the rest of the body is getting hotter, will selectively reduce brain temperature. This entails a fascinating process. Cooled blood from the skin of the face drains into the angularis oculi vein passing at the side of each eye at the bridge of the nose. The vein travels through the bony orbit of the eye and into the cranial cavity, where it joins the jugular vein—the main vein taking blood from the brain. The cool jugular vein runs alongside the carotid artery carrying blood to the brain, allowing blood about to enter the brain to be cooled a little, and the brain's temperature can be kept down. A method for measuring brain temperature is to place a thermocouple carefully down the auditory canal up to the eardrum, as just behind the eardrum is the small tympanic artery that has a temperature close to that of the brain. We measured this tympanic temperature in some of our subjects, and found that during high intensity exercise the facial cooling kept the brain temperature rise down to 0.5°C, compared with a rectal temperature rise of 1.0°C.

I suspect, but cannot prove, that rather than a general body temperature rise being behind the SWS increases following exercise, it is the increase in brain temperature that really matters. Technological problems have prevented us from going further along these lines for the moment. But there is something else to report. I have proposed that the reason why unfit subjects fail to show obvious SWS increases after exercise is that they cannot exercise for long enough to get sufficiently hot. But we can increase their body temperature by putting them in a bath of warm water, exactly the same as the passive heating condition of the earlier experiment, where fit subjects were used. So we asked a group of healthy but unfit volunteers to sit in the bath of warm water, just as before, for the same duration, and at the same time of day (during the afternoon)[65]. Rectal temperatures were measured during the bathtime, and subjects slept in the sleep laboratory the following nights.

After each half-hour in the bath, they left the bath for a 10-minute cool down—it is dangerous to allow people to overheat (so I must stress that readers should not attempt this themselves). There was also a control condition, of again sitting in the bath, but this time with the water temperature at a luke-warm 35°C. It was not unpleasant, and left rectal temperature unchanged, as can be seen in Fig. 4.8. Contrast this with the rises in body temperature shown for the warm bath condition, punctuated by the

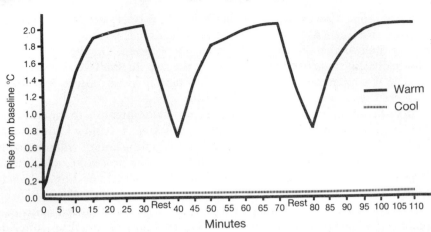

Fig. 4.8 Effect of a warm (40 °C) bath on rectal temperature—three half-hour sessions with two 10-minute rest periods. As a control condition, subjects sat in a luke warm (35 °C) bath, and rectal temperature remained unchanged. Both conditions were given in the after-noon. After the warm bath, sleep the following night contained more SWS, and subjects were sleepier at bedtime. See text for details.

falls during the two rest periods. Note how quickly the subjects cooled down, even in the short rest periods. Within half an hour of the session ending, body temperature was back to normal.

As one might expect, the cool bath had no effect on sleep that night, and in particular SWS was the same as usual. But as in the case of the fit subjects earlier, the hotter bath not only caused a rectal temperature rise of around 2.0°C, but also led to a 30 per cent increase in SWS. However, unlike the fit subjects, these people also found that the hotter bath made them much more sleepy at bedtime, and they fell asleep more quickly. Even lying in the warm bath made the subjects sleepy (which is something most of us experience), but this soon passed after the bath session had ended, only to return again in the evening. One spin-off from the study seems to be that a warm bath may well be an aid for poor sleepers.

Let me now give an overall summary of this section. The body restitution and sleep hypothesis explains the SWS rise after exercise in terms of a genera-lized increase in body tissue repair (especially for muscles). I argue that this SWS increase has little or nothing to do with the body directly. Firstly, because SWS (or rather the delta EEG activity of SWS) is produced by the cerebrum, we must consider how this organ itself is influenced by exercise, and not so much how the rest of the body is affected—especially as we have no evidence to show that body restitution is heightened during sleep after exercise. Secondly, increases in SWS following exercise seem to depend on the extent to which the brain gets hot during the exercise. So the exercise itself seems immaterial to this issue, and should perhaps be considered simply as another method for increasing brain temperature, like passive heating. Exactly why a warmer brain leads to increased SWS is still a matter for debate. One reasonable explanation for me is that rises in brain temperature increase brain metabolism and speed up the various processes of wakefulness that promote SWS. Maybe this increased metabolism heightens cerebral 'wear and tear', or causes a more rapid accumulation of some substance in the brain that regulates SWS.

4.12 Conclusions—does sleep promote enhanced body restitution?

My answer is no—case not proven. Following on from the previous chapter, where I concluded that there were few, if any, adverse effects of sleep deprivation on body functioning, I have now proposed that there is no evidence to support a body restitutive theory for *human* sleep. My main points are as follows:

1. *The stimulus to body restitution is not sleep but food intake* (i.e. amino acid absorption from the gut). Consequently, the usual fasting state of sleep would not support an overall increase in the protein content of tissue. The reverse seems more likely—tissue dissolution during sleep. The few studies measuring protein turnover in humans over 24 hours endorse these conclusions.
2. *Increases in rates of mitosis during sleep are not stimulated by sleep, but are just a circadian phenomenon concomitant with sleep.* The hormones cortisol and adrenaline have a major influence here, and their release is independent of sleep.
3. *The low metabolic rate of sleep would be incompatible with the relatively high energy costs of any substantial rise in protein synthesis.* This low metabolic rate again points to decreased synthesis. Arguments based on increases in cell energy charge during sleep are misleading and lack the necessary evidence.
4. *Reasons for the sleep-related hGH output are unclear.* For example, it may be a preventative measure for sparing tissue protein during the long fast of sleep. Our feeding style and diet could well have some impact here, and contrasts with the high protein diet and 'gorging' of carnivores, where there is no sleep-related GH release.
5. *The SWS increase after exercise has little to do with body functioning and seems to be the result of a raised cerebral temperature.*
6. *Physical rest facilitates body restitutive processes.* Humans usually have adequate rest for such purposes during wakefulness.

Points 1, 2, and 6 also very much apply to mammals in general, including rodents. But rodents, like other less advanced small mammals, do not have the capacity for relaxed wakefulness. Because of their *ever-active wakefulness, sleep is their only immobilizer*. Therefore, various restitutive processes that would otherwise happen during wakefulness may be delayed until sleep. By default, sleep will allow increases in these restitutive processes, but will not be their cause. This situation does not apply to carnivores, primates, and other mammals with a well-developed cerebrum that allows them to have extended periods of relatively inactive wakefulness (e.g. lying, sitting, and slow walking). However, there are other aspects to the function of sleep in various mammalian groups, and these will be covered in Chapter 7.

My case against heightened body restitution occurring during human sleep rests here. It excludes the cerebrum of course, where the likelihood for a restitutive role for sleep seems much stronger, and this is what I shall be looking at in the next chapter. SWS may be the particular candidate for cerebral restitution, especially as it is central to core sleep.

References

1. Adam, K. and Oswald, I. (1983). Protein synthesis, bodily renewal and the sleep–wake cycle. *Clinical Science*, **65**, 561–567.
2. Bullough, W.S. (1948). Mitotic activity in the adult male mouse, *Mus musculus L.* The diurnal cycles and their relation to waking and sleeping. *Proceedings of The Royal Society B*, **135**, 212–233.
3. Rennie, M.J., Edwards, R.H.T., Krywawych, E.S., Davies, C.T.M., Halliday, D., Waterlow, J.C. and Millward, D.J. (1981). Effect of exercise on protein turnover in man. *Clinical Science*, **61**, 627–639.
4. Dohm, G.I., Kalsperek, G.J., Tapscott, E.B. and Beecher, G.R. (1980). Effect of exercise on synthesis and degradation of muscle protein. *Biochemical Journal*, **188**, 255–262.
5. Borbély, A.A. and Neuhaus, H.U. (1979). Sleep deprivation: effects on sleep and EEG in the rat. *Journal of Comparative Physiology*, **133**, 7–87.
6. Waterlow, J.C., Garlick, P.J. and Millward, D.J. (1978). *Protein Turnover in Mammalian Tissues and in the Whole Body*. North Holland, Amsterdam.
7. Clugston, G.A. and Garlick, P.J. (1982). The response of protein and energy metabolism to food intake in lean and obese man. *Human Nutrition: Clinical Nutrition*, **36C**, 57–70.
8. Golden, M.H.N. and Waterlow, J.C. (1977). Total protein synthesis in elderly people: a comparison of results with (15N) glycine and (14C) leucine. *Clinical Science and Molecular Medicine*, **53**, 277–288.
9. Clugston, G.A. and Garlick, P.J. (1982). The response of whole-body protein turnover to feeding in obese subjects given a protein-free, low energy diet for three weeks. *Human Nutrition: Clinical Nutrition*, **36C**, 391–397.
10. Scheving, L.E. (1959). Mitotic activity in the human epidermis. *Anatomical Record*, **135**, 7–20.
11. Clausen, O.P.F., Thorud, E., Bjerknes, R. and Elgjo, K. (1979). Circadian

rhythms in mouse epidermal basal cell proliferation. *Cell and Tissue Kinetics*, **12**, 319–337.

12. Gillberg, M., Anderzen, I., Åkerstedt, T. and Sigurdson, K. (1986). Urinary catecholamine responses to basic types of physical activity. *European Journal of Applied Physiology*, **55**, 575–578.

13. Vonnahme, F.J. (1974). Circadian variation in cell size and mitotic index in tissues having a relatively low proliferation rate in both normal and hypophysectomised rats. *International Journal of Chronobiology*, **2**, 297–309.

14. Fisher, L.B. (1968). The diurnal mitotic rhythm in the human epidermis. *British Journal of Dermatology*, **80**, 75–80.

15. Durnin, J.G.V.A. and Passmore, R. (1967). *Energy, Work and Leisure*. Heinemann Educational Books, London.

16. Bullough, W.S. (1948). The effects of experimentally induced rest and exercise on the epidermal mitotic activity of the adult mouse, *Mus musculus* L. *Proceedings of the Royal Society B*, **135**, 233–242.

17. Bullough, W.S. and Laurence, E.B. (1966). Accelerating and decelerating actions of adrenalin on epidermal mitotic activity. *Nature*, **210**, 715–716.

18. Bullough, W.S. and Laurence, E.B. (1961). Stress and adrenaline in relation to the diurnal cycle of epidermal mitotic activity in adult male mice. *Proceedings of The Royal Society B*, **154**, 540–556.

19. Bullough, W.S. and Laurence, E.B. (1964). Mitotic control by internal secretion: the role of the chalone-adrenaline complex. *Experimental Cell Research*, **33**, 176–194.

20. Bullough, W.S. and Laurence, E.B. (1968). The role of corticosteroid hormones in the control of epidermal mitoses. *Cell and Tissue Kinetics*, **1**, 5–10.

21. Jazwinska, E.C. (1986). Sleep deprivation alters the cell population kinetics in the jejunum of the male Syrian hamster (*Mesocricetus auratus*). *Cell and Tissue Kinetics*, **19**, 335–360.

22. Shapiro, C.M., Goll, C.C., Cohen, G.R. and Oswald, I. (1984). Heat production during sleep. *Journal of Applied Physiology*, **56**, 671–677.

23. Adam, K. (1980). Sleep as a restorative process and a theory to explain why. *Progress in Brain Research*, **53**, 289–305.

24. Atkinson, DE. (1977). *Cellular Energy Metabolism and its Regulation*. Academic Press, New York.

25. Karlsson, J. and Saltin, B. (1970). Lactate, ATP, and CP in working muscles during exhaustive exercise in man. *Journal of Applied Physiology*, **29**, 598–602.

26. Flatt, J.P. (1978). The biochemistry of energy expenditure. In: Bray, G.A. (ed.) *Recent Advances in Obesity Research II*. Newman Publishing, New York. pp. 211–228.

27. Van den Noort, S. and Brine, K. (1970). Effect of sleep on labile phosphates and metabolic rate. *American Journal of Physiology*, **218**, 1434–1439.

28. Reich, P., Geyer, S.J. and Karnovsky, M.L. (1972). Metabolism of brain during sleep and wakefulness. *Journal of Neurochemistry*, **19**, 487–497.

29. Durie, D.J.B., Adam, K., Oswald, I. and Flynn, I.W. (1978). Sleep: cellular energy charge and protein synthetic capability. *IRCS Medical Science*, **6**, 351.

30. Chapman, A.G., Fall, L. and Atkinson, D.E. (1971). Adenylate energy charge in

Escherichia coli during growth and starvation. *Journal of Bacteriology*, **108**, 1072–1086.

31. Ayuso-Parrilla, M.S. and Parrilla, R. (1975). Control of hepatic protein synthesis. *European Journal of Biochemistry*, **55**, 593–599.

32. Mendelsohn, S.L., Nordeen, S.K. and Young, D.A. (1977). Rapid changes in initiation-limited rates of protein synthesis in rat thymic lymphocytes correlates with energy change. *Biochemical and Biophysical Research Communications*, **79**, 53–60.

33. Takahashi, Y., Kipnis, D.M. and Daughaday, W.H. (1968). Growth hormone secretion during sleep. *Journal of Clinical Investigation*, **47**, 2079–2090.

34. Mendelson, W.B., Jacobs, L.S. and Gillin, J.C. (1983). Negative feedback suppression of sleep-related growth hormone secretion. *Journal of Clinical Endocrinology and Metabolism*, **56**, 486–488.

35. Jefferson, L.S. (1980). Role of insulin in the regulation of protein synthesis. *Diabetes*, **29**, 487–495.

36. Parker, D.C., Rossman, L.G., Kripke, D.F., Gibson, W. and Wilson, K. (1979). Rhythmicities in human growth hormone concentrations in plasma. In: Kreiger, D.T. (ed.), *Endocrine Rhythms*. Raven Press, New York, 143–173.

37. Minuto, F., Underwood, L.E., Grimaldi, P., Furlanfo, R.W., van Wyck, J.J. and Giordano, G. (1981). Decreased serum somatomedin C concentrations during sleep: temporal relationship to the nocturnal surges of growth hormone and prolactin. *Journal of Clinical Endocrinology and Metabolism*, **52**, 399–403.

38. Kawakami, M., Kimura, F. and Tsai, C-W. (1984). Relationship between the three-hour-period sleep–wakefulness cycle and growth hormone secretion in the immature rat. *Journal of Physiology*, **348**, 271–283.

39. Kimura, F. and Tsai, C-W. (1984). Ultradian rhythm of growth hormone secretion and sleep in the adult male rat. *Journal of Physiology*, **353**, 305–315.

40. Parker, D.C., Morishima, M., Koerker, D.J., Gale, C.C. and Goodner, C.J. (1972). Pilot study of growth hormone release in sleep of the chair-adapted baboon: potential as a model of human sleep release. *Endocrinology*, **91**, 1462–1464.

41. Quabbe, H-J., Gregor, M., Bumke-Vogt, C., Witt, I. and Giannella-Neto, D. (1983). Endocrine rhythms in a non-human primate, the rhesus monkey. *Advances in Biological Psychiatry*, **11**, 48–59.

42. Horne, J.A. (1985). Sleep function, with particular reference to sleep deprivation. *Annals of Clinical Research*, **17**, 199–208.

43. Valk, I.M. and van den Bosch, J.S.G. (1978). Intradaily variation of the human ulnar length and short term growth—a longitudinal study of eleven boys. *Growth*, **42**, 107–111.

44. Moldofsky, H., Lue, F.A., Einsen, J., Keystone, E. and Gorczynski, R.M. (1986). The relationship of interleukin-1 and immune function to sleep in humans. *Psychosomatic Medicine*, **48**, 309–318.

45. Åkerstedt, T., Palmblad, J., de la Torre, B. and Gillberg, M.R. (1980). Adreno-cortical and gonadal steroids during sleep deprivation. *Sleep*, **3**, 23–30.

46. Åkerstedt, T. (1979). Altered sleep–wake patterns and circadian rhythms. *Acta Physiologica Scandinavica*, Supplement **469** (entire).

47. Weitzman, E.D., Zimmerman, J.C., Czeisler, C.A. and Ronda, J. (1983). Cortisol secretion is inhibited during sleep in normal man. *Journal of Clinical*

Endocrinology, **56**, 352–358.
48. Åkerstedt, T. (1984). Hormones and sleep. In: Borbély, A.A. and Valatx, J-L. (ed.). *Sleep Mechanisms*. Springer-Verlag, Berlin. pp. 193–203.
49. Wurtman, R.J., Baum, M.J. and Potts, J.T. (1986). The medical and biological effects of light. *Annals of the New York Academy of Sciences*, **453** (entire).
50. Martin, C.R. (1976). *Textbook of Endocrine Physiology*. Williams and Wilkins, Baltimore.
51. Kales, A., Heuser, G., Jacobson, A., Kales, J.D., Hanley, J., and Zweizig, J.R. (1967). All night sleep studies in hypothyroid patients, before and after treatment. *Journal of Clinical Endocrinology*, **27**, 1593–1599.
52. Ruiz-Primo, E., Jurado, J.L., Solis, H., Maisterrena, J.A., Fernandez-Guardiola, A. and Valverde, R. (1982). Polysomnographic effects of thyroid hormones in primary myxedema. *Electroencephalography and Clinical Neurophysiology*, **53**, 559–564.
53. Dunleavy, D.L.F., Oswald, I., Brown, P. and Strong, J.A. (1974). Hyperthyroidism, sleep and growth hormone. *Electroencephalography and Clinical Neurophysiology*, **36**, 259–263.
54. Horne, J.A. (1981). The effects of exercise on sleep. *Biological Psychology*, **12**, 241–291.
55. Griffin, S.J. and Trinder, J. (1978). Physical fitness, exercise and human sleep. *Psychophysiology*, **15**, 447–450.
56. Ryback, R.S., Lewis, O.F. and Lessard, C.S. (1971). Psychobiologic effects of prolonged bedrest (weightlessness) in young healthy volunteers. *Aerospace Medicine*, **42**, 529–535.
57. Adey, W.R., Bors, E. and Porter, R.W. (1968). EEG sleep patterns after high cervical lesions in man. *Archives of Neurology*, **19**, 377–383.
58. Åstrand, P.-O. and Rodahl, K. (1977). *Textbook of Work Physiology*. McGraw Hill, New York.
59. Maloletnev, V.I. and Chachanaschvili, M.G. (1979). Changes in sleep structure in athletes after rapid weight reduction in steam bath. (In Russian.) *Bulletin of the Academy of Sciences of the Georgian SSR*, **96**, 690–2.
60. Horne, J.A. and Staff, L.H.E. (1983). Exercise and sleep: body heating effects. *Sleep* **6**, 36–46.
61. Horne, J.A. and Moore, V.J. (1985). Sleep effects of exercise with and without additional body cooling. *Electroencephalography and Clinical Neurophysiology* **60**, 33–8.
62. Torsvall, L., Åkerstedt, T., and Lindbeck, G. (1984). Effects on sleep stages and EEG power of different degrees of exercise in fit subjects. *Electroencephalography and Clinical Neurophysiology*, **57**, 347–53.
63. Shapiro, C.M., Bortz, R., Mitchell, D., Bartell, P., and Jooste, P. (1981). Slow wave sleep: a recovery period after exercise. *Science*, **214**, 1253–4.
64. Cabanac, M. and Caputa, M. (1979). Natural selective cooling of the human brain: evidence of its occurrence and magnitude. *Journal of Physiology* **286**, 255–64.
65. Horne, J.A. and Reid, A.J. (1985). Night-time sleep EEG changes following body heating in a warm bath. *Electroencephalography and Clinical Neurophysiology*, **60**, 154–7.

5. Waking awareness, subsequent sleep, and cerebral 'restitution'

5.1 Background

Impairments to behaviour and to performance at psychological tests are the most apparent findings with human subjects during sleep deprivation. This indicates that the organ most affected by sleep loss is the cerebrum. I have suggested (Section 3.9) that these impairments are partly due to a build-up of some sort of behavioural drive to sleep. I have called this *optional sleepiness*, which can be counteracted to a large extent by the sleep deprived subject applying more effort. However, I believe there is another component to sleepiness, *core sleepiness*, which is due to increasing wear and tear on the cerebrum, which requires a special form of sleep, *core sleep*, for its restitution. Core sleep seems to be reflected mostly in the delta EEG activity of SWS, particularly in the 'deeper' form of stage 4 sleep, found during the first few sleep cycles of a normal night's sleep. Only a portion of the lost sleep needs to be regained following sleep deprivation, and stage 4 sleep occurs in abundance here. However, there seems to be more to core sleep than simply delta activity, as REM sleep also plays a role. About half of our nightly REM sleep can be considered as core sleep, and the remainder as *optional sleep*. The topic of REM sleep is covered more fully in Chapters 6 and 8.

For me, the concept of 'cerebral restitution' during sleep is more than just the reversal of a behavioural drive to sleep, or of the elimination of some biochemical substance within the brain for keeping us asleep. Instead, these latter two phenomena may well underlie optional sleep. Although the cerebrum probably needs off-line repairs and adaptations to nerve networks following wakefulness, I have also proposed (Section 2.12) that there is some spare capacity within the cerebrum to withstand a degree of disrepair, with spare networks able to be switched in during wakefulness as others fail. A fundamental reason why I consider that the cerebrum is in particular need of off-line repair is that, unlike many other organs in the body, it cannot really rest during wakefulness, as it has to be in a high state of quiet readiness—vigilant and ready to respond quickly to new situations.

The term 'cerebrum' is rather vague, and definitions vary amongst neuroanatomists as to what exactly is meant. Obviously, it relates to the two cerebral hemispheres, and includes both the cerebral cortex (the grey matter —the neuronal cell bodies) and various inner structures (including the white matter—the axons). Although I believe that the 'cerebral restitution' to which I have just referred, relates mostly to the cerebral cortex, I really do not know whether these inner structures should be excluded or included. So I shall purposely remain a little vague and keep to using the term 'cerebral' rather than 'cerebro-cortical'.

I would like briefly to repeat an important point I made earlier (Section 3.9), concerning the 'lower' parts of the brain, particularly the brain stem. These regions look after the vital basic functions such as respiration, which must obviously continue throughout sleep and wakefulness. Their inbuilt routines are inflexible and preprogrammed. For them, repairs must occur on-line, with sleep not specifically being required for this purpose. One of the first people to make this point, over 20 years ago, was Professor Guiseppi Moruzzi, from the University of Pisa[1]. He was one of the discoverers of the brain's reticular formation. This, and other subsequently found brain regions that regulate sleep and wakefulness, mostly lie in the more 'basic' parts of the brain, and Moruzzi pointed out that, paradoxically, these sleep centres do not need sleep themselves.

'Slow wave sleep' (SWS) is a term that is also applied to the sleep of other mammals like the rodent and cat. But this time it is used as an alternative name for non-REM sleep in its entirety. Human SWS is, of course, not synonymous with non-REM sleep, but a 'deeper' variety of it. In fact, these other animals seem to have an equivalent to our SWS within their non-REM sleep, which has been clearly shown for the rat by investigators at the University of Chicago Sleep Laboratory[2], and more recently in further detail, by Borbély[3]. But this animal has a poorly developed cerebrum and, whereas human SWS is produced wholly by the cerebrum (specifically the cerebral cortex), for the rat this 'deeper' non-REM sleep also seems to come from structures outside the cerebrum. Consequently, the rat's equivalent of our SWS may have a different role to that of the human. On the other hand, the cat's cerebrum is much larger and more complex, and bears a greater resemblance to ours than that of the rat. The cat's deeper variety of non-REM sleep[4] is indeed mostly centred on the cerebrum, and may have a similar significance to that of humans. As to what the significance of SWS may be? Well, that is the central theme of this chapter.

5.2 Influences of wakefulness on subsequent sleep

Increase the length of wakefulness, as in sleep deprivation, and sleep will lengthen. There seems to be nothing remarkable about this, and it can be explained in a host of ways. However, of greater interest is that only a portion of the total lost sleep is made up, around 30 per cent, which consists of most of the lost SWS (particularly stage 4 sleep), and about half of the lost REM sleep. All of the lost stages 1 and 2 sleep seem to be lost for good. Stage 4 sleep is highly positively correlated with the length of prior wakefulness, more so than is REM sleep. Because of this, stage 4 sleep seems the most likely candidate of all the sleep stages to be associated with some sort of cerebral recovery from wakefulness. Of course such a correlation does not necessarily indicate causation, but it certainly warrants more careful enquiry.

Some of the earliest work on the effects of different lengths of wakefulness on stage 4 and REM sleep was done in the early 1970s by Webb (whose experiments on sleep deprivation I mentioned in Chapter 2). In one series of studies, he and his assistant, Harmon Agnew[5,6], requested their subjects to go to bed at 11 p.m., following periods of wakefulness ranging from 5 to 70 hours. Webb and Agnew only presented their findings for the first 4 hours of this sleep, and Fig. 5.1 has been adapted from these. Levels of stage 4 sleep rose steeply from 5 to 24 hours wakefulness, and then showed a shallower

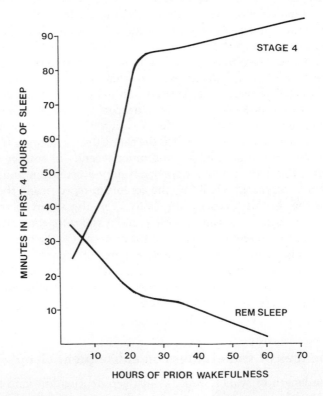

Fig. 5.1 Effects of different lengths of wakefulness and sleep deprivation on stage 4 and REM sleep in the first 4 hours of recovery sleep. Note the opposite trends. Stage 4 sleep shows the positive recovery effect, not REM sleep. See text. (Adapted from Webb and Agnew[5,6])

increase. This 'ceiling effect' was because there is a limit to the amount of stage 4 that can be contained in the first 4 hours of sleep, and the rest spills over into later hours. With very long periods of wakefulness, as for example in the 205-hour sleep deprivation study (Section 2.7), excess stage 4 sleep was carried over into the following night (Table 2.3). Webb and Agnew found quite a different recovery pattern for REM sleep. Its levels fell in these first 4 hours, to almost nothing after 60 hours of wakefulness.

Obviously, when wakefulness goes beyond 16 hours or so, one begins to enter sleep deprivation. So the findings of Webb and Agnew could be interpreted from the perspectives of either prolonged wakefulness or stage 4 sleep deprivation. Although both are in effect the same thing, we can avoid any confusion by considering the influence of prior wakefulness alone, without stage 4 deprivation. This can be done by looking only at the left half of the graph in Fig. 5.1, with wakefulness going from 5 to 16 hours. Here, there is a linear rise in stage 4 sleep, contrasting with a linear fall in REM sleep.

Later work by Dr Ken Hume and Professor John Mills, who at the time were in the Physiology Department at Manchester University[7], looked in more detail at the effects of varying the lengths of wakefulness on SWS and REM sleep (results for stage 4 alone were not given). Wakefulness did not exceed 16 hours (i.e. there was no sleep deprivation). The contrasting trends for SWS and REM sleep were quite striking and are shown in Fig. 5.2, and

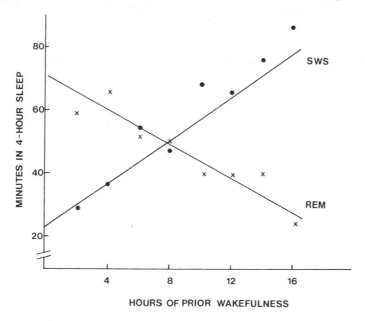

Fig. 5.2 SWS (•) and REM sleep (X) during 4 hours of sleep following different lengths of wakefulness, without sleep deprivation. The straight lines give the best fits, and again show opposite trends. (Adapted from Hume and Mills[7])

support Webb and Agnew's findings. One important point that I have not
mentioned about Webb and Agnew's experiment is that they also looked at
the time of day at which sleep was taken. This was also done by Hume and
Mills. It was clear from both studies that the time of the day of sleep had little
impact on SWS—it was just the length of prior wakefulness that mattered.
On the other hand, there was a major time-of-day effect on REM sleep.
Unlike SWS, REM sleep has an obvious circadian rhythm in its propensity,
peaking around 11 a.m., and troughing at midnight. I will not go into this last
point now, except to say that Fig. 5.2 just gives the findings for sleep
averaged over all times of the day. I will be taking up this time-of-day effect
with REM sleep again, in Section 6.6.

There have also been a few reports giving details of the SWS content of
much shorter daytime sleeps, that is naps. Often these are not long enough to
enable all of the accumulated SWS need to be 'paid off', but the positive
correlation between SWS levels and length of prior wakefulness is again
clear[8]. However, what is particularly interesting are the changes in SWS
during the following night's sleep. What happens is that the amount of SWS
in a nap is naturally subtracted from the following night's usual SWS level.
On the other hand, the amount of REM sleep at night is not reduced in this
way, but remains the same. These points are reflected in Table 5.1 of the
findings taken from a well-known study[9] by Dr Ismet Karacan and colleagues
from the Baylor College of Medicine at Houston. It shows the effects of 1–2
hour morning (10 a.m.) or afternoon (4 p.m.) naps on night-time sleep,
averaged for 11 young adults.

These naps affected neither the total length of night-time sleep nor the
amount of REM sleep at night, but just increased the daily amounts of each.
However, the minutes of SWS over 24 hours stayed remarkably constant,
regardless of whether SWS was confined solely to the night (baseline), or
taken in two parts—in a nap, and at night. It should be noted that these
subjects were not sleep deprived in any way beforehand. It is very easy for
most people to nap in the daytime, even though this may not be their usual
habit. Note also how the afternoon nap contained more SWS compared with

Table 5.1 Morning (a.m.) or afternoon (p.m.) naps and night-time sleep. Note
how SWS levels rise with increasing wakefulness, from the a.m. to the p.m. nap,
and how this SWS subtracts from the usual night's quota. In both respects, the
reverse occurs to REM sleep. See text for details. (From Karacan et al.[9])

Type of sleep	a.m. nap	Night	Total	p.m. nap	Night	Total	Baseline night (no nap)
SWS	4	74	78	26	52	78	80
REM	43	97	143	22	101	123	91
Total sleep	107	372	479	113	375	488	369

that of the morning nap, because more wakefulness elapsed before the after-noon nap.

Dr Bob Feinberg, working until recently at the Veterans Administration Medical Center in San Francisco, is a well-known and rather outspoken sleep researcher who has been arguing for many years that we should be devoting more attention to the much overlooked SWS. Among the numerous experi-ments he has run was a nap study, similar to the one above, but where the EEG was examined in a much more precise way. He was also one of the first to point out the problems associated with the visual scoring method of the sleep EEG in relation to delta EEG waves. For example, some delta waves occur outside SWS, in stage 2 sleep. These are 'missed' by the conventional rules for scoring stages 3 and 4 sleep (Section 1.3), and this stimulated Feinberg into becoming one of the pioneers in developing computer tech-niques for measuring the EEG slow (delta) waves of sleep. Several mathe-matically based methods originating from fields outside that of the EEG could potentially do this. I will not go into these, except to mention that, although they are an improvement on the visual scoring method, they do have some pitfalls of their own when applied to the EEG, because it is a very changeable waveform. Feinberg's system uses 'period analysis', which is one of the best at overcoming these difficulties.

In their nap experiment, Feinberg and colleagues[10] first obtained baseline sleep recordings from ten young adult subjects, who were then given up to 2 hours for a nap the next afternoon. The subjects returned to bed for their usual sleep later that night. EEG records were visually scored into sleep stages and then analysed by his computer-based period analysis technique. In what is really an oversimplification of the procedure, delta waves are iden-tified, measured for size, and the values summated to produce an 'integrated amplitude', registered as volts per second. Using conventional sleep staging, the baseline night contained an average of 42 minutes of SWS, the naps 13 minutes, and the ensuing night-time sleep 19 minutes. So, the value for nap plus nighttime sleep, at 32 minutes, fell short of the normal baseline level. However, computer analysis showed how constant SWS really was. The inte-grated amplitude of delta waves averaged 0.194 volts per second during the baseline night, 0.044 for the nap, and 0.146 for the subsequent night. These two latter values combined to 0.190 volts per second—only 2 per cent dif-ferent from the baseline.

5.3 SWS changes over the night, and 'models' of SWS

Feinberg uses these nap sleep findings to support further his proposals that delta EEG activity reverses in some way the effect of wakefulness on the brain. He had already pointed out in 1974[11] that the decline in SWS over a night's sleep (see Fig. 1.2) seems to reflect the decay of some factor that has

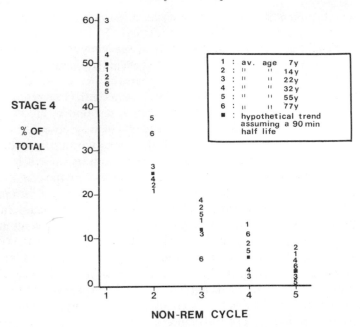

Fig. 5.3 Trends in stage 4 sleep for successive sleep cycles over the night, in six age groups—given as percentages of the night's total. Note the similarity between all the trends, and that all values fall by half for each successive cycle, i.e. stage 4 sleep has a 'half-life' of 90 minutes. See text for details. (Calculated from the findings of Feinberg[11])

built up steadily during wakefulness. Partly to illustrate this, he presented detailed findings on the sleep stage characteristics of six age groups, averaging 7, 14, 22, 32, 55 and 77 years of age. He emphasized then, and still does, that we should look at the progress of sleep over the night not in hours, but in terms of the 90-minute cycles of REM and non-REM sleep, which is in effect the 'biological hour', and I agree with him. This work was done before the advent of his computer technique. So, as a guide to the changes in delta activity over the night in these subjects, I have plotted out in Fig. 5.3 the values of stage 4 sleep for each 90-minute sleep cycle, but have given them as a percentage of the total amount for the whole night. For any age group, the percentages across all five cycles add up to 100 per cent. Remember though, in absolute terms stage 4 sleep declines with age, and that this diagram only gives relative changes over the night.

It can be seen that each age group shows similar trends over the night, with the value for each cycle being roughly half that of the one before (i.e. it is an 'exponential decay' process), with a half-life of 90 minutes. That is, half of the stage 4 sleep disappears every 90 minutes. In Fig. 5.3, I have also shown what a true decay of 90 minutes would look like, and this fits Feinberg's data almost exactly.

Professor Alex Borbély (see also see Section 4.2) and colleagues[12], have developed a mathematical model to describe the SWS changes over the night. He also uses computer analysis of the EEG to measure delta wave changes, but this technique is different from that of Feinberg as it is based on what is known as frequency analysis, and uses the Fourier method. Borbély considers the fall in SWS over the night to represent 'process S', a mechanism or substance like that of Feinberg's, which builds up over wakefulness and is reversed or decays exponentially during sleep. However, Borbély's model is more advanced as it also takes into consideration factors other than just the length of prior wakefulness and the shape of the decay of SWS over the night. It also incorporates a powerful circadian influence on sleep length (not on SWS though), which he calls 'process C', linked to the circadian change in body temperature. In his model, the two processes, S and C, interact in precise ways to allow various predictions to be made, for example, about the length and timings of sleep. Not surprisingly, his model is very attractive to sleep researchers. But in view of its complexity, I will not describe it further, but recommend the reader to read about it in Borbély's own excellent book '*Secrets of Sleep*'[12]. By the way, my categories of core and optional sleep are in effect subdivisions of Borbély's process S. For me, his process C is the circadian temperature rise that normally determines the ending of optional sleep (see Section 6.6).

Other sleep researchers apart from Feinberg and Borbély have suggested that SWS represents some sort of recovery relating to wakefulness. Returning to the last section, there is Webb and his work on the relationship between SWS and the length of prior wakefulness. Then there are the authors of the first nap study I described[9], who concluded that 'stage 4 sleep is the manifestation of a consummatory process which runs its course to completion' (p. 398). I have been writing over the last 10 years about SWS reflecting some form of recovery of the cerebrum from the effects of wakefulness[13]. There are even pertinent reports going back a hundred years—not describing SWS of course, but not far off the mark. Dr John Hughlings Jackson, the eminent neurologist of the Victorian era, wrote in 1884 that as a result of wakefulness:

'There is what I will call internal evolution, a process which goes on most actively in the higher centres. On account of its great preponderance in the highest centres of man, he differs so greatly from lower animals . . . Manifestly new, although evanescent combinations are made during dreaming; but I contend that permanent rearrangements (internal evolutions) are made during so-called deep dreamless sleep'[14]

But for Feinberg, Borbély, and other contemporary sleep researchers, including myself, what SWS truly represents is another matter. None of these theories and observations tell us what is really going on inside the brain during SWS, particularly whether SWS is essential for the repair of the cerebral 'wear and tear' that occurs during wakefulness, as I have speculated. It will be seen in the rest of this chapter that all I have to go on in this respect is circumstantial evidence. One could argue, rather like Webb does for example[15], that a build up of a need for SWS during a period of wakefulness could simply represent the accumulation of a behavioural drive to sleep, controlled perhaps by some chemical substance within the brain for inducing and maintaining sleep. Both mechanisms are bound to decline over time otherwise we would never wake up! I must admit that this seems a fair and parsimonious view given the state of the art so far. For Webb then, sleep is just a 'non-behaviour' solely for the purpose of occupying unproductive hours, with no restorative benefit for the cerebrum or any other organ.

In my terms, Webb sees all of sleep as optional sleep, and sleep deprivation effects on behaviour are caused by a very large accumulation of some substance, or of a behavioural drive to sleep. If this is true, then conceivably one day an antidote to the drive or substance may be discovered that would enable us to stay awake permanently without suffering any impairment to behaviour or cerebral activity. But I do not think that this will ever be entirely possible, as I believe the cerebrum needs some sleep (core sleep) for restitution. Cerebral impairment will still appear—as reflected in core sleepiness (see Section 2.14). On the other hand, optional sleep and sleepiness could conceivably be eliminated by a chemical antidote. Although there are natural substances within the brain that induce sleep (see Section 5.12), none seems to be *the* sleep substance, and as yet there are certainly no antidotes. The substances identified so far seem only to be modulators of sleep—that is they modify sleep. An analogy for what I mean by modulation can be seen in hunger. Despite a recent filling and satisfying meal, the unexpected smell of a freshly baked cake will modulate feeding behaviour by making us want to eat a slice of it. Hunger pangs and salivation probably occur, but such a desire to eat does not mean that we really need this food.

5.4 Brain work during wakefulness

Increasing the length of wakefulness is not the only way of elevating SWS, and we have already seen (Section 4.11) that rises in body temperature, or more likely in brain temperature, lead to more SWS. There are, no doubt, many possible explanations for this temperature effect, and several lines of argument can be made from the knowledge that a raised brain temperature will speed up cerebral metabolic rate (CMR). This is simply because chemical reactions within the cerebrum, like all chemical reactions, will naturally increase their rates when the system they are part of warms up. The repercussions, though, can be varied.

For example, let us for argument's sake take the sleep substance perspective, regardless of whether it is the direct cause of SWS or merely modulates it. Levels of this substance seem to build up within the brain during wakefulness. Increasing the brain's metabolism by heating may accelerate such a build-up, and in effect simulate an increase in the length of wakefulness. The warmer the brain, and the longer it remains warmer, the greater is the build-up of this substance. Another line of argument comes from the cerebral restitution perspective—that as nerve activity has a chemical basis increased cerebral temperature and CMR will also speed up this activity, and thus heighten wear and tear on nerve networks.

CMR is relatively high during wakefulness. Even during relaxed wakefulness with the eyes shut, when we have 'nothing on our minds', there is still much neural activity going on, as the cerebrum remains alert and in a state of quiet readiness. Nevertheless, CMR can rise a little further, by about another 15–20 per cent. Apart from bringing this about by heating up the brain or by giving certain drugs, there are other, natural ways. These come under the heading of 'brain work', for example the heightening of various mental events. Anything that increases alertness or makes one more aware of the environment will increase brain work. Pain, anxiety, and emotion are very effective at doing this, but we need not go to this extent, as curiosity and fascination in some external event are almost as good. Increasingly sophisticated but harmless ways for looking inside the human brain to measure CMR have been developed (see below), and show how heightened mental activity leads to rises in CMR. If the increased mental activity is limited to certain parts of the cerebrum, then there will only be a localized or 'regional' rise in CMR. However, if all of the cerebrum is involved through a generalized rise in behaviour and arousal, then the metabolism of most of the cerebrum will increase.

The first indications of how CMR might change in humans under various states of arousal came from measuring changes in cerebral blood flow (CBF). Work on animals has shown that there is a high positive correlation between the amount of blood passing through cerebral tissue and the tissue's metabolic rate. Several methods for measuring CBF have been used, with the most popular using a mildly radioactive isotope of the inert gas xenon, injected into the bloodstream and 'traced' by a special camera that can spot regional changes in CBF. Although this method has advanced over recent years, it has been superseded by techniques that assess how fast glucose or oxygen from the blood are metabolized in the brain. Glucose, which is the brain's main source of fuel, or the oxygen needed to oxidize this glucose, can be 'labelled' radioactively, injected into the bloodstream, or breathed in as in the case of oxygen, and then traced within the cerebrum using a PET (positron emission tomography) scanner located outside the head. This method can accurately measure the rate of glucose or oxygen usage within even very small regions in the cerebrum. Both the xenon and PET methods have been used with waking subjects under various states of alertness, and in studies of the sleeping brain. I will describe what happens during sleep later (Section 5.10) because for the moment, I want to continue with the topic of waking alertness and how this influences CMR and CBF.

One of the most famous institutes that has studied the relationship between brain activity and CBF is the Department of Clinical Neurophysiology at the University Hospital, Lund, Sweden. Amongst the principal investigators are Drs David Ingvar and Neils Lassen. For their original experiments using the xenon technique[16], they required their subjects to lie on a comfortable bed and undergo various mental states, which I will shortly outline. The part of the cerebrum they showed to have the highest blood flow during wakefulness, and presumably the greatest neural activity, was the frontal area—a finding confirmed many times since, and called by Ingvar and coworkers the 'hyper-frontal' pattern. It will be remembered (Section 2.13) that this brain area is particularly associated with conscious awareness and the planning of behaviour in the widest sense, including many aspects of 'thinking'.

When Ingvar's subjects looked at various objects, the most apparent rises in regional CBF (up to 20 per cent above resting levels) were in the posterior part of the cerebrum which handles visual information (the visual cortex), and also in a part of the frontal cortex concerned with eye movements (the 'frontal eye fields'). On the other hand, sounds and speech produced regional CBF increases in the auditory areas of the cortex, and when subjects touched and felt objects there were rises in the 'somatosensory' areas. More interestingly, when subjects were given psychological tests there was a general rise in CBF over the cortex. However, the extent of this depended on how much effort the subjects were applying to the task. The more they had to 'understand' and be aware of the task, the more CBF rose.

Subsequently, detailed studies of the frontal areas of the cerebral cortex have been carried out at the Karolinska Hospital in Stockholm, using the PET scanner[17]. The hyperfrontal pattern showing a high CMR is clearly evident with subjects lying awake, relaxed, motionless, and having closed eyes and plugged ears. It rises further as brain work and alertness increase, but, interestingly, it disappears entirely during sleep. These remarkable studies also showed that the frontal areas can be subdivided into various functional zones—for example, those that deal with input from the senses that require searching, comparisons, and decisions (superior prefrontal areas), those associated with the analysis of patterns, and the recollection and description of visual scenes (midfrontal areas), those looking after the voluntary control of eye movements (posterior prefrontal areas), and finally those involved with the verbal recollection of stories (intermediate prefrontal area).

To conclude, there is strong evidence that increased brain work during wakefulness, typically brought about by a heightening of thought processes and increased awareness of what is happening in the environment, will elevate CMR. This is obviously associated with increased neuronal activity. But whether or not these physiological signs also suggest increased cerebral 'wear and tear', or an accelerated build-up of a sleep-promoting substance, are matters which cannot be resolved at present. In the next section I shall show how such increased awareness also leads to more SWS in the subsequent night's sleep. We do not really know why this is so—only that it is associated with increased brain work during wakefulness. However, even more fascinating is the fact that SWS is found predominately in the frontal areas of the brain (Section 5.10), and it is in these areas where much of the increase in brain work occurs.

5.5 Increased awareness during wakefulness and subsequent sleep

In Section 2.18 I reported that sleep deprivation under more 'real life' conditions, compared with staying in the laboratory, produced greater feelings of fatigue, and more SWS in the recovery sleep. From what we have seen in the previous section, it is quite likely that those realistic conditions would have produced more brain work. There is a lot more to be said about this topic—not only how heightened awareness during wakefulness affects human sleep, to be discussed here, but how it may lead to contrasts between mammals in the function of sleep, as will be seen in Chapter 7.

Let me describe what I mean by 'awareness'. It is a general concept covering all those events within the cerebrum which are associated with the assimilation and understanding of what is going on in the environment. This involves recognizing information from all the senses, deciding what it means, selecting which part of this large sensory input should really be attended to, and arriving at courses of action that involve planning and drawing on old memories. The more of the environment we have to attend to, and the more this changes from minute to minute, the greater is the awareness and the greater the brain work involved.

There are differences between mammals in the importance of the various senses. For many of the more 'primitive' mammals, such as insectivores and rodents, the sense of smell is dominant, for others like whales it is hearing, and for a minority including humans it is vision. What may be a stimulating environment for the rat with its acute sense of smell, like a garbage tip at night, would be very dull, almost invisible, and even offensive for us. So, 'awareness' has to be understood from the different sensory viewpoints of each group of mammals. For humans and most other primates, most of the awareness of the environment comes through vision. Of the entire number of nerve fibres entering the brain from all our senses (e.g. vision, hearing, touch, etc.) one-third comes from the eyes. Unlike most other mammals, primates have evolved a visual system that is remarkable for its high contrast colour vision, fine visual acuity, stereopsis, eye movement control, and superb eye–hand coordination. Therefore, our visual system and our visual perception of what is going on is ideally suited to an environment possessing colour, detail, depth, and panorama. We are also naturally curious, and a continually changing visual environment maintains interest and heightened awareness, and of course keeps brain work elevated.

Very few studies on human sleep have manipulated sensory stimulation during wakefulness, and, apart from our own experiments that I shall come to shortly, all have used situations quite remote from anything found in the real world. Such studies have required their subjects to wear, for example, red-tinted lenses, lenses that narrowed the field of vision, or distorting prisms. Whilst I am tempted to point out how inappropriate these devices seem for natural behaviour, I must add that the experiments were taking another approach to sleep, and were usually concerned with REM sleep. They were testing the hypothesis that REM sleep consolidates the previous day's learning—the more this learning, the more the REM sleep (a quite unconvincing idea in my opinion, as I shall be discussing in Section 8.4). Subjects had to learn to see the world through distorting prisms, etc., and this was expected to lead to more REM sleep. But none of the experiments found any such effect. These devices will not increase daytime awareness—quite the converse as they reduce perception of the environment. We discovered this during one of our own pilot studies carried out on distorting prisms. Not only was vision very restricted, but several people experienced vertigo and had to spend much of the time sitting down.

In Section 2.18 I described a sleep deprivation experiment of ours that manipulated the amount of the subjects' awareness in the visual environment. Natural and unstressful methods were used, such as sightseeing, visits to museums, etc., and seeing epic cinema films. These events incorporated plenty of colour, complexity, and variety. Games were played, for example table tennis, which involved eye–hand co-ordination, depth, and movement. These also helped maintain the subjects' motivation.

Sleep loss under the stimulating conditions produced greater feelings of sleepiness, and more SWS in the recovery sleep. But because of the sleep deprivation we were unable to examine the effects of the stimulation alone. So we carried out two further studies that did not involve deprivation[18,19]. To avoid repetition, I will only describe the more recent of the two[19]. Nine young adults volunteered to spend five consecutive nights in the sleep laboratory. They were expecting to participate in a short study that was just looking at sleep following normal everyday behaviour, and to see how sleep varied from night to night under normal living routines. During the daytimes they had to stay in their usual home environment, and not do anything out of the ordinary or exciting. Also, they had to keep a half-hourly diary of their daily activities. Daytime naps were forbidden, and regular, normal meals were eaten. Alcohol was avoided, as was coffee and other stimulants. The subjects were told to expect that on the morning of one of these days, they would be asked to come to the laboratory and do a series of pencil and paper psychological tests designed to test reading skills, as part of another study. Actually, this was untrue. We had something much more interesting in store, but did not want them to know about it beforehand.

Neither did the experimenters know exactly on which of the 5 days this special day was to be. It was chosen randomly by an independent person, in order to avoid any anticipatory effects in the results. However, the experimenters were aware what was really going to happen. When the day arrived, the subjects were told that we had changed the plan, and instead they were invited to spend the day out, at our expense, accompanied by us. After hearing the proposed itinary they readily accepted this alternative to what would have been a relatively dull day, and an air of excitement prevailed. They were to be kept occupied throughout the day, from 10 a.m. to 10 p.m. Exercise was kept to a minimum and they ate normally. The day started with a scenic drive to a city they were not very familiar with, where they visited a new exhibition and shopping centre and a museum. Another car journey followed, to a large amusement park and zoo at a 'stately home'. Then came more sightseeing of the countryside on the return journey, and the evening was spent in the local cinema. The subjects arrived at the sleep laboratory that night feeling very sleepy. When they were eventually allowed to go to sleep, at their normal bedtime, all fell asleep rapidly.

Compared with the other nights, the most significant effect on sleep was an increase in SWS, particularly in stage 4 sleep. Sleep length was not affected, and they woke up naturally at their usual times, feeling quite refreshed. REM sleep remained unchanged, although from the 'learning' hypothesis for REM sleep (Section 8.4), one might have expected a sizeable increase here. The only other point of note was a small increase in SWS on the following night.

This was an unusual day for our subjects, and it had to be safe as well as enjoyable. Ideally, we would have liked to have given them something more appropriate to everyday life. Driving a car is a good example, particularly around a city or along winding country roads, as the driver has constantly to be fully aware of what is happening in the complex and ever changing visual scenes. To balance out any effect of driving itself, another driving session would be needed, though this time under the unstimulating and monotonous conditions of a motorway. Obviously, the first condition might be more stressful. But this would be to our advantage as it would increase brain work—provided that the driving was not too demanding to cause distress. The problem with this type of study, though, is that there is always the risk of an accident, albeit small, which presents great difficulties for experimenters from the viewpoint of subject safety, insurance, etc. Therefore, we had to keep to something safe for our subjects, and that is why we arranged the day out. It was not too unrealistic as it simulated what many of us experience when holidaymaking or on a day's sightseeing, or shopping in another city. As many of us have noticed ourselves, such days usually bring on the desire for an 'early night', and it is interesting how many anecdotes there are of people 'sleeping like a log' on holiday. There are other possible reasons for this, of course, apart from vague remarks like 'it's the sea air'. Increased alcohol consumption, and getting away from the pressures of home and work, must have important roles to play.

If several hours of urban driving were to increase the need for SWS, then I would speculate that heightened feelings of sleepiness experienced after the driving would be due to *core* sleepiness (see Section 2.14). So the best way for overcoming this sleepiness would be to sleep, and not for example to try and overcome it by further stimulation. This would contrast with motorway driving where the feeling of sleepiness would more likely be due to monotony and boredom, that is *optional* sleepiness. This is counteracted not necessarily by sleep, but by stimulation—such as a walk around the motorway service area. The point I am making is that sleepiness during or after driving may not always be the same phenomenon, and could well lead to quite alternative methods of treatment.

I would like to end by briefly mentioning animal studies where laboratory rodents are exposed to 'enriched environments'. Instead of being confined to the dull monotony of a cage, they are allowed to explore a larger and more stimulating environment. Like the inverting prism experiments on humans, these studies have been conducted within the context of the assumed association between REM sleep and learning, and none has looked at 'deeper' varieties of non-REM sleep. For this reason, I shall cover them in detail in Chapter 8, dealing with REM sleep.

5.6 Reduced sensory stimulation during wakefulness

Reduced sensory stimulation does not necessarily mean that awareness or brain work should fall, as many of the processes of thinking still continue. It should be remembered that even when subjects relax with their eyes shut, the 'hyperfrontal' pattern of CBF and CMR remain (Section 5.4). Consequently, whereas it is relatively easy to increase CMR above these relaxed waking levels, a reduction to below these levels is difficult to attain within the sphere of wakefulness.

There are a few findings relating to sleep during or following periods of sensory reduction. These can be subdivided into short-term reductions lasting a day or so, or long-term, as in blindness. In the first category, there is a report on the effects on the following night's sleep of 12 hours of relaxation with the eyes shut or staring at a blank wall[20]. The outcome was minor—a 10 per cent reduction in sleep length, and no changes in SWS or any of the sleep stages. A more extreme experiment put volunteers under conditions of perceptual isolation[21]. For 4–7 days subjects spent 20 hours a day lying on a bed in a soundproof room, listening to white noise (a 'hissing' sound). They wore gloves and cardboard cuffs to reduce touch, and light-diffusing goggles to prevent them seeing anything clearly. Breaks occurred only for eating and toilet activities. For the first day or so, much of the time was spent sleeping—for about 12 out of 24 hours. This extra sleep consisted of REM and stage 2 sleep, and from my perspective had the characteristics of extended optional sleep. Whilst SWS fell on the first night, this was probably due to a reduction in the length of the preceding wakefulness (Section 5.2). By the fourth isolation day sleep had returned to its usual 8 hours a day, and SWS was also the same as normal.

These two sleep studies are the only ones I know that produced short-term sensory reductions. But before I go on to the long-term studies, there is another short-term experiment that is of some relevance. It was really concerned with the effects of weightlessness on sleep[22]. For 5 weeks, four healthy young adults had to lie flat on their backs on beds. They only left these to go to the toilet, and then they were carried. When lying, they wore prisms over their eyes to allow them to see around their room, and especially TV—but their vision would have certainly been restricted. They were prevented from napping in the daytime. I mentioned this experiment briefly, in Section 4.10, within the context of exercise and sleep, and I stated that this led to no fall in SWS. But this is not the full story as SWS apparently increased! I have not mislead you, though, as this apparent increase was in relation to a single baseline sleep taken one night before the experiment began. But the baseline SWS levels of 69 minutes were suspiciously low for such an age group (see Fig. 5.4). During bedrest, SWS averaged 91 minutes, which was much more typical. Interestingly, two sleep recordings were made 2–4 weeks into recovery when the subjects were back on their feet and into their normal routines—again SWS averaged 91 minutes. I believe that this was the more realistic baseline value with which to compare the bedrest condition, and that for unknown reasons the initial value was unusually low. So there was no effect on SWS.

There have been two studies on sleep in the blind that have provided information on SWS. But whether or not long-term sensory restriction in the form of blindness leads to an eventual reduction in SWS is a matter that cannot be fully resolved, as these two studies seem to come up with contrasting findings. One[23] was only a brief report, really concerned with the 24-hourly output of the hormones hGH and cortisol. For six out of eight subjects these outputs turned out to be normal. The investigators gave no details on sleep stages except to say that for most subjects these were also apparently normal. The other study was more detailed[24] and had a different outcome. Five subjects, who had been blind since childhood or later, and in four cases blind for over 8 years, had their night-time sleep EEGs recorded for three nights, and hGH output monitored for one night. In several respects their sleep was normal for their ages—particularly for the total amounts of sleep and the number of awakenings during the night. There was one very obvious finding—a substantial reduction in SWS in all subjects. The youngest person, at 24 years, averaged 54 minutes SWS per night (compared with about 85 minutes of SWS expected for this age), a 37-year-old subject showed no SWS (about 60 minutes would be expected at this age), a 45-year-old averaged only 6 minutes SWS (about 45 minutes expected), and the two older subjects, at 60 and 63 years, also had no SWS (about 25 minutes expected). Further details of SWS changes with age are given in Fig. 5.4.

REM sleep was difficult to measure as two subjects had no eyes. However, the investigators had the impression that there was a general reduction in REM sleep across the group. These subjects spent most of their nights in stage 2 sleep, and, needless to say, the usual SWS-related hGH output was reduced, being absent in the three subjects without SWS. The investigators were perplexed by these findings and gave no reason for the low SWS values. They stressed that their subjects had not taken daytime naps, nor were they on any drug, nor did they have any medical condition such as hypothyroidism that would reduce SWS. One speculative explanation of mine is that the long-term loss of the *main* sensory input to the cerebrum of these blind people might well reduce their overall awareness of the environment, leading perhaps to less brain work, and a lessened need for cerebral restitution. But as we know nothing about CMR or other indices of brain work during wakefulness in blind people, I stress that my explanation is pure speculation.

5.7 SWS reductions in psychiatric disorders

There are some psychiatric disorders where SWS is often remarkably low, and for this reason worth mentioning. These are schizophrenia and the more severe forms of depression. Both can be present in a patient for very long periods of time. Whilst each is a complex illness, where there could well be various reasons to explain the low SWS values, I cannot help but mention that both usually have as a major symptom a loss of interest in the outside world, and a preoccupation with one's own thoughts. Such a decline in awareness of the environment points to lowered brain work during wakefulness, which might be the link with the low levels of SWS. Again, this is a tentative line of reasoning for such a little understood phenomenon and I shall not dwell on it for too long.

In recent years the most prolific reports on the sleep patterns of patients suffering from depression have come from Dr David Kupfer and colleagues at the Western Psychiatric Institute and Clinic of the University of Pittsburg. Not only do these patients have decreased SWS, but there is an earlier appearance of REM sleep after sleep onset (a shorter 'REM latency'), a

Table 5.2 Main sleep characteristics in a group of young depressed patients. Compared with healthy subjects of similar ages. See text for details. (From Kupfer et al.[26])

Minutes	Depressed	Normal
Time actually asleep	338	396
Time taken to get to sleep	42	15
Time in SWS	6	22
Time in REM sleep	91	91
Time to REM sleep from sleep onset	46	73
No. of eye movements per minute REM sleep	130	87

greater than usual amount of REM sleep during the first half of the night, and more eye movements during REM sleep[25]. These characteristics apply to both younger and older patients, and are not just due to natural ageing effects on sleep, when SWS happens to decline anyway.

The main sleep characteristics in depression are shown in Table 5.2 taken from one of Kupfer's studies[26] of a group of 22–44-year-old medication-free, mostly 'unipolar', depressed patients (i.e. they did not also suffer from periods of mania—this would be 'bipolar' depression), compared with an age-matched healthy control group. Although in the normal subjects the amounts of SWS seem lower than usual (see Fig. 5.4), the sleep records of both groups were scored in the same way, by the same people, and on a 'blind' basis. So we should use the relative differences in SWS. The depressed patients had about one-third the SWS compared with the control subjects. The delta EEG activity of sleep was also analysed by the computer analysis techniques of Borbély (see Section 5.3), which verified the low amounts of delta activity for the patients.

There has been much debate about whether the greater preponderance of REM sleep at the beginning of the night in depressed patients is due to: (a) the reduced SWS, (b) an inexplicable increase in REM sleep need at the beginning of sleep that suppresses SWS, or (c) distortions in the circadian rhythms of REM sleep and body temperature. An excellent review[27] of these alternatives has been written by Drs Hartmut Schulz and Reimer Lund, respectively from the Max Planck Institute for Psychiatry, at Munich, and the University of Munich. Schulz is particularly well known for his work on the 90-minute cycling of REM sleep. Whilst these reviewers do not dispute the findings of low SWS levels in such patients, their favoured explanation for the early onset of REM sleep is a flattening of the circadian rhythm of body temperature, which prematurely triggers REM sleep.

Concerning the sleep patterns of schizophrenic patients, about half of them seem to have no SWS. Schizophrenia is a general term covering certain personality and thought disorders. There is usually emotional detachment, with the sufferers absorbed in their own inner life. The outside world is usually blocked out to the extent that grossly abnormal thoughts, such as delusions and auditory hallucinations (usually voices) may gain control of the individual. Although the literal translation of the word 'schizophrenia' from its greek basis is 'split mind', many psychiatrists would view a more appropriate interpretation to be 'split from reality'.

First reports of a dearth of stage 4 sleep in such patients came 20 years ago, and there have been several more since then, reviewed more recently by Feinberg and his colleague Dr John Hiatt[28]. In their latest study[29] the computer-controlled period analysis technique (Section 5.3) was applied to the sleep EEGs of five medication-free, 26–31-year-old patients. The findings were compared with a group of similarly aged healthy individuals. Of the various sleep characteristics, the main differences between the two groups of subjects again lay with stage 4 sleep (SWS findings were not given), which averaged 47 minutes for the control group over the night, but only 11 minutes for the patients. These differences were reflected in the computer analysis, particularly in the average amplitude of the delta waves, which was 30 per cent less for the patients over the whole night. For both this delta amplitude and the visual scoring of stage 4 sleep, the portion of sleep containing the greatest difference between the groups was the first period of non-REM sleep.

Interestingly, recent findings[30] from careful psychological assessments of the problems encountered by schizophrenic patients have shown that the functions of the frontal and temporal areas of the cerebrum are particularly impaired. This is also borne out by xenon tracer measures of CBF[31] and PET scans[32], which show low CMR levels for the frontal region. These techniques were described in Section 5.4, and both have shown that such patients have *hypo*frontal patterns of CBF and CMR during wakefulness, rather than the usual hyperfrontal pattern seen in normal individuals. Intriguingly, and as will be seen in Section 5.9, it is this frontal area of the cerebrum where the delta EEG activity of SWS is the most prolific. So it is possible that the low SWS levels in schizophrenia are somehow associated (but not necessarily causally related) to the hypofrontal blood flow, and with what seems to be the low brain work of this area, also shown by the psychological impairment[30]. Such a line of thinking could apply to depressed patients, as PET scans on them are beginning to show that they also seem to have a hypofrontal CMR pattern[32,33].

5.8 SWS and ageing

One of the most detailed accounts of the changes in sleep with age has been provided by Dr Robert Williams and others in their book, *EEG of Human Sleep*[34]. I have taken some of their data and plotted out the changes in certain sleep characteristics (Fig. 5.4). Delta activity and SWS are at their most

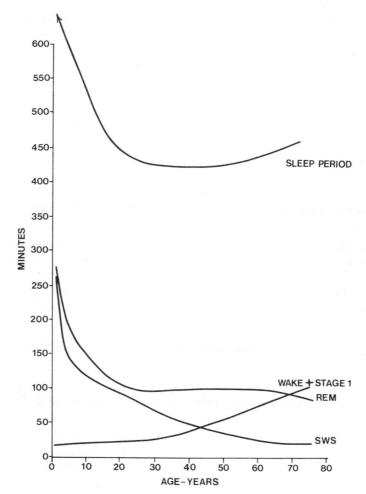

Fig. 5.4 Changes of certain sleep characteristics with age. 'Sleep period' is the time from sleep onset to final awakening in the morning, and includes any wakefulness during the night. The most noticeable changes in the first 10 years of life are sizeable falls in the sleep period, REM sleep, and SWS. Old age brings increases in lighter (stage 1) sleep and wakefulness, and a further fall in SWS. There are few differences with age between the sexes for these characteristics, and the data for the sexes have been averaged. (Based on data from Williams et al.[34])

prolific during infancy, and likewise the amounts of total daily sleep and REM sleep. CMR is also at its greatest at this time of life, and of course so is the development of the cerebrum. These two latter factors, together with the wealth of new sensory experiences bombarding the infant's cerebrum, must have some direct impact on sleep—but how all these variables interact is still a mystery.

SWS tends to occupy about 20–25 per cent of sleep from the first year of life until about the mid twenties. REM sleep changes more over this period, from about 35 per cent of total sleep to about 25 per cent. However, because the length of sleep ('sleep period') also falls over this time, from about 800 minutes to about half this amount, the actual minutes per night of both SWS and REM sleep drop substantially, as can be seen in Fig. 5.4. Beyond about 20 years of age, the daily sleep period remains fairly stable until retirement age, and so does both the percentage and absolute number of minutes of REM sleep per night. However, for SWS the picture is different. It can be seen that from the third decade the number of minutes of this type of sleep fall quite noticeably. According to Williams and colleagues, in percentage terms the nightly SWS drops to about 13 per cent by the mid thirties, and then to about 5 per cent by the sixties. These changes are reciprocated by increases in stage 1 sleep and wakefulness. Of the two components of SWS, stages 3 and 4 sleep, the latter virtually disappears by about the sixties. If SWS is related to the levels of waking awareness and brain work, and perhaps some form of cerebral recovery at night, as I have proposed, then on face value these findings suggest that all these phenomena decline quite substantially with age.

However, the fall in SWS with age is not really as great as it seems, and is partly based on a technicality. In order for SWS to be scored, the amplitude of the delta waves on the EEG record must be greater than 75 microvolts. As one gets older, the amplitude of delta waves falls to below this level. Consequently, when scoring SWS, these lower amplitude waves have to be discounted as SWS and are included within stage 2 sleep. Webb and Feinberg have particularly criticized this aspect of sleep stage scoring. So for example, using the usual sleep stage criteria, seventy-year-old people only seem to have about a quarter of the SWS to that of young adults. But the actual number of delta waves drops to only three-quarters of the level in young adults[35]—most of these waves are under the 75 microvolt threshold. If this threshold is lowered to 50 microvolts for the purposes of scoring SWS, as Webb recommends[36], then SWS values are also about three quarters of the young adult values. Nevertheless, whatever ways one looks at SWS or delta waves in the elderly, these do fall with age. By the way, this explanation does not apply to the low amounts of SWS for the patients I described in the previous section (e.g. schizophrenia). Delta waves are far fewer, although there is some reduction in amplitude.

Dr René Spiegel, working at the Sandoz Laboratories in Basle, has devoted considerable time to the study of sleep patterns in the elderly, particularly those that are demented, and he is one of Europe's leaders in this field. It appears that, in both the elderly and the demented, SWS bears less of a relationship to wakefulness than it does in younger people. For example, increasing the length of wakefulness in such subjects does not necessarily elevate SWS as it does for young adults (see section 5.2). Therefore, Spiegel and colleagues[37] propose that SWS duration is not of any particular significance for normal or demented elderly people. This may well be so, and I am cautious in extending my views on SWS to the elderly. But there are particular problems encountered in looking at sleep and wakefulness in both these groups of the elderly. For example, if wakefulness is lengthened, then they tend to spend more of wakefulness in a drowsy state, attending to little that is going on around them. And of course, in the case of demented patients, there is generally a gross impairment of the cerebrum, where delta wave generation is quite abnormal anyway, often appearing in large quantities throughout wakefulness.

5.9 SWS deprivation

To see whether SWS is a special form of sleep different from other sleep stages, for example, in providing particular benefits to the cerebrum, the most obvious test would be to deprive people of SWS and see what happens. In comparison, there should be a similar amount of deprivation of say, stage 2 or REM sleep. But, as one might guess, such an experiment is exceedingly difficult to perform as SWS deprivation alone cannot be achieved without complications, and few studies have pursued this difficult area.

The best known investigation of this type came from Webb's laboratory[38], where a technique was developed for giving the sleeper a small electric shock to the foot, sufficient only to shift him into another sleep stage, but not enough to cause waking. Two groups of six young adults were deprived of either stage 4 sleep or REM sleep by this method for seven nights. However, the deprivation distorted sleep in more ways than expected. Stage 4 sleep deprivation usually shifted the sleeper into stage 2 sleep, leading to larger than normal amounts of this sleep, whilst REM sleep deprivation usually produced more stage 1 sleep. There was an added problem. Since the number of minutes of stage 4 sleep over the night in this age group comes to about half that of REM sleep, one might expect that stage 4 deprivation would require fewer arousals. But this was not the case, as the average number of stimulations per night needed for the deprivation of stage 4 sleep came to 217 against only 44 for REM sleep. I emphasize that these are averages over the seven nights, as the number of stimulations had to increase for both types of deprivation over the nights. Obviously, stage 4 sleep deprivation produced much more sleep disturbance. The larger number of stimulations required for stage 4 sleep deprivation suggests a considerable need for this type of sleep—seemingly much greater than that for REM sleep. On the other hand, maybe the re-entry into SWS is just an easier process than is the re-entry into REM sleep.

Both SWS and REM deprivation effects may have been masked by other factors that were different for the two conditions, hence preventing true comparisons to be made. Psychological performance tests were carried out in the daytime, but these tended to be measures of general motivation and sleepiness (e.g. reaction times and addition tests), rather than of higher levels of cerebral function for example (see Section 2.13). Both types of deprivation led to similar decrements in these tests, with the chief complaint by all the subjects being sleepiness. However, interesting changes in personality were found.

During stage 4 sleep deprivation subjects became:

'physically uncomfortable, withdrawn, less aggressive, and manifested concern over vague physical complaints and changes in body feelings. Overall, the impression suggested a depressive and hypochondriacal reaction.'

On the other hand, during REM sleep deprivation they were:

less well integrated and less personally effective. They tended to show signs of confusion, suspicion, and withdrawal. These subjects seemed anxious, insecure, introspective, and unable to derive support from other people (p. 856).

In view of the unwanted other factors that may well have affected the two types of sleep deprivation, especially the generalized sleep disruption, it is difficult to make much more out of these findings. Such problems were also encountered in a more recent experiment by Dr Michael Bonnett, now at the Veterans Administration Medical Center at Loma Linda, California. For many years he has been looking at the effects of sleep disturbance. One of his meticulous studies incorporated a night of SWS deprivation[39], achieved by arousing subjects via a loud sound. This had to be done for an average 63 times over the night, and then only an 80 per cent elimination of SWS could be achieved. A control condition, run on a separate occasion, gave a similar number of arousals, but randomly and outside of SWS. On the morning after both conditions, subjects were tested at the Wilkinson Auditory Vigilance Task, and performance had deteriorated to similar levels. Subjects were allowed a nap shortly afterwards, and were very sleepy, judging by the rapidity with which they fell asleep on both occasions. It could be argued that, fundamentally, SWS deprivation is no different in its effects than the deprivation of any other form of sleep. But we are still left with the problem that a severe disruption of sleep would overwhelm more subtle changes (perhaps due to the loss of SWS).

I would like to end by returning to the study from Webb's laboratory[38], as there was another interesting finding. Surprisingly, the experimenters received very few complaints from both groups of subjects about the electric shocks as these seemed to go unnoticed. Also, few subjects reported being awakened during the nights. This and other work outside the field, in the area of sleep disorders, clearly show that unless arousals from sleep last for more than 10–15 seconds, then there is no recollection of the event the next morning—even if these arousals number in the hundreds, as may happen with sleep apnoea. Here, breathing ceases for about 15 seconds at a time, followed by a brief arousal that allows breathing to return to normal. Usually sufferers report uninterrupted, often good sleep, and are perplexed as to why they are so sleepy in the daytime.

5.10 Brain and behaviour during SWS

In Section 5.2 I briefly mentioned computer methods for analysing EEG activity more precisely. The rapid development of computer technology has enabled certain of these techniques to be advanced further, by being incorporated into what is known as 'topographical mapping' of the EEG over the cerebral cortex. That is, EEGs are obtained from many electrodes over the scalp, and every few seconds this activity is analysed into its component frequencies (usually by the Fourier method). The distribution of these frequencies over the cortex is then mapped out as a changing colour picture on a TV screen. A particular EEG frequency can be homed in on, and shown in greater detail. One of the first people to use this remarkable method was Dr Monte Buchsbaum, from the Department of Psychiatry, at the University of California at Irvine. In a collaborative investigation with colleagues from elsewhere[40], he produced a series of topographical maps, and those for delta activity are shown in Fig. 5.5.

The left side of the cerebrum is displayed going from awake through all the sleep stages. The darker the shading, the more intense is the delta power. I have simplified matters, as Buchsbaum and colleagues actually give a greater range of shading than that presently shown, as well as numerical values for the power depicted by each shade. Little sign of delta activity can be seen in wakefulness, stages 1, and REM. It begins to make its appearance in stage 2 sleep, and is shown as a light zone on the crown. The investigators described the progressive appearance of this activity, from stages 2 to 4 sleep, to be like the pulling-on of a night-cap, moving down from the crown and becoming substantial in stage 4 sleep. In this latter stage, the regions of greatest intensity are found frontally.

Because of technological limitations, we still know little of what is going on inside the human brain during SWS, or, for that matter, during any other form of sleep. All we can do, metaphorically speaking, is to scratch the surface. SWS is, in behavioural terms, a deep form of sleep, when arousal of the sleeper is usually the most difficult to accomplish of all the sleep stages. Some qualification of this statement has to be made with respect to REM sleep, and I will return to the topic very shortly. Studies of EEG-evoked potentials (see Section 2.21) taken during the various sleep stages indicate that SWS, particularly stage 4 sleep, is rather unusual from the rest as in

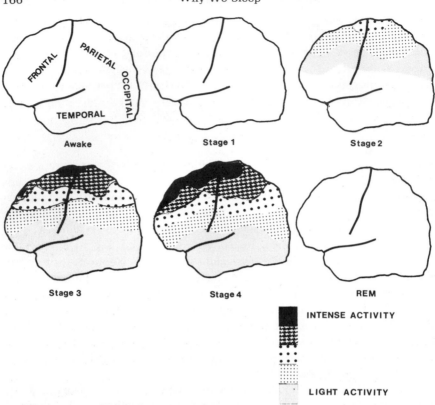

Fig. 5.5 Topographical maps of the development of delta EEG activity over the cerebral cortex during sleep stages. The left side is shown. The progressive appearance of delta activity over the cortex can be likened to the pulling on of a night-cap. This activity is more concentrated in the frontal regions. White indicates a relative absence of delta waves. See text for details. (Adapted from Buchsbaum et al.[40]. Reproduced by permission of Raven Press)

many respects the cerebrum seems to be disconnected from much of its sensory input, and from certain influences of the lower brain areas[41]. Also, during stage 4 sleep, new and unique components occur in these potentials[42], the meaning of which are unknown. However, there seems to be no difference between SWS (or other sleep stages) and wakefulness in the processing of sensory information at levels below the cerebrum[43].

Arousability from the various sleep stages depends on the magnitude of the stimulus and its significance to the sleeper. In the case of sounds, the factors are loudness and meaning. So, if the sound is merely noise, without any personal significance to the sleeper, then descending from sleep stages 1 to 4, increased loudness is required for an arousal[44,45]. REM sleep is similar to stage 4 sleep in this respect. However, if the sound has personal significance, for example calling the sleeper's name, or the crying of a sleeping mother's child, then REM sleep is as light as stages 1 and 2 sleep, requiring only a whisper or whimper. SWS on the other hand is not so discriminative, and still requires loudness. It is as if some form of monitoring of the environment is going on in REM sleep, with the sleeper easily awoken when necessary. During SWS even this monitor seems mostly asleep, but it is not totally unreactive. Simple acts such as pushing a microswitch attached to the hand in response to a loud buzzer, to avoid a small electric shock, can still be accomplished[46], albeit to a more limited extent than in stages 1 and 2 sleep (REM sleep was not tested).

Children are particularly difficult to arouse from SWS, and even very loud (personally insignificant) sounds of up to 123 decibels are reported to have no effect[47]. On the other hand, awakenings occurred for about half the occasions at this level during REM sleep, and for one-third of the occasions during stage 2 sleep.

When sleepers are awoken out of non-REM sleep, 'thinking' is often reported, and contrasts with the much greater visual imagery, unrealism, and more vivid actions of dreaming usually found (but not wholly) in REM sleep (see Section 8.1). Such thinking seems to be prevalent in stage 2 sleep and declines somewhat in stage 4 sleep. Sometimes, disturbing mental events can occur during SWS, with the most notable being sleepwalking ('somnambulism') and night terrors ('*pavor nocturnus*'), which are distinct from the nightmares found during dreaming sleep. These SWS phenomena can be found together, mainly occur in childhood, and tend to run in families. Anxiety seems to set these episodes off, and there have been various theories about their underlying psychological meaning—whether, for example, they are an expression of deep and repressed emotional conflicts.

In both sleepwalking and night terrors the mind is only partly responsive to what is going on in the environment, and seems to be concerned with its own internal events. The sleepwalker behaves like an automaton with a limited repertoire of behaviour. Sleepwalking episodes can last up to 30 minutes, but usually average 5–15 minutes. Several years ago Dr Roger Broughton, one of Canada's leading sleep researchers, proposed that sleepwalking and night terrors, together with nocturnal bedwetting (enuresis), all reflect some form of disordered arousal from stage 4 sleep[48]. But such a conclusion is contested by Dr Anthony Kales and colleagues from the State University College of Medicine at Hershey, Pennsylvania, who have made detailed sleep EEG recordings of sleepwalkers[49]. These researchers found that such sufferers usually remain in SWS whilst sleepwalking, etc. and show few signs of arousal.

Excellent descriptions of sleepwalking and night terrors have been given by Broughton[48], for example:

In a typical sleepwalking attack the individual sits up quietly, generally an hour or two after falling asleep, gets out of bed, and moves about in a confused and clumsy manner. Soon his behaviour becomes more coordinated and complex. He may avoid objects, dust tables, go to the bathroom, or utter phrases which are usually incomprehensible. It is difficult to attract his attention. If left alone he goes back to bed. A great deal of stimulation is required to awaken him. And when he is awakened he has little if any recollection of his sleepwalking activities, and no recollection of dreaming. Nevertheless, these remarkable acts are almost universally interpreted as an acting out of dream activity. The sleep terror attack (typically) of children is very different. The child abruptly sits up in bed and screams. He appears to be staring wide-eyed at some imaginary object; his face is covered with perspiration and his breathing is laboured. Consoling stimuli have no effect. After the attack, dream recall is rare and usually fragmentary. The child has no recollection of the episode next morning (p. 2).

It is difficult to come to any definite conclusion from these various limited findings about what, exactly, is going on inside the cerebrum during SWS. What does emerge is that the cerebrum becomes more oblivious to sensory input. But as to why—that is another matter.

5.11 Cerebral restitution during SWS?

Because we cannot really get inside the human brain, I cannot really address the topic of whether SWS or any other form of sleep provides the cerebrum with heightened levels of restitution and repair following the impositions of wakefulness. All I have is incidental information that can be interpreted to favour this restitution role, or, to be quite frank, the alternative position that sleep has no restitutive benefit for the brain, and that all the behavioural and EEG phenomena of SWS are simply the consequence of some sleep drive/sleep factor that is at its most intense during SWS. That is, SWS is simply a more intense form of optional sleep. Even studies on higher mammals, where electrodes can be placed inside neurones within the cerebrum, shed little extra light on this particular topic.

CMR and CBF (see Section 5.4) during sleep show progressive falls over most areas of the cerebrum from wakefulness through the sleep stages to stage 4 sleep, where the levels are about 25 per cent lower than those for wakefulness[50]. The frontal and central areas of the cerebrum show the greater declines. During REM sleep, CBF rises by about 40 per cent above waking levels for most parts of the cerebrum, particularly in the frontal areas. PET scans (Section 5.4) of glucose uptake in the cerebrum support all these findings, and again for both SWS and REM sleep the major changes seem to be within the frontal and central areas of the cerebrum[51].

Although there have been several studies of CMR and neuronal activity in the cortex during sleep in the cat and monkey, most have generally looked at REM and non-REM sleep, but have not selected the deeper form of non-REM sleep—the equivalent of human SWS. One of the most notable investigations of non-REM sleep in the cat was by Drs Margaret Livingstone and David Hubel at Harvard Medical School[52]. I briefly mentioned it at the end of Chapter 3, and now I would like to describe their study in a little more detail, as it was so remarkable. Before I begin, I must stress that we do not know to what extent their findings and conclusions apply to the deeper variety of non-REM sleep, or apply to all of non-REM sleep.

The investigators concentrated on the visual cortex. During wakefulness, the neuronal firing patterns in this area were smooth and regular, but during non-REM sleep firing was much more spontaneous and irregular. Livingstone and Hubel observed that in the awake animal these neurones are 'slaves to sensory input', which are 'held in quiet readiness'. But during non-REM sleep they are 'less fettered by sensory constraints, but more at the mercy of events related to the still all-too-mysterious slow waves' (p. 560). During non-REM sleep, then, visual sensory input into these areas of the cortex seemed to be dampened, and CMR measurements showed that deeper layers of the visual cortex appeared to shut down. Livingstone and Hubel were clearly puzzled by these findings, and were unable to determine whether:

the muffling of sensory input during sleep serves to insulate the animal from its environment, to permit uninterrupted sleep, or whether sensory systems also need to rest, and the deceased responsiveness we see reflects whatever recuperative processes the brain undergoes during sleep (p. 561).

Another fascinating study of the regional CMR in 75 areas of the brain in sleeping monkeys compared non-REM sleep levels with those of wakefulness[53]. CMR fell in all areas of the cerebrum during non-REM sleep by an average of 30 per cent. But such findings have been questioned by other investigators looking at the cat[54]. Here, throughout much of the cerebrum, there was no change in CMR levels during non-REM sleep when compared with those of wakefulness. These researchers considered that the waking levels registered in the previous study were abnormally large to start with, owing to the methods used to keep the monkeys awake. One reason, they claim, why CMR should not fall during non-REM sleep is that the energy demand on the brain switches from the processes associated with the high neuronal firing of wakefulness, to those of non-REM sleep that facilitate raised protein synthesis in neurones and neuroglial cells (cerebral restitution?). Certainly, there is increasing evidence from animal studies that during non-REM sleep certain aspects of RNA and protein synthesis in the cerebrum increase to beyond waking levels[55]. But little is known about protein turnover rates, as protein breakdown is difficult to measure (see Section 4.1).

So far, I have paid little attention to neuroglial cells. In fact, they make up much of the mammalian brain, and are particularly prolific in the cerebrum, increasingly so with mammalian advancement. In the human cerebrum, neuroglia far outnumber neurones. The term 'neuroglia' comes from the Greek, meaning 'nerve glue', and although these cells seem largely to support and protect neurones, little is understood about their function. But we should not underestimate their roles, especially in the light of developments I shall be describing in the next Section. With respect to the topic of cerebral restitution during SWS, I have so far only related this to cerebral neurones, but it may be just as important to cerebral neuroglia. There are several types of neuroglia: oligodendrocytes and Schwann cells, which help to manufacture the myelin sheaths around neurones, astrocytes, which maintain the structural support for neurones, are in close contact with capillaries, and may well be a central part of the 'blood–brain barrier', ependymal cells, which form the linings of the ventricles within the brain and the spinal canal, and last, but certainly not the least, the microglia—they are particularly fascinating in relation to the processes of sleep, as will now be seen.

5.12 Sleep 'substances' and immunoenhancement

Microglia are modified monocytes (another white blood cell that is part of the immune response—see Section 3.8) that have become incorporated into the brain during its development. Microglia move around the cerebrum, presumably to protect the brain against pathogens, and remove dead cells. Microglia can take on various forms, and there is evidence that they are able to turn into a form of astrocyte. Microglia, probably astrocytes, and monocytes in the blood, produce interleukin-1, which is one of a group of substances that stimulate lymphocytes and other white cells into action, including the production of antibodies. However, IL-1 is not an antibody itself. It has a variety of actions, and is also known as an 'endogenous pyrogen'. When released in relatively large quantities it raises body temperature and causes fever. Of even more interest is that IL-1 is a potent sleep inducer.

Let me start a more detailed account of this intrigue by going back to the work of Moldofsky and colleagues[56], briefly mentioned in Section 4.7. They are among a growing number of sleep researchers who believe that SWS is associated with some sort of boost to the immune system. But whether or not this boost is also related to the SWS-related hGH release, and/or the associated depression of cortisol output, is a matter that must remain open for the time being. Moldofsky and co-workers took frequent blood samples via a venous catheter in the arm, from six healthy, sleeping subjects during EEG monitoring. Onset of SWS was associated with a rise in certain aspects of immune activity, which seemed to be at least partly stimulated by a surge in blood levels of IL-1. There were increases in lymphocyte responses to certain antigens, and in natural killer cell activity. Afternoon naps containing SWS were also associated with these immunological changes and the rise in IL-1.

The physiological and clinical significance of this sleep-related immuno-enhancement still have to be assessed. From what has been found so far, these changes would not warrant any statement to the effect that sleep is necessary for the successful combat of infectious diseases, etc.—only that the immune system seems to be given a boost. This does not mean that the immune system will be impaired without SWS. Remember, from the little evidence we have from the effects of sleep deprivation on the immune system (Section 3.8), nothing of clinical significance was reported. It could be argued that SWS potentially leaves us more vulnerable to infection, perhaps because of the fall in body temperature accompanying SWS. Therefore, as a countermeasure, the immune system is boosted. Given that IL-1 can increase body tempera-ture, maybe the rise of this substance in the blood during SWS ensures that body temperature does not fall too far?

There are other indications of a link between sleep and the immune system, although this comes from animal studies and may be circumstantial. Certain brain centres helping to regulate sleep also influence the immune response. For example, lesions in the hypothalamus causing insomnia or excessive sleep (depending on where the lesion is) also alter the immune response. However, the hypothalamus looks after many aspects of homeostasis, and such lesions have additional effects, especially on thermoregulation.

Much of the remarkable research on animals into IL-1, sleep, and the immune system is now being performed by Dr Jim Krueger and colleagues, working until recently at The Chicago Medical School and now at the Depart-ment of Physiology and Biophysics at the University of Tennessee. Krueger originally came from the laboratory of Dr John Pappenheimer, at Harvard Medical School. For many years until his retirement, Pappenheimer had been carrying out pioneering research into sleep substances—naturally occurring chemicals within the brain that induce sleep. In one of his famous experi-ments[57] Pappenheimer sleep deprived goats, and extracted a then unknown substance, 'Factor S', from their cerebrospinal fluid. When given to other animals it readily produced sleep. Recently[58], Factor S has also been extracted from human urine—3 000 litres of urine being required to produce 7 millionths of a gram of Factor S. Nevertheless, this was potent enough to be divided up into 500 doses which, when given to rabbits, produced large increases in non-REM sleep lasting for about 6 hours. The extended sleep seemed natural enough, although much of it was the deeper form of non-REM sleep, possibly equivalent to our SWS. Animals could be woken up without difficulty in these circumstances, and then might eat or groom them-selves for a short while, only soon to return to sleep.

Factor S has now been identified as a muramyl peptide, a substance that closely resembles components of bacterial cell walls. Obviously, the first thought was that Factor S was simply some form of bacterial contamination. But further work by Krueger and colleagues[59] has shown that although this substance may have come originally from bacteria, perhaps from those living in the gut and lungs, Factor S has been adopted by the brain as part of its own biochemistry.

Muramyl peptide was subsequently synthesized, and one of its variants, muramyl dipeptide (MDP) was shown to produce excessive amounts of non-REM sleep when injected into a variety of mammals—rats, rabbits, cats, and monkeys. There was some delay in this effect after the injection, and sleepiness did not reach its peak until after about 3 hours. I should add that REM sleep is usually unaffected. MDP has other actions—it stimulates the immune system, and causes fever. Its actions on humans have not been fully investigated yet, but in rabbits, body temperature rises by 1–2°C. As most of us know with influenza, etc., sleepiness often accompanies fever. So the question obviously arises whether the sleepiness produced by MDP is simply a by-product of the fever? This is where IL-1 comes into the picture again, as Krueger believes that MDP acts through stimulating IL-1 production by lymphocytes in the blood, and by certain neuroglia.

As I have mentioned, IL-1 is an endogenous pyrogen. However, the sleepiness produced by IL-1 is probably not just a by-product of the fever. Krueger's group have now shown[60] that if the fever is prevented by other drugs then the sleepiness still occurs—suggesting that fever and sleep are independent effects of IL-1. Besides, there are varieties of MDP that cause fever but not sleepiness. I should add, as an aside, that the sleepiness produced by a warm environment is a different phenomenon, and body temperature does not usually increase.

IL-1 levels rise during very heavy exercise, and this may be partly responsible for the continuation of a high body temperature for a while after the exercise has ceased[61]. So it is possible that this delayed fall in body temperature could enhance the SWS increases following heavy exercise, described in Section 4.11. But there are problems with this argument. Animal studies show that the sleep and temperature-raising effects of IL-1 only last for about 2 hours after injection (there are no equivalent human studies). If parallels can be drawn with my own experiments, when night-time increases in SWS were found after afternoon exercise, then it should be remembered that the raised body temperature during the exercise returned to normal within half an hour of the end of exercise, and sleep did not occur until about 8 hours later—presumably when any exercise-related rises in IL-1 would have long since disappeared.

I could go on looking at the possible associations between IL-1, sleep, immunoenhancement, body temperature, and exercise. However, much is still unknown, especially about IL-1. Another tantalizing role for this substance seems to be the stimulation of nerve growth factors within the brain[62]. We do not know whether IL-1 is central to the regulation of sleep, or is just part of a complex network of influences on sleep. There are increasing signs that IL-1 is not the final link in a chain of chemicals affecting sleep. For example, Krueger's group point out[60] that it promotes the release of prostaglandin D2 (see below).

Sleep substances could be the simple answer to why we sleep—sleep is due to their accumulation. Destroy one, or break a link in the chain, and we would become permanently sleepless. But what would be the consequences— nothing, or would cerebral impairment set in? My own suspicions are that these substances are only modulators of sleep, unrelated to the underlying functions of sleep. In the same way, mealtimes and the smell of food encourage us to eat, but do not explain why we have to eat.

Other natural sleep substances have been discovered within the mammalian brain. But it is not known whether or to what extent they might act through IL-1, or through other routes. 'Delta-sleep-inducing peptide' (DSIP), found in the blood of sleeping rabbits, was amongst the first to attract attention about 20 years ago[63]. When given to other mammals such as rats, it rapidly produces a deep form of non-REM sleep, containing many delta waves, and also increases REM sleep. Although DSIP is potent, its effects seem not to last for very long[64]. Japanese researchers are now figuring prominently in the area of sleep substances, and they have identified several more compounds. One of their leading investigators is Professor Shojiro Inoué, from the Tokyo Medical and Dental University. He and colleagues have recently compared and evaluated these compounds[64]. 'Sleep-promoting substance' (SPS) and prostaglandin D2 seem to be the most notable. The former was extracted from the brain stem of sleep-deprived rats, and contains four components each with sleep-promoting properties of its own. The most promising of these is uridine, which has long-acting sleep effects, particularly the prolongation of REM sleep.

Inoué and coworkers[64] emphasize that all the various sleep substances, including MDP and IL-1, act on sleep in different ways. DSIP seems mainly to be a good at inducing sleep, whereas MDP and prostaglandin D2 have delayed actions, and respectively either increase non-REM sleep or generally help to maintain sleep. SPS and uridine have steady and longer-lasting sleep-promoting effects. The impact of all these compounds on body temperature still remains to be fully explored. DSIP will decrease body temperature if the animal is in a cold environment, but increases it in a hot one. Prostaglandin D2, on the other hand, may well reduce body temperature. Generally speaking, all these findings suggest, like those of Krueger, that the temperature and sleep-inducing effects of sleep substances are independent of each other, and particularly that increased sleep is not due to a raised body temperature.

As well as increasing either or both REM and non-REM sleep, some of these sleep substances will enhance the deeper form of SWS in animals. In terms of my core and optional division of sleep, it seems that both can be influenced by sleep substances. What is very much a mystery, especially to me, is to what extent these substances are influencing the fundamental functions of sleep, or just the control mechanisms of sleep.

5.13 Conclusions

Of the various parts of the brain, it is the cerebrum that is most likely to require sleep for some form of off-line restitution—for example for the repair of neural circuits, and consolidation of the waking day's events. One reason for this is that the cerebrum remains working at a high rate throughout wakefulness, and is in a near-continuous state of 'quiet readiness'—unable to relax outside sleep. Also, it was shown in Chapters 2 and 3 that cerebral function is more profoundly impaired by sleep deprivation than is the function of any other organ or part of the brain. Unfortunately, we have neither the way of harmlessly getting inside the human cerebrum, nor the technology for studying nerve growth and the activities of the neuroglia within the living human brain. Thus there is no firm evidence from which I can establish whether or not cerebral restitution is taking place during SWS or during any other form of sleep. All I have been able to present is circumstantial findings and a line of argument that, to be quite frank, only suggests cerebral restitution. Of all the arguments presented in this book, this is the weakest in terms of hard factual support.

A window on the sleeping cerebral cortex is provided by the EEG, which shows clear changes during sleep. One type of electrical activity seems to reflect a recovery role more closely than others—the delta EEG waves of human SWS, particularly of stage 4 sleep. This EEG activity is produced by the cerebral cortex, and in the case of humans is particularly evident in the frontal regions (the behaviours associated with these areas are described in Section 2.10). Although SWS has been claimed to be associated with heightened tissue repair in the rest of the body, I have argued strongly against this notion (Chapters 3 and 4). So I re-emphasize that SWS only reflects events within the cerebrum.

Stage 4 sleep, more than any other type of sleep, is influenced by the length of prior wakefulness, and to this extent best fits any restitutive role. Also, it is the sleep having the most cerebral shutdown and isolation. There seems to be a great pressure to obtain stage 4 sleep, taking priority over all other sleep states. Such sleep is central to my concept of core sleep. When brain work and cerebral metabolism are elevated during wakefulness, either through brain heating or by heightening one's awareness of the environment, during wakefulness, then the greatest impact on sleep is an increase in stage 4 sleep. Certain clinical states, such as schizophrenia, are associated with decreased stage 4 sleep, a lower cerebral metabolism (particularly in the frontal areas), and less awareness of the environment. Although I have speculated that there may be causal links between these features, they may all simply be an effect of an unknown common factor.

Stage 4 sleep could be just a deeper form of non-REM sleep, where the processes that occur during non-REM sleep happen more intensely. Therefore, when a certain 'depth' is reached certain other events are triggered, such as the hGH release. However, stage 4 sleep is not simply a driving process or momentum to ensure that sleep is able to coast along for a preset number of hours. For example, we have seen from daytime nap studies that SWS can be 'subtracted out' from night-time sleep without affecting total sleep time—an afternoon nap absorbs some of that night's stage 4 sleep.

There are several ways whereby stage 4 sleep can be increased, with some influencing its control mechanisms rather than affecting any underlying function. Sleep substances may be working through the former route. A good analogy relates to feeding—there are substances that will stimulate the appetite, but this does not mean that we need more food, only that feeding control mechanisms and eating behaviour have been affected.

The fascinating findings that SWS may have a connection with immuno-enhancement is still somewhat of an enigma. The SWS-related hGH release may be related to this in some way, although I suspect that this release has several roles, and I particularly favour it having a protein-sparing effect owing to the sleep fast (Section 4.7). Changes to the immune system during SWS can be viewed in several ways. One is that the immune system is rejuvenated somehow, to the benefit of our everyday health. Another is that perhaps SWS leaves us more vulnerable to pathogens that happen to be around, and so some immunoenhancement is required as a precaution. If the former condition were true, then many fascinating ideas develop. For example, here may be another link between psychological well-being and the effectiveness of the immune response to ward off infection. Increased interest and awareness in one's surroundings will lead to more SWS, and a greater night-time boost to the immune system. This assumes that such a lifestyle is not stressful, otherwise there will be counterproductive effects. For example, cortisol levels will rise, and as this hormone tends to dampen the immune response the overall outcome may be detrimental to health. On the other hand, loss of daytime interest, particularly in the long term, as in depression perhaps, is associated with less SWS and maybe a greater liability to infection. But these are flights of fancy—it is now time to take up a more substantive theme.

References

1. Moruzzi, G. (1966). The functional significance of sleep with particular regard to the brain mechanisms underlying consciousness. In: Eccles, J.C. (ed.) *Brain and Conscious Experience*. Springer-Verlag, Berlin. pp. 345–388.

2. Rosenberg, R.S., Bergmann, B.M. and Rechtschaffen, A. (1976). Variations in slow wave activity in the rat. *Physiology and Behaviour*, **17**, 931-938.
3. Borbély, A.A. and Neuhaus, H.U. (1979). Sleep-deprivation: effects on sleep and EEG in the rat. *Journal of Comparative Physiology*, **133**, 71-87.
4. Ursin, R. (1971) Differential effect of sleep deprivation on the two slow wave sleep stages in the cat. *Acta Physiologica Scandinavica*, **83**, 352-361.
5. Webb, W.B. and Agnew, H.W. (1971) Stage 4 sleep: influence of time-course variables. *Science*, **174**, 1354-1356.
6. Agnew, H.W. and Webb, W.B. (1973). The influence of time course variables on REM sleep. *Bulletin of the Psychonomic Society* **3**, 131-133.
7. Hume, K.I. and Mills, J.N. (1977). Rhythms of REM and slow wave sleep in subjects living on abnormal time-schedules. *Waking and Sleeping*, **3**, 291-296.
8. Maron, L., Rechtschaffen, A. and Wolpert, E.A. (1964). Sleep cycle during napping. *Archives of General Psychiatry*, **11**, 503-508.
9. Karacan, I., Williams, R.L., Finley, W.W. and Hursch, C.J. (1970). The effects of naps on nocturnal sleep: influence on the need for stage-1 REM and stage 4 sleep. *Biological Psychiatry*, **2**, 391-399.
10. Feinberg, I., March, J.D., Floyd, T.C., Jimison, R., Bossom-Demitrack, L. and Katz, P.H. (1985). Homeostatic changes during post-nap sleep maintain baseline levels of delta EEG. *Electroencephalography and Clinical Neurophysiology*, **61**, 134-137.
11. Feinberg, I. (1974). Changes of sleep cycle patterns with age. *Journal of Psychiatric Research*, **10**, 283-306.
12. Borbély, A.A. (1986). *Secrets of Sleep*. Basic Books, New York.
13. Horne, J.A. (1976). Hail slow wave sleep: goodbye REM. *Bulletin of the British Psychological Society* **29**, 74-79.
14. Jackson, J.H. (1958). Evolution and dissolution of the nervous system. In: Taylor, J. (ed.) *Selected Writings of John Hughlins Jackson*. Staples, London: pp. 45-75.
15. Webb, W.B. (1975). *Sleep The Gentle Tyrant*. Prentice-Hall, New Jersey.
16. Lassen, N.A., Ingvar, D.H. and Skinho, E. (1978). Brain function and blood flow. *Scientific American*, **239** (October), 50-59.
17. Roland, P.E. (1984). Metabolic measurements of the working frontal cortex in man. *Trends in Neurosciences*, **7**, 430-435.
18. Horne, J.A. and Walmsley, B. (1976). Daytime visual load and the effects upon human sleep. *Psychophysiology*, **13**, 115-120.
19. Horne, J.A. and Minard, A. (1985). Sleep and sleepiness following a behaviourally 'active' day. *Ergonomics*, **28**, 567-575.
20. Regestein, Q.R., Buckland, G.H. and Pegram, G.V. (1973). Effect of daytime alpha rhythm maintenance on subsequent sleep. *Psychosomatic Medicine*, **35**, 415-418.
21. Potter, W. and Heron, W. (1972). Sleep during perceptual deprivation. *Brain Research*, **40**, 434-439.
22. Ryback, R.S., Lewis, O.F. and Lessard, C.S. (1971). Psychobiologic effects of prolonged bed rest (weightlessness) in young healthy volunteers. *Aerospace Medicine*, **42**, 529-535.
23. Weitzman, E.D., Perlow, M., Sassin, J., Fukushima, D., Burack, B. and

Hellman, L. (1972). Persistence of the episodic pattern of cortisol secretion and growth hormone release in blind subjects. *Transactions of the American Neurological Association*, **97**, 197–199.

24. Kreiger, D.T. and Glick, S. (1971). Absent sleep peak of growth hormone release in blind subjects. *Journal of Clinical Endocrinology*, **33**, 847–850.

25. Kupfer, D. (1984). REM activity and delta wave abnormalities in affective states. *Research Communications in Psychology, Psychiatry and Behaviour*, **9**, 149–175.

26. Kupfer, D., Ulrich, R.F., Coble, P.A., Jarrett, D.B., Grochocinski, V.J., Doman, J., Matthews, G. and Borbély, A.A. (1985). Electroencephalographic sleep of younger depressives. *Archives of General Psychiatry*, **42**, 806–810.

27. Schulz, H. and Lund, R. (1985). On the origin of early REM episodes in the sleep of depressed patients: a comparison of three hypotheses. *Psychiatry Research*, **16**, 65–77.

28. Feinberg, I. and Hiatt, J.F. (1979). Sleep patterns in schizophrenia: a selective review. In: Williams, R.L., Karacan, I. and Frazier, S.H. (ed.) *Sleep Disorders, Diagnosis and Treatment*. Wiley, New York. pp. 205–231.

29. Hiatt, J.F., Floyd, T.C., Katz, P.H. and Feinberg, I. (1985). Further evidence of abnormal non-rapid eye movement sleep in schizophrenia. *Archives of General Psychiatry*, **42**, 797–802.

30. Taylor, M.A. and Abrahams, R. (1984). Cognitive impairment in schizophrenia. *American Journal of Psychiatry*, **141**, 196–201.

31. Ariel, R.N., Golden, C.J., Berg, R.A., Quaife, M.A., Dirksen, J.W., Forsell, T., Wilson, J. and Graber, B. (1983). Regional cerebral blood flow in schizophrenics. *Archives of General Psychiatry*, **40**, 258–263.

32. Buchsbaum, M.S. *et al.* (1984). Anteroposterior gradients in cerebral glucose use in schizophrenia and affective disorders. *Archives of General Psychiatry*, **41**, 1159–1166.

33. Baxter, L.R., Phelps, M.E., Mazziotta, J.C., Schwartz, J.M., Gerner, R.H., Celin, C.E. and Sumida, R.M. (1985). Cerebral metabolic rates for glucose in mood disorders. *Archives of General Psychiatry*, **42**, 441–447.

34. Williams, R.L., Karacan, I. and Hursch, C.J. (1974). *Electroencephalography (EEG) of Human Sleep: Clinical Applications*. Wiley, New York.

35. Blois, R., Feinberg, I., Galliard, J-M., Kupfer, D.J. and Webb, W.B. (1983). Sleep in normal and pathological aging. *Experientia*, **39**, 551–558.

36. Webb, W.B. and Drebelow, L.M. (1982). A modified method for scoring slow wave sleep of older subjects. *Sleep*, **5**, 195–199.

37. Spiegel, R., Koberle, S. and Allen, S.R. (1986). Significance of slow wave sleep: considerations from a clinical viewpoint. *Sleep*, **9**, 66–79.

38. Agnew, H.W., Webb, W.B. and Williams, R.L. (1967). Comparison of stage four and 1-REM sleep deprivation. *Perceptual and Motor Skills*, **24**, 851–858.

39. Bonnet, M.H. (1986). Performance and sleepiness following disrupted sleep allowing or prohibiting slow wave sleep. *Sleep Research*, **15**, 68.

40. Buchsbaum, M.S., Mendelson, W.B., Duncan, W.C., Coppola, R., Kelsoe, J. and Gillin, J.C. (1982). Topographical cortical mapping of EEG sleep stages during daytime naps in normal subjects. *Sleep*, **5**, 248–255.

41. Sato, S., Dreifuss, F.E. and Penry, J.K. (1975). Photic sensitivity of children

with absence seizures. *Electroencephalography and Clinical Neurophysiology*, **39**, 479–489.

42. Velasco, F., Velasco, M., Cepeda, C. and Munoz, H. (1980). Wakefulness-sleep modulation of cortical and subcortical somatic evoked potentials in man. *Electroencephalography and Clinical Neurophysiology*, **48**, 64–72.

43. Campbell, K.B. and Bartoli, E.A. (1986). Human auditory evoked potentials during natural sleep: the early components. *Electroencephalography and Clinical Neurophysiology*, **65**, 142–149.

44. Williams, H.L., Hammack, J.T., Daly, R.L., Dement, W.C. and Lubin, A. (1964). Response to auditory stimulation, sleep loss and the EEG stages of sleep. *Electroencephalography and Clinical Neurophysiology*, **16**, 269–279.

45. Bonnet, M.H. (1986). Auditory thresholds during continuing sleep. *Biological Psychology*, **22**, 3–10.

46. Granda, A.M. and Hammack, J.T. (1961). Operant behaviour during sleep. *Science*, **133**, 1485–1486.

47. Busby, K. and Pivik, R.T. (1985). Auditory arousal thresholds during sleep in hyperkinetic children. *Sleep*, **8**, 332–341.

48. Broughton, R. (1968). Sleep disorders: disorders of arousal. *Science*, **159**, 1070–1078.

49. Kales, A., Soldatos, C.R., Caldwell, A.B., Kales, J.D., Humphrey, F.J., Charney, D.S. and Schweitzer, P.K. (1980). Somnambulism. *Archives of General Psychiatry*, **37**, 1406–1410.

50. Sakai, F., Meyer, J.S., Karacan, I., Derman, S. and Yamamoto, M. (1979). Normal human sleep: regional cerebral haemodynamics. *Annals of Neurology*, **7**, 471–478.

51. Heiss, W.D., Pawlick, G., Herholz, K., Wagner, R. and Weinhard, K. (1985). Regional cerebral glucose metabolism in man during wakefulness, sleep, and dreaming. *Brain Research*, **327**, 362–366.

52. Livingstone, M.S. and Hubel, D.H. (1981). Effect of sleep and arousal on the processing of visual information in the cat. *Nature*, **291**, 554–561.

53. Kennedy C. *et al.* (1982). Local cerebral glucose utilisation in non-rapid eye movement sleep. *Nature*, **297**, 325–327.

54. Petitjean, F., Seguin, S., Des Rosiers, M.H., Salvert, D., Buda, C., Janin, M., Debilly, M., Jouvet, M. and Bobillier, P. (1982). Local cerebral glucose utilisation during waking and slow wave sleep in the cat. A^{14}C deoxyglucose study. *Neuroscience Letters*, **32**, 91–97.

55. Guiditta, A., Rutigliano, B. and Vitale-Neugebauer, A. (1980). Influence of synchronised sleep on the biosynthesis of RNA in neuronal and mixed fractions isolated from the rabbit cerebral cortex. *Journal of Neurochemistry*, **35**, 1267–1272.

56. Moldofsky, H., Lue, F.A., Eisen, J., Keystone, E. and Gorczynski, R.M. (1986). The relationship of interleukin-1 and immune function to sleep in humans. *Psychosomatic Medicine*, **48**, 309–318.

57. Pappenheimer, J.R., Miller, T.B. and Goodrich, C.A. (1967). Sleep promoting effects of cerebrospinal fluid from sleep deprived goats. *Proceedings of the National Academy of Sciences USA*, **58**, 513–517.

58. Garcia-Arraras, J.E. (1981). Effects of sleep-promoting factor from human urine on sleep cycle of cats. *American Journal of Physiology*, **241**, E269–E274.

59. Krueger, J., Walter, J. and Levin, C. (1985). Factor S and related somnogens: an immune theory for slow wave sleep. In: McGinty, D.J., Drucker-Colin, R., Morrison, A. and Parmeggiani, P.-L. (ed.). *Brain Mechanisms of Sleep*. Raven Press, New York. pp. 253–269.

60. Walter, J., Davenne, D., Shomam, S., Dinarello, C.A. and Krueger, J.M. (1986). Brain temperature changes coupled to sleep states persist during interleukin 1 enhanced sleep. *American Journal of Physiology*, **250**, R96–R103.

61. Cannon, J.G. and Kluger, M.J. (1983). Endogenous pyrogen activity in human plasma after exercise. *Science*, **220**, 617–619.

62. Giulian, D. and Lachman, L.B. (1985). Interleukin-1 stimulation of astroglial proliferation after brain injury. *Science*, **228**, 497–499.

63. Monnier, M. and Hosli, L. (1964). Dialysis of sleep and waking factors in blood of the rabbit. *Science*, **146**, 796–798.

64. Inoué, S., Honda, K., Komoda, Y., Uchizono, K., Ueno, R. and Hayaishi, O. (1984). Differential sleep-promoting effects of five sleep substances nocturnally infused in unrestrained rats. *Proceedings of the National Academy of Sciences USA*, **81**, 6240–6244.

6. Core and optional sleep

6.1 Introduction

It will be remembered that following sleep deprivation only about 30 per cent of the total sleep lost seems to be reclaimed, with most of the lost stage 4 sleep and about half the REM sleep returned. When subjects have their daily sleep reduced for at least a few days (Section 2.15), psychological performance is not noticeably impaired until sleep is down to 4–5 hours per day. I see these findings as strong evidence for there being an essential component of sleep that I have called core sleep, centring on SWS, particularly stage 4 sleep, and to some extent on REM sleep. During a normal night's sleep, core sleep occupies about the first three sleep cycles—the initial 4–5 hours of sleep. This gives way to optional sleep, which makes up the remainder of sleep. I use the term optional with some caution, as we clearly cannot just dispense with this sleep overnight, although, as will be seen, a few weeks of careful adaptation will allow a sizeable proportion of this sleep to be removed without producing increased daytime sleepiness or other ill-effects.

Fig. 6.1 shows the time courses for these two types of sleep over the night. It applies to the sleep of mammals in general, and this is why I have indicated how optional sleep changes with safety, danger, and boredom. Boredom affects human sleep, as will be seen shortly, whereas safety and danger are more applicable to the sleep of other mammals—a theme that will be dealt with in the next chapter. Core sleep increases as prior wakefulness lengthens, and I covered this topic in Section 5.2. In the next chapter I shall be discussing more fully why I believe that core sleep will also increase with mammalian evolution, specifically with increasing cererebral development. Fig. 6.1 shows optional sleep to be present at the beginning of the sleep period, in addition to core sleep. The reasons for this are given in Section 6.9, dealing with stage 2 sleep—in effect, stage 2 sleep is optional sleep. But there will be more about this later.

All mammals sleep, even those in the most dangerous sleeping conditions. Such findings are difficult to explain from the viewpoint that sleep is wholly a non-restitutive drive or instinct. Instead, this provides strong support in favour of at least some of sleep (core sleep) having an essential role, probably of a restitutive nature, which as I have suggested, is mainly for the cerebrum. Optional sleep seems to be controlled by some form of drive behaviour, influenced by a circadian rhythm that regulates both the length of sleep and the onset of waking. This rhythm is adaptable of course, and in those mammals

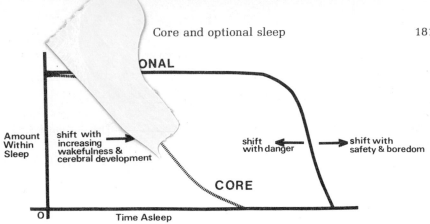

Fig. 6.1 Core and optional sleep in mammals—general trends over the daily sleep period, and factors influencing them. See text for details.

dependent on daylight or darkness and living naturally in the wild, where daylight varies in length with the seasons, the rhythm may change accordingly. So, one role for optional sleep may be as a time filler when the mammal has little else to do, for example, when the animal is constrained by darkness. Another role relates to energy conservation, particularly as an immobilizer in smaller mammals unable to exhibit relaxed wakefulness. If, on the other hand, sleep leaves the animal vulnerable to danger, then sleep will be shorter and approaches a minimum core amount, with little or no optional sleep.

In this chapter I am going to describe more findings favouring my core–optional sleep hypothesis, with respect to humans. The next chapter deals with this topic in relation to other mammals. Human sleep not only provides a good basis for the understanding of mammalian sleep function, but it also acts as a good example for illustrating core and optional sleep.

6.2 Natural long and short sleepers amongst humans

Within any age group of good sleepers the total amount of sleep per day follows a normal distribution, and I am excluding those people suffering from insomnia. In young adults, for example, the average sleep length is about 7.5 hours, with a standard deviation of about 1 hour. That is, around 65 per cent of young adults sleep between 6.5 and 8.5 hours, and about 95 per cent between 5.5 and 9.5 hours. One of the first investigators to compare the sleep structure of long and short sleepers was Webb. He ran two major investigations on healthy young adults who had been carefully screened for personality and medical problems. The first study, on a total of 28 subjects[1] compared sleepers above and below one standard deviation from the average sleep length, and the second study, involving 54 subjects[2] went further and

Table 6.1 Sleep stage characteristics for different groups of sleepers. (Adapted from the studies by Webb and Agnew[1] and Webb and Friel[2])

	Duration (minutes)			
	Long (over 8.5 h)	Control (7.5 h)	Short (under 6.5 h)	Very short (under 5.5 h)
Wake + stage 1	40	26	14	16
Stage 2	277	215	168	118
Stage 3	22	29	18	23
Stage 4	72	81	81	70
SWS (stages 3 + 4)	94	110	99	93
REM	155	101	96	60
Total	566	452	377	287

compared sleepers above and below two standard deviations. Both studies included a third group of subjects whose sleep length was at the average of 7.5 hours.

Table 6.1 gives the findings for the three groups (long, control, and short) in the first study, and for the very short sleepers in the second study. In the first group of short sleepers it can be seen that the main difference between them and the control group lies with reductions in stage 2 sleep. The amounts of SWS and REM sleep are about the same. Longer sleepers differed from these two other groups in having more REM and stage 2 sleep, and again SWS remained constant. The very short sleepers not only had very low levels of stage 2 sleep, but REM sleep was now also reduced. SWS, though, was unchanged. In fact, the most interesting finding across all subjects is that the amounts of SWS seem to be approximately equal.

What appears to be happening to the very short sleepers is that rather than their sleep being compressed into 5.5 hours from the average 7.5 hours, with proportional reductions across all sleep stages, instead the normal last 2 hours of sleep disappear. So their sleep has the same sleep stage characteristics to the first 5.5 hours of sleep of the 7.5-hour sleeper. The hypnogram given in Fig. 1.2 helps illustrate this point. There it can be seen that these latter 2 hours of sleep are made up of REM and stage 2 sleep—the 'missing' sleep in the very short sleepers. Long sleepers, on the other hand, seem to have an additional sleep cycle similar to that normally found at the end of sleep in the 7.5-hour sleeper—hence the additional stage 2 and REM sleep for the former sleeper. Finally, an interesting finding for both groups of short sleepers was that they had little wakefulness and stage 1 sleep, suggesting that their sleep was less disturbed and more efficient.

The subjects of the second study, who usually slept outside the range 5.5–9.5 hours, were given a battery of personality, scholastic, and medical tests to see whether there were any differences between the groups. Nothing of great note was found, except for some possible signs of hypomania (a very mild type of mania) amongst the very short sleepers. As will be seen shortly, for those rare sleepers who naturally need only 3 hours sleep or less a day, the hypomania can be more evident. Other researchers have reported that longer sleepers seem to be 'worriers', with a more depressive outlook on life[3].

In Section 2.19 I discussed whether long and short sleepers differ in their recovery sleep after sleep deprivation, and described the findings of Benoit, Foret, and colleagues[4]. Long sleepers, who averaged 9 hours sleep a night, seemed to be able to absorb the extra demand for SWS into their recovery sleep. The short sleepers, averaging 5 hours sleep a night, had to add this SWS to their recovery sleep—that is, their recovery sleep was longer than their usual sleep. Further details of their baseline and recovery sleep patterns are given in Fig. 2.6. Separate information on stages 3 and 4 sleep was not available. Their baseline sleep patterns were very similar to those of Webb's subjects, shown in Table 6.1. Again, SWS remains fairly constant, REM sleep increases from short to long sleepers, and the shorter sleepers seem to have more efficient sleep, with much less wakefulness and stage 1 sleep.

A few genuine cases of extremely short sleepers have been documented. Although there are other unsubstantiated claims coming from newspapers, etc., these usually turn out to be bogus or gross distortions[5]. Many extremely short sleepers examined at sleep laboratories turn out to be people who are chronically fatigued and sleep deprived, who have forced themselves into taking little sleep. Others are quite frankly liars, out for the publicity. The majority though seem to be quite honest and are just grossly mistaken. A case comes to mind where a lady claimed not to sleep 'a wink' at night, and supported her claim by being able to hear a nearby church clock strike each hour. It turned out that, unknown to her, she regularly awoke throughout the night a few minutes before the hour (to hear the clock strike), returning to sleep a few minutes later!

One of the best accounts of genuine extremely short sleepers came from a study carried out 20 years ago in Australia by Dr Henry Jones and Professor Ian Oswald (who was working there at the time). Following the help of the press, they located two healthy men who habitually slept for about 3 hours a night[6]. One, identified as 'McK', a 54-year-old very active businessman, 'conveyed an impression of vigor and restlessness, though not of hypomania'. The other, called 'H', a 30-year-old draughtsman, had decided to cut down his sleeping 6 years previously because he was 'too busy' as he had many outside interests. Jones and Oswald described him as 'a vigorous and over meticulous man and not hypomanic'. Both McK and H came to the laboratory for 6 to 7 nights of sleep recordings, and on average they slept about 2.75 hours per night. The findings are given in Table 6.2. I have also included for comparison (in brackets) the minutes of sleep stages etc. that might be expected for approximately the first 2.75 hours of sleep in normal-

Table 6.2 Sleep patterns of two extremely short sleepers (from Jones and Oswald[6]). Compared with the first two sleep cycles of age-related normal sleepers (from Feinberg[7]).

Age (years)	Duration (minutes)			
	Mr McK	(Normal)	Mr H	(Normal)
	54		30	
Wakefulness	0?	(13)	0?	(5)
Stage 1	4		3	
Stage 2	39	(79)*	41	(48)*
Stage 3	52	(25)	33	(24)
Stage 4	32	(13)	48	(47)
SWS (Stages 3 + 4)	84	(38)	81	(71)
REM	40	(37)	38	(39)
Total	167	(167)	163	(163)

* Stages 1 & 2 combined

length sleepers of similar ages. This latter information has been extracted from the first two complete sleep cycles given in Feinberg's detailed account of sleep cycle patterns in various age groups.[7].

The similarity of Mr H's sleep with the age-related norm is quite impressive, indicating that his sleep may represent the first part of normal sleep. However, this does not apply to the older McK, as there are clear differences. Nevertheless, both men spent half of their sleep in SWS, which is several times the proportion found in normal-length sleepers of the same age. On the other hand, the proportion of REM sleep for these two men is normal, at around 25 per cent. Although I suggest that Messrs McK and H are down to their core sleep, I should add that their 2.75 hours of sleep seems low, and I consider core sleep in most people to be longer than this, at around three sleep cycles (about 4.5 hours of sleep). Interestingly, Mr H claimed that when he took the occasional holiday he could sleep for longer.

In Ottawa, Dr Roger Broughton (whose other work is described in Section 5.10) and a colleague, Dr Donald Stuss, located five healthy men (aged from 23 to 57 years) and one woman (39 years), who were extremely short sleepers[8]. Sleep ranged from 1.5 to 4.0 hours a day, and had been at this level for an average of 15 years. Unfortunately, sleep laboratory records could only be obtained from one individual, the 57 year old. Other subjects' claims were verified by relatives and through questioning by the investigators. Personality tests on all subjects showed that for four of them there was what Stuss and Broughton described as, 'a moderate to marked drive level, a gregarious personality, relative freedom from reporting medical symptoms, and a tendency to use repression and denial'. Assessments on the Minnesota Multiphasic Personality Inventory (MMPI), a well-known personality test, showed their highest scores to be on the hypomania scale. The other two subjects were quite different, and were described as having 'a tendency to withdrawal, and perhaps depression, more of a willingness to admit psychological weakness, and a less marked level of activity'.

The man from whom the investigators obtained sleep EEG records claimed to have slept less than 2 hours a night for the previous 25 years. This was his regular sleep pattern and there was no 'catching up' at weekends. He spent several periods in the laboratory of four nights each, which included: sleeping at his usual level of about 95 minutes, a shortened sleep at half this amount, and an extended sleep of around 2.5 hours. On each of these occasions, an hour after awakening, he was given a series of psychological tests that included prolonged vigilance, addition, calculations, card sorting, and visual-motor memory.

The results can be seen in Table 6.3, and again I have included values based on Feinberg's data[7] that would be expected from the first 95 minutes of a normal sleeper of the same age. Differences between the two are apparent. The increase in SWS with lengthened sleep is a puzzle. Whilst most performance tests showed little effect of one night's sleep reduction, card sorting and calculations were impaired somewhat. On the other hand, extended sleep led to grogginess and a worsening performance for most tests—a strong indication that 95 minutes of sleep was indeed his true amount, and he was not cutting down to impress the experimenters.

There is one other study of an extremely short sleeper—a 70-year-old lady (a retired nurse), living alone, and claiming to sleep for only 1 hour a night. She was investigated by a colleague of mine, Dr Ray Meddis[9], who is now at Loughborough University, but at the time was based at Bedford College, University of London. She came to his laboratory for night-time EEG measurements, on one occasion for three nights and on a second occasion for

Table 6.3 Sleep patterns in an extremely short sleeper — normal, restricted, and extended sleep (see text) (from Stuss and Broughton[8]). In brackets are the values expected in the first sleep cycle of a similarly aged, normal-length sleeper (based on data from Feinberg[7])

| | Duration (minutes) | | |
	Usual	Shortened	Lengthened
Stage 1 + wakefulness	14 (10)	2	19
Stage 2	28 (51)	4	36
Stage 3	20 (10)	5	23
Stage 4	27 (10)	31	50
SWS	47 (20)	36	73
REM	6 (14)	0	24
Total	95 (95)	42	152

five nights. Her oral temperature was taken periodically during the daytime and evenings. Although she said that she did not sleep in the daytime, this was not able to be verified. The circadian rhythm of her body temperature showed a peak between 10 p.m. and 2 a.m. and a trough between 8 a.m. and 2 p.m. These values are about 10 hours out of phase with the values one would normally expect from a person of this age, and suggest that her best time for sleep was during the mid morning, and time of least sleep and most alertness was around midnight.

During the initial run of nights in the laboratory, she stayed awake for the first two nights, and then only slept for 99 minutes on the third night. This consisted of 13 minutes of stage 2 sleep, 31 and 18 minutes respectively of stages 3 and 4 sleep, and 37 minutes of REM sleep. Feinberg's data for the first 99 minutes of sleep from a similar-aged normal-length sleeper, gives about 9 and 8 minutes for stages 3 and 4 respectively, and 18 minutes for REM sleep. These are noticeably different from those of this lady, and suggest that she had more pressure for SWS. We cannot rule out the possibility that unbeknown to the experimenters she sleep deprived herself on the first two nights. This would have led to a recovery sleep of unusually high SWS. Nevertheless, it is likely that she was indeed a short sleeper, but the question remains, how short?

Her sleep was quite erratic during the second series of nights, with sleep lengths of 0, 82, 204, 19, and 29 minutes successively. It is difficult to make much out of these findings, and they left Meddis rather perplexed. She was a very active lady who 'despised inactivity' and 'rarely experienced tiredness'. I spent an afternoon visiting her, and although Meddis considered her not to be hypomanic, I am not so certain. Erratic sleep of this type can accompany hypomania, where the circadian timing of sleep can become greatly disrupted. She was an endearing lady, involved in several grand projects including writing a book and painting many pictures. None of these works was completed, and she seemed to have the habit of starting ambitious ventures but never finishing them. She talked almost continuously and drank much tea. She said she drank about 20 cups a day, and from what I saw and tasted, it was strong—probably enough to have had some stimulating effect on her behaviour, and may have been partly responsible for her short sleep.

These facinating studies on very short sleepers produce as many questions as answers. All three studies only cover a total of four subjects, and there is very little of this type of research to draw on. Obviously, these people are exceedingly rare, perhaps to the point of abnormality. So, such findings might be viewed as the exception rather than the rule, and of questionable relevance to the understanding of sleep in the other 99.9 per cent of the population. These people seem to be fairly normal in other respects, or are they?

Cases of healthy non-sleepers have never subsequently been verified. The only well-documented report[10] of a non-sleeper was of a 27-year-old man who was admitted to hospital with a total inability to sleep, and suffering from an involuntary control of limb muscles, pain in the extremities, and diarrhoea. Recordings in the sleep laboratory confirmed this absence of sleep, and a diagnosis of the rare neurological disease Morvan's chorea was made. His condition for the following 9 months was monitored. He claimed never to feel sleepy, and apparently there was no 'intellectual disorder'. But actual neuropsychological assessment of his cerebral functioning was not reported on. At night, particularly between 9 p.m. and 11 p.m., he experienced dramatic hallucinations involving all the senses, and great pain in the extremities. These episodes lasted between 20 minutes and an hour, and the EEG at the time showed him to be either awake or in stage 1 sleep.

Sleeping tablets had no effect, and he was treated with 5-hydroxytryptophan (5-HTP)—a substance that naturally occurs in the brain, and is part of the biochemical pathway leading to serotonin. At this time, in the early seventies, serotonin was thought to be a substance central to the biochemical processes controlling sleep in humans and other mammals, but nowadays its role is more debatable. The patient improved dramatically at first, and normal sleep began to return. Withdrawal of 5-HTP therapy worsened his condition, and the therapy was again attempted. But this time it was ineffective and he died—11 months after the disorder appeared.

At autopsy there were no obvious brain damage or lesions, although there were very small haemorrhages in several brain areas. The cause of his death was not fully known, and it is difficult for me to comment much further, except to say that although these findings might suggest that the cerebrum does not need sleep after all, as this man appeared to live an apparently 'normal' life for a while, little is known about how his cerebrum was really functioning at this time. The extent to which zero sleep contributed towards his death will remain a mystery.

I believe that short sleepers are down to their core sleep and have very little or no optional sleep. This may be due to their genes, or to a gradual process of learning to sleep less, or perhaps, as I think more likely, to both mechanisms. Some of these people may even have a defect in their sleep regulation centres that may also be responsible for peculiarities of mood such as hypomania. In this latter respect, it should be noted that it is common for patients suffering from true mania to take little or no sleep, and when they do sleep this is on a very irregular basis. However, for the short sleeper with a normal mood, less than 3 hours sleep a night (say the first two sleep cycles) does seem to be remarkably short, even for core sleep. But core sleep should follow a normal distribution in its length, with people varying in the amount they need. Maybe then, the extremely short sleeper is someone without optional sleep, who is also at the low end of the normal distribution for core sleep. This would be a very rare combination of events, but of course, extremely short sleepers are indeed exceedingly rare.

6.3 Can the normal sleeper adapt to less sleep?

Given the opportunity, most people can eat and drink more than their true physiological needs, and cut down food and water intake say by 15–20 per cent without any harmful effects[11]. In the case of food limitation, body weight will fall a little and then stabilize at a new weight. Obviously time is required for adaptation and there will be some hunger at first, but there would not be starvation, providing that the food restriction is not too great. In effect there are also core and optional requirements for food and water —why not the same principles for sleep?

What constitutes a reasonable sleep 'diet'? There is good evidence that, given the time to adapt, the average 7.5 hours a night sleeper can reduce sleep by about 1.5–2 hours, on a more or less permanent basis, without having excessive daytime sleepiness or impaired psychological performance. It is unlikely, however, that the majority of us could go down to 3 hours sleep a night, to the levels of the natural extremely short sleeper. The 'rule' is obvious: the greater the sleep reduction, the more is the difficulty in adapting. Nevertheless, as I mentioned in Section 2.15 and will pick up again shortly, we can cope quite well on about 4 hours sleep for a few nights. We can even manage without any sleep for one night, as was found with the total sleep deprivation studies (Section 2.12).

Not only can we take less sleep, but it is very easy to sleep longer than normal. This was demonstrated earlier (Section 5.2), when I discussed how daytime naps are not subtracted from the following night's sleep length, but are in effect an addition. It is also relatively easy for most of us to 'sleep in' in the mornings by a further 1–2 hours, without any reduction in the amount of the following night's sleep. I will develop the theme of 'extra' sleep further in the next section. What I am arguing at the moment is that, given time to adapt, the latter part of our normal sleep can quite easily be reduced or extended by 1–2 hours.

One of the earliest well-reported investigations of long-term sleep reduction was in 1935, by Dr Richard Wellington Husband from the University of Wisconsin[12]. Only one subject was used—introduced at the beginning of Husband's paper as, 'Miss Helen Rose, a final year student, who offered to sacrifice herself physically and socially to carry out a fairly lengthy and rigid routine of sleep regulation'. Initially she slept for 1 month at her normal 8 hours a night, followed by another month sleeping 6 hours a night in two blocks of 3 hours each, separated by 3 hours of wakefulness. This period of wakefulness was from 2 a.m. to 5 a.m., and she spent it 'writing, studying and sewing'. These times were kept very regular. Each Saturday morning she was given a medical check-up and a battery of 11 tests that included: hand steadiness, finger-tapping speed, card sorting, tracking, reaction time, a coding task, grip strength, body sway, and IQ measurement. Nothing of note was found apart from what Husband described as, 'suggestions as to very slight loss of efficiency in body sway and speed of tapping, but these were slight and inconsistent'. However, he wisely observed that practice effects with certain tasks could have counteracted some detriment due to sleepiness.

Practice effects also leave some question marks over three more recent and well known investigations, starting with that of Drs Laverne Johnson and William Macleod, which was conducted at the Naval Hospital in San Diego[13]. In this study three young adult volunteers, two men and a woman, reduced their total sleep time by 30 minutes a night every 2 weeks, from their usual 7.5 hours sleep a night. The whole regimen lasted 5 months, and then they were allowed to sleep as much as they wanted to. One man pulled out at the 4.5-hour point and he was dropped from the study, but the others continued down to 4 hours and stayed at this level for 3 weeks. Daytime napping was discouraged but not forbidden. Throughout the study they kept daily diaries of their sleep times, sleepiness during the day, and difficulty in getting up in the mornings. Twice weekly they rated their mood. During the baseline period and at the 5.5-hour and 4.0-hour levels they underwent psychological performance tests and had sleep EEG records taken at night.

Whilst performance tests showed little or no change from the baseline values until around the 4–5-hour sleep level, practice effects may have crept in to counteract any decline. No control group was run in order to measure these effects, although the subjects' diaries and mood scores tended to confirm that real problems did not begin until around the 5-hour point. Then they began to become irritable and experienced obvious daytime sleepiness. The sleep patterns of the two remaining subjects showed that, as one might expect, SWS remained unchanged. For the woman, over the baseline, 5.5-, and 4-hour nights respectively, the SWS levels were 96, 84, and 95 minutes, and for the man these values were 114, 85, and 103 minutes. REM sleep values were respectively, 71, 39 and 22 minutes for the woman, and 105, 68 and 30 minutes for the man. Sleep became less disturbed for both of them. One of the key findings of this study resulted from a follow-up of the subjects' sleep taken about 8 months afterwards, during which time they were free to sleep as they wished. The woman reported that 6 hours of sleep a day was now quite adequate, and the man 5 hours—these were sleep reductions of 1.5 and 2.5 hours respectively below their original levels.

A related and larger study was carried out a few years later, in a collaborative investigation between the Naval Health Research Centre at San Diego and The University of California at Irvine[14,15]. This time, the volunteers were four couples (four men and four women) averaging 25 years of age. Usual sleep lengths were 8 hours per night for three couples, and 6.5 hours for the other couple. Following a 3-week baseline period, all reduced their sleep in a similar manner to before. Initially by 30 minutes at a time for every 2 weeks, and then every 3–4 weeks as the reductions got harder. When each couple felt they had gone far enough, they stayed within half an hour of that point for a further 3 months. Again, daily diaries were kept, together with daytime sleepiness ratings.

They went to the laboratory for a whole day of psychological testing, once during the baseline, at the end of each reduction level, and once after a 6-month follow-up. This included the Wilkinson Auditory Vigilance Task, memory and addition tests, as well as personality measurement. But, as in the previous investigation, there was no control group and no account could be taken of practice effects. Such improvements may have been partly responsible for the findings of no decline in any of the performance measures, even at the lowest reduction levels. I suspect that some impairment was probably present, as the subjects did report increasing sleepiness towards the final phases of reduction. The 8-hour sleepers began to find difficulties in getting up in the mornings when sleep reductions went below 6 hours. However, daytime sleepiness, efficiency at work, and irritability were not much of a problem for most subjects until sleep was down to about 5 hours.

Of the 8-hour sleepers, two reduced their sleep to 5.5 hours, two to 5.0 hours, and two reached 4.5 hours. The couple that usually slept for 6.5 hours got down to around 5 hours. Over the following year, whilst they were free to sleep for as long as they wanted to, their sleep habits were still monitored. All the 8-hour sleepers voluntarily remained at sleep lengths 1–2.5 hours below their original baseline levels. Their daytime alertness, efficiency at work, and all other aspects of behaviour were quite normal. Interestingly though, the two 6.5-hour sleepers reverted back to their original sleep lengths.

During this study sleep EEG recordings were taken at home for every level of reduction. Table 6.4 gives the sleep stage characteristics of the 8-hour sleepers, at the various sleep reductions, and at a follow-up several months later. Adaptations to the reductions seem to have been made through the progressive loss of stage 2 and REM sleep—seemingly from the sleep cycles at the

Table 6.4 Sleep characteristics during gradual sleep reduction for the 8-hour sleepers in the study by (Friedmann et al.[15])

Sleep reduction (hours)	Sleep stages (minutes)					
	Wake + 1	2	3	4	SWS	REM
8.0	34	228	32	48	80	116
7.5	27	213	37	40	77	113
7.0	24	200	40	43	83	99
6.5	21	163	38	58	96	101
6.0	27	138	37	54	91	91
5.5	13	147	31	56	87	83
5.0	15	111	30	51	81	80
4.5	14	123	27	35	62	68
Follow-up	23	155	35	57	92	88

end of sleep. SWS rose slightly, probably because of the extended day (see Section 5.2), although at the lowest reduction level SWS did fall. Wakefulness and stage 1 sleep were reduced, indicating better sleep. Also, subjects fell asleep more rapidly, especially when sleep was below 5.5 hours.

A much more drastic sleep reduction experiment was run by Webb and Agnew[16]. The sleep of their 15 subjects was cut down literally overnight from their usual 7.5–8 hours to 5.5 hours for 60 days. Subjects kept sleep logs, and at weekly intervals sleep EEGs were recorded and measurements made of vigilance performance, addition, memory, and mood. Of the performance tests only vigilance was impaired, with a gradual decline over the weeks, but again there was no control group for practice effects to be determined. Sleep diaries initially showed that most subjects had difficulty arising in the mornings and felt sleepy during the day. However, after the first week or two much of this seemed to pass. Some changes in mood occurred at first, but soon returned to normal. Sleep onset at night became more rapid, and again stage 4 sleep remained stable, with REM sleep falling by about 25 per cent. Webb and Agnew concluded that, 'a chronic loss of sleep by as much as 2.5 hours a night is not likely to result in major behavioural consequences' (p. 265). In my view, the sleepiness experienced by these subjects during the first week or so would have been optional sleepiness, able to be countered by the subjects applying more effort (see Section 2.14).

Such a sudden cut-back of sleep is a rather drastic approach, and the more gradual methods of reduction employed by other studies seem to produce much less daytime sleepiness. Another short investigation[17] also cut sleep back to 5 hours a night, suddenly and overnight, from the normal 8 hours per night. Very noticeable amounts of daytime sleepiness were found for at least a week—the duration of the reduction period.

Whilst it seems fairly certain that over a few weeks we can adapt to 1–2 hours less sleep (i.e. the initial daytime sleepiness disappears), there are still some doubts. The use of psychological tests that are very sensitive to sleepiness is so crucial to these sleep reduction studies. One can never be certain that personal claims by the subjects are really accurate. So the key issue is whether improvements with practice at these tests really do counteract decrements due to sleepiness. In order to resolve this issue, we ran our own experiment[18].

Twelve volunteers, six men and six women, in their mid twenties were selected from a larger group of people. To make the study more attractive, our subjects were paid moderately well. Although we do get volunteers who are prepared to be subjects for no payment, they often tend to be unreliable, and are sometimes rather odd people, out to 'prove' themselves. Our subjects normally slept 7.75–8.25 hours a night, and were healthy, good sleepers, known to be reliable, and could keep honest and accurate records of their sleep and daytime activities. They were randomly placed in one of two groups: (1) sleep reduction, or (2) normally sleeping control.

The control group had to do everything that the reduction group did, except the sleep restriction. The reduction group were required to keep strict bedtime and awakening times, as well as to undergo sleep restriction. So the control group also had to keep to a strict sleeping schedule. It was very important for us to have a good rapport with our subjects. We asked all of them to do their best, but not to worry unduly if they could not keep to the schedules—we wanted to know whether or not people could keep to these arrangements. There was no pressure on the subjects to misrepresent sleep times and sleepiness ratings in their diaries. Alarm clocks had to be used every morning, but placed away from the bed to force the sleeper to get up to turn the alarm off. They had to avoid daytime naps, and were asked not to drink more than their usual amounts of tea and coffee. Alcohol intake had to be kept to a minimum.

Both groups began with a baseline week of familiarization with the various tests and a full briefing. The sleep reduction consisted of an initial week of 1 hour less sleep a night, down to an average of 7 hours sleep a night, followed by 3 weeks at 6.5 hours sleep a night, and finally 2 weeks at 6.0 hours sleep. The method of reduction could be individually planned for each subject according to their wishes, that is they could go to bed later, rise earlier, or do some of both. Once the method was agreed on, it had to be followed strictly. A similar programme was arranged with the control group concerning the fixing of their exact bedtimes and arising times. Neither group were allowed days off from their regimens, especially at weekends.

At the end of each week, at a set day and time (i.e. 5 or 6 days into any new sleep reduction), a pair of subjects, one from each group, came into the laboratory for one hour of the Wilkinson Auditory Vigilance Test, followed by an EEG measurement of sleepiness. The tedium of such a long time at this vigilance test makes it very sensitive to sleepiness. For the EEG assessment, subjects were wired up for a normal sleep recording. Each laid on a comfortable bed in a warm, darkened, and sound-damped individual bedroom for 30 minutes. Purposely, this was very conducive to sleep, but we wanted our subjects to try and stay awake with their eyes open for as long as possible. The more sleepy the subject, the shorter the time they can do this before their eyelids close and the eyes roll upwards, with the EEG showing stage 1 sleep. We also monitored this eye 'rolling', as it is a very useful measure of sleepiness. The number of minutes that the EEG and eye movement activity showed the subject to be fully alert, with no signs of drowsiness, gave us a sleepiness score—the greater the sleepiness, the shorter this time. During the baseline and final reduction weeks, subjects came to the sleep laboratory in the evenings for all-night sleep EEG recordings.

Sleep reduction turned out to be quite uneventful. No one pulled out, and all managed to complete the series of reductions successfully. When sleep was down by 1.5–2 hours, subjects experienced some difficulties waking up in the mornings, but none reported any increased daytime sleepiness after the first few days of each reduction period. The control group had little problem in keeping to their schedules. Over the weeks, both groups showed identical changes with vigilance performance. Indeed, there was a noticeable practice effect in both groups, as both showed the same improvement in performance. There was no sign of any performance loss during sleep reduction. However, it must be remembered that this testing did not take place until each reduction period had been going for some days—seemingly after any sleepiness on the initial days had passed.

The daytime EEG measures of sleepiness showed no differences between the groups. Night-time sleep EEGs on the last week of sleep reduction produced the familiar pattern of no change to stage 4 sleep or to SWS, but significant reductions to REM sleep, wakefulness during the night, and to stages 1 and 2 sleep. The time to fall asleep at night fell by more than half, again indicating that sleep reduction seems to be a useful aid to 'better' sleep.

By the last week of reduction most subjects felt that they could continue on at the 2-hour reduced sleep level with little difficulty. All our evidence supported this view, and so we called a halt to the experiment, as there seemed little point in continuing. We asked the reduction group whether they had made any use of the extra wakefulness, as apart from the payment the other usual reason for volunteering for this study was so that they could spend more time at various projects. But most found that, to be quite frank, this did not happen, as they tended to spend more of the day wasting time. This is a case of 'Parkinson's Law', I'm afraid—the time taken for a task expands to fit the time available. Maybe long sleepers are efficient people, able to do a day's work quickly and then have more time to sleep!

I must emphasise that in all these sleep reduction studies the sleep taken was uninterrupted. Sleep that is frequently disturbed produces considerable sleepiness the next day, no matter how long the sleep time. This point was made in Section 5.9, where I gave as an example the sleep disorder apnoea. Here, unknown to the sleeper, there are numerous brief arousals during the night, producing profound sleepiness the next day, despite what might seem to have been a good 8 hours or more of sleep.

The ability for us to adjust sleep length (i.e. optional sleep) by a few hours gradually over time makes sense when one considers how dependent we used to be on daylight and darkness until the comparatively recent appearance of artificial lighting. Because we are so reliant on our eyes, and since our eyes need good light to see, we had little else to do in the dark except to sleep. Seasonal changes in daylight and darkness, which become more profound the further away from the equator, would encourage us to develop the ability to adjust sleep length according to the seasons. It is a good principle to be able to extend sleep during the winter to while away the long nights. But it was not a good idea to have to sleep for 10 hours during the precious daylight hours of the summer when there was a harvest to be gathered for the winter, or when there were predators around that also relied on daylight.

6.4 Sleep extension

It is relatively easy for us to take more than our usual daily sleep 'quota'. For example, it will be remembered that people in perceptual isolation (Section 5.6) will sleep much more, and, as we all know, daytime boredom can soon lead to an unscheduled nap even though sufficient sleep may have been taken the previous night. Such naps usually do not lead to similar reductions in sleep length the following night (Section 5.2). I should add though that for people who nap every day, particularly those who take an afternoon siesta, this habitual sleep will eventually become part of the total daily sleep need, so that less sleep is taken at night. But for those of us who take the occasional afternoon nap this is usually surplus to any sleep requirement.

Napping behaviour has been studied in some detail by researchers at the Institute of Pennsylvania Hospital[19]. They divided nappers into two main types—'appetitive' and 'replacement' nappers. Appetitive nappers were described as those who, 'nap primarily for reasons other than sleep need, and derive psychological benefits from the nap not directly related to the physiology of sleep' (p. 687). This contrasts with the replacement nappers, who nap to make up for previously lost sleep at night. A third group of individuals was identified—the non-napper, for whom, 'the aftermath of napping seems to be sufficiently unpleasant that it is actively avoided'.

One of their studies, run by Dr David Dinges and colleagues[20], looked at total daily sleep amounts in two groups of appetitive or replacement nappers who napped on average two to three times a week. No sleep EEG recordings were made, but for about a month subjects kept detailed diaries of their sleep habits and completed questionnaires. Both groups typically napped for about 60–75 minutes, and almost invariably around mid afternoon. The results can be seen in Fig. 6.2, giving the outcome for both groups. Total daily sleep lengths are shown for: (a) nap days; (b) the night before, and for comparison (c) nights that were not followed by a nap the next day. As expected, replacement nappers were compensating for sleep lost the night before, and appetitive nappers simply added the nap time on to their night-time sleep.

The more interesting group for me were the appetitive nappers, whose nap sleep, I argue, is an example of how our daily (optional) sleep can be extended by an hour or so. Although the appetitive nappers felt that they 'needed' these naps a few times during the week, the investigators reported that the reason behind these naps was not so much increased sleepiness, but differences in mood on the day of the nap. Dinges and colleagues were particularly

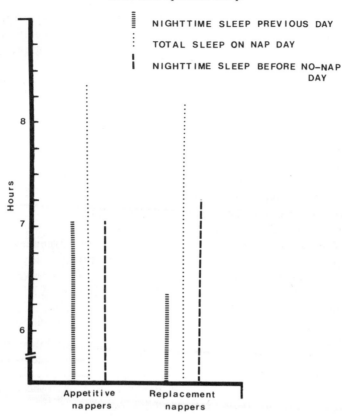

Fig. 6.2 Total daily sleep in 'appetitive' and 'replacement' nappers—showing: (a) total sleep on the nap day, (b) sleep length on the previous night, and (c) night-time sleep before a no-nap day. Note how total sleep is increased on the nap day for appetitive nappers. See text for details. (From Dinges *et al.*[20])

impressed by the afternoon preponderance of naps, and supported the view that our internal sleep–wake clock is designed naturally for two sleeps a day —a long one at night and a short one during the afternoon. This is exactly what happens to people living in hot climates, of course. The siesta is partly a cultural phenomenon, but is probably more of a reflection of the internal clock. In northern Europe, the cultural pressure is against this siesta, even though many of us still notice the feeling of sleepiness after lunch and during the afternoon.

The extent to which we can increase daily sleep has been demonstrated from another perspective, through looking at something most of us can do—'oversleeping' in the morning. Two of the earliest investigations were run by Dr Eugene Aserinsky, working at Jefferson Medical College[21, 22]. In both experiments, subjects had to remain on a bed, in a quiet and darkened room for 30 hours[21] or 54 hours[22], and sleep as much as they could. They were allowed to get up only to eat and go to the toilet, but had to spend the rest of the time either sleeping or with their eyes shut. The total sleep taken in the first study averaged 20 hours—equivalent to about 14 hours per 24-hour day. For the second investigation, 32 hours were spent asleep, which is again about 14 hours sleep per day. Most of this sleep was taken at night, with intermittent naps during the daytime.

Of particular interest to Aserinsky was the density of eye movements during REM sleep (i.e. the number of eye movements per minute of REM sleep). Similar findings were noted for both studies. During the first night, REM density increased progressively with each period of REM sleep, until about 10 hours of sleep had elapsed, and then remained at this relatively high level, or rose even slightly higher. This plateau in REM density appeared to Aserinsky as a sign of sleep satiety.

Aserinsky's methods of confinement seem rather extreme, too unlike everyday life. I did not incorporate his work into Section 5.6 (under the topic of sleep and SWS during reduced sensory stimulation) as he gave no details about SWS or other sleep stages, apart from REM and non-REM sleep in their entirety. Other investigators have been less stringent, simply asking their subjects to 'sleep on' in the morning for as long as possible. Subjects are then allowed to get up and carry on with their normal activities. Two hours sleep extension, of uninterrupted sleep, seem to be quite easily accomplished. If subjects remain in bed longer, then sleep usually becomes fitful and increasing amounts of wakefulness and drowsiness appear. One of the first studies of this type was by Dr Paul Verdone at the National Institute of Mental Health, Bethesda[23]. Twenty-two young adult volunteers slept for an average of three nights in the laboratory. Typically, they spent around 10.5 hours in bed, sleeping for about 9.5 hours—about 2 hours longer than normal. Like Aserinsky, Verdone was only interested in REM sleep, and gave no information on other sleep stages.

Feinberg and colleagues have also looked at extended sleep[24, 25]. As one might expect (see Section 5.3), they were particularly interested in SWS and stage 4 sleep. Twenty-one young adult volunteers who normally averaged 7 hours sleep a night had to remain in bed for 12 hours, from 11 p.m. to 11 a.m. They obtained an extra 210 minutes of sleep on the extended night. This did not lead to any reduction in total sleep the next night—that is, the extended sleep was indeed extra sleep. REM density showed the same steady increase over the first 10 hours of sleep as that seen by Aserinsky. The proportion of REM sleep in this oversleep was about 35 per cent higher than the usual level of around 25 per cent. There was no sign of SWS in the oversleep, and I stress this point because, as will be seen shortly, other research shows a small return of SWS if sleep is extended for longer. By the way, all these findings with SWS were confirmed by Feinberg's computer analysis technique (Section 5.3).

Bedtime the next night was the same as usual. Consequently, the waking day had been shortened by about 20 per cent owing to the extra sleep. Interestingly, during the next night there was an 18 per cent fall in SWS, particularly in stage 4 sleep—confined to the first period of SWS, soon after sleep onset. Such findings further confirm the relationship between the length of wakefulness and the amount of subsequent SWS, described in Section 5.2.

When sleep is extended beyond about 11 hours, SWS often makes a reappearance. This was first noticed about 15 years ago by Dr Bendrich Roth and colleagues from the Charles University, Prague[26]. He is a leading authority on the disorder 'hypersomnia'—an inherited syndrome of excessive sleep length accompanied by a type of drunkenness and confusion on awakening. Such sufferers can sleep up to 20 hours a day. Roth and colleagues found that, typically, SWS reappears after about 12 hours of sleep, in short episodes totalling about 15–20 minutes.

More detailed investigations into this SWS reappearance in healthy normal sleepers have been carried out recently by Dr Pierre Gagnon and colleagues from the School of Psychology at the University of Ottawa[27]. Ten young adults who normally averaged 8 hours sleep a night were asked to sleep for 15 hours from midnight. Eight subjects were able to sleep most of this time, although wakefulness became increasingly prevalent towards the end—averaging just over an hour during the last 6 hours of extended sleep. These findings can be seen in Fig. 6.3. Of great interest to Gagnon and colleagues was the reappearance of an average of 17 minutes of SWS (11 minutes of stage 4 sleep) during the last 3 hours of extended sleep, and this was thought to be due to a 12-hour rhythm of SWS, with peaks around midnight and midday.

I have a supplementary explanation for these findings, coming in two parts. Firstly, given that wakefulness leads to more SWS (Section 5.2), some of the SWS return can be accounted for as a 'paying off' the wakefulness within the oversleep. During 8 hours of normal sleep the subjects had about 103 minutes of SWS, following 16 hours of wakefulness. That makes around 6.5 minutes of SWS per hour of wakefulness. Around one-third of the 17 minutes of SWS in the oversleep might be accounted for by the 1 hour of wakefulness in the oversleep. The remaining two-thirds of this SWS can, I believe, be explained by the second part of my argument. In many respects REM sleep is very much like wakefulness—a case I make in depth in Section 8.10. Therefore, REM sleep may also create a need for SWS, especially if much REM sleep accumulates over the night, as in extended sleep. Let us go back to the data of Gagnon's team, and assume that all of the REM sleep in the first part of normal sleep up to the usual last SWS period is paid off by that SWS. The remaining REM sleep from the sixth hour of sleep onwards, until the reappearance of SWS, comes to about 2 hours. On a rough basis of 6.5 minutes of SWS per hour of wakefulness or REM sleep, the result can account for the remainder of the SWS return.

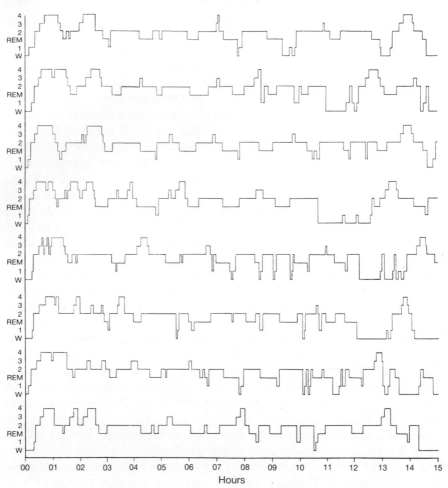

Fig. 6.3 Sleep hypnograms in eight subjects sleeping for 15 hours from midnight. Note that stage 4 sleep is uppermost in each profile. Waking becomes more apparent during the last 3 hours of sleep, and there is a SWS return here. (From Gagnon *et al.*[27]. Reproduced by permission of Raven Press)

Gagnon and colleagues carried out two other extended-sleep experiments, to examine more closely the timing of the SWS reappearance. In one of these[27], the same subjects repeated the sleep extension, but delayed their sleep onset to 4 a.m., sleeping on to 7 p.m. Again, eight out of ten subjects were able to extend their sleep beyond 12 hours. This time SWS reappeared twice—an average of 22 minutes around noon (remember, bedtime was delayed), and another 25 minutes after about 12 hours of sleep. Once more, the investigators explained the latter reappearance in terms of a 12-hourly rhythm in SWS. But in this experiment there were 47 minutes of SWS in the oversleep—30 minutes more than in the first study—how was this? This time the amounts of interim wakefulness and REM sleep came to about 2.5 hours, and on a reckoning of 6.5 minutes of SWS per hour, it would account for only around 20 minutes of the extra SWS. For the remainder, the simplest explanation it seems to me is because the subjects had extended their prior wakefulness (Section 5.2) by going to bed 4 hours later. This would produce another 26 (4 × 6.5) minutes of SWS!

6.5 Are we chronically sleep deprived?

An interesting view on sleep extension was raised by Webb and Agnew after they had also carried out one of these studies[28]. Subjects were allowed to sleep on until awakening spontaneously. Up to this point the sleep contained little wakefulness, and the subjects obtained an extra 126 minutes of sleep (there was no return of SWS). Because of this ease in oversleeping, Webb and Agnew proposed the provocative question, 'are we chronically sleep deprived?' That is, maybe we should be sleeping for about 9–10 hours a night rather than the average 7.5 hours. They backed up this notion by going back in the scientific literature to a report written in 1910 on the sleep habits of young adults. Then sleep normally lasted for 9 hours a night.

Another good point Webb and Agnew made is that many of us do not feel fully refreshed on awakening, and need to use alarm clocks. From their own survey of over 1000 young adults, less than one-third reported that they 'typically wake up in the morning feeling fresh and rested', and another third 'found it hard to get it up in the morning'. But I must stress that such reports only related to a short period of time after awakening, and we do not know how these people felt for the rest of the day.

Some people do wake up in the mornings feeling fully alert and able to get out of bed immediately, but why should this be the normal state of affairs? Should we really expect to be asleep one moment and fully awake the next? Most people experience a gradual transition from alertness to sleepiness during the hour or so around bedtime. Even sleep onset from 'lights out' takes some minutes. So why cannot the reverse process the next morning also take a little time? The fact that arousal from sleep may take a while is not enough evidence to imply insufficient sleep. More support for Webb and Agnew's idea needs to come from other sources, such as whether there is sleepiness during the rest of the day. After all, sleepiness on awakening in the mornings usually soon disappears following arising and walking around the house for a short while.

No long-term research has been done on sleep extension to see whether extended sleep can become a regular habit or wanes after a while, with people waking up at their old time. From the short-term studies, there is little evidence to show that 2 hours of extra sleep improves daytime alertness and performance at work. In fact the evidence points to a fall in daytime performance. The natural timing of sleep and wakefulness has its own circadian rhythm, linked to the circadian rhythm of body temperature (see Section 1.2). Sleeping outside our normal hours, even taking 2 hours of oversleep, seems to disrupt the normal sleep–wake rhythm, and paradoxically daytime sleepiness is increased—at least for the first few days.

Dr John Taub, from St Louis University, has looked at the effects of oversleep on daytime psychological performance, although his studies have usually been for only a single night and day. In one of his most recent reports[29], subjects overslept for an average of an extra 2 hours. Half an hour after arising, following breakfast, they did an hour of performance testing, including a short-time memory test and 30 minutes at the Wilkinson Auditory Vigilance Task. The same procedures were adopted for a further (control) day of normal-length sleep. The findings were quite clear—performance deteriorated significantly at all tasks. For example, memory scores fell by 15 per cent, and missed signals at the vigilance task rose by 60 per cent. From Taub's other work, the signs are that this apparent daytime sleepiness continues for much of the day, and is perhaps something many of us have also experienced after a 'sleep in'. I see this increased sleepiness to be due to the disturbed timing of optional sleep.

Two hours of oversleep usually shows little sign of being light or fitful. Going beyond this amount, sleep becomes more disturbed and wakefulness increases, as was seen in the Gagnon study. Webb has written an interesting account of how normal sleep naturally ends[30], that is, without any intervention by an alarm clock for example. He noted that less than 0.5 per cent of research papers on sleep give any account of the process of awakening, and that many people held to Kleitman's conclusions[31] that, 'partial or even complete awakenings . . . become more frequent toward the end of customary periods of sleep; finally, because of increasing difficulties in lapsing back to sleep, they culminate in overt termination of sleep' (p. 127). Webb expressed strong doubts about this, and examined his own findings, particularly those from his sleep extension study that I have just mentioned.

He analysed the last hour of the 2 hours of extended sleep from 16 subjects. Of the total of 960 minutes (i.e. 16 × 60), there were only 16 minutes of wakefulness. Although 105 minutes of light (stage 1) sleep were found, half of this came from three subjects. Another index of sleep disturbance is the number of sleep stage changes per hour. But this remained the same as for a normal night's sleep (5.7 and 6.1 per hour respectively). There were large differences between individuals—not only in the capacity for oversleep, but from what sleep stage subjects awoke. Webb concluded that, whilst Kleitman's views might be correct when applied to sleep going beyond 2 hours of oversleep, until this point is reached Kleitman was probably wrong—sleep will continue in an orderly way.

6.6 The circadian timing of sleep

This is a key area of sleep research that throws more light on daytime sleepiness, sleep extension, and the control of waking up. I have already described within the context of sleep deprivation (Chapter 2), how there is a clear circadian rhythm of sleepiness, reaching a peak around 2–4 a.m., and a trough around 6–8 p.m. I see the sleep-wakefulness rhythm as a regulator of optional sleep rather than of core sleep, as the main influence on the latter is not the time of the day, but the length of prior wakefulness (Section 5.2).

During the early 1980s three research groups, in Sweden, West Germany, and the USA, simultaneously produced substantial reports[32-34] showing how the length of sleep is linked to the circadian rhythm of body temperature. Even though they took different approaches, all the groups were in close agreement with each other with their findings. Two studies isolated their subjects, one at a time, for a month or so, in environments completely free of all time cues, and with little social contact. The third, by Drs Törbjorn Åkerstedt (whose other work was described in Sections 3.7, and 4.8) and Mats Gillberg from Stockholm, kept this isolation down to 1 day, and it was the most 'natural' of the three studies. I will begin with this one.

Six subjects averaging 37 years of age took part. Every week, over a series of weeks, they went to the sleep laboratory for 2 days and the interim 'night'. On each occasion there was a different starting time for sleep, numbering seven in all. The subjects always took as much sleep as they wanted. The day prior to each sleep was spent in the laboratory, with the subjects isolated from daylight, clocks, radios, and other sources of time. They were not told what the time was when they were sent to bed. For the baseline night, sleep began at 11 p.m., following 16 hours of wakefulness. Other bedtimes were delayed by 4 hours at a time, to 3 a.m., 7 a.m., and so on, up to 11 p.m. Such delays meant that sleep deprivation was also involved. The ordering of these sleep times was varied from subject to subject.

The outcome was quite clear—the longest sleep, of around 10 hours, occurred after evening bedtimes, and the shortest after morning bedtimes. Interestingly, as the awake time increased with the postponement of sleep from 11 p.m. towards 11 a.m., sleep length decreased. As usual, SWS appeared in the first few hours of sleep, and increased with the lengthening of prior wakefulness. SWS was not affected by the time of day of sleep. Åkerstedt and Gillberg believed that the most feasable explanation for their findings was that there is a 'block' to sleep or a sleep 'terminator' at around noon, which pays only some heed to the time of the day when sleep begins. The terminator seems to be triggered at a certain point on the circadian rise in temperature. However, there is one proviso for this concept, as later work of theirs has shown that a sleep episode is not terminated until at least a baseline night's worth of SWS has been obtained[35].

The two other studies, by Dr Juergen Zulley and coworkers[33] at the Max

Planck Institute for Chronophysiology at Andechs near Munich and by Dr Charles Czeisler and colleagues[34] at the New York Montefiore Hospital, kept their volunteers alone in individual isolation units for usually at least a month. In both studies, subjects ate and drank when they wished, but had no communication with the outside world. Contact with the experimenters was minimal, and there were no clues to the time. Sleep, body temperature, and various other physiological functions were monitored continuously. Both studies found that under these time-free conditions, and after varying intervals, circadian rhythms tended to break out of the normal 24-hour day and 'free run'. Whereas the body temperature rhythm soon started to cycle at its natural period of slightly longer than 24 hours, at about 24.5 hours, the circadian rhythm of sleep and wakefulness continued roughly on a 24-hour cycle for about 2 weeks. As a result, the relationship between the circadian rhythms of body temperature and sleep altered. At first the difference was small. The trough in body temperature, normally found during the middle of night-time sleep, now occurred just before sleep onset. But after about 10–14 days in isolation, the synchrony between these two rhythms often broke up, or, to use the correct terms, they became 'uncoupled' or 'desynchronized' to go their separate ways. However, this only happened in about half the subjects, whereas for the remainder the sleep and temperature rhythms continued to remain fairly synchronized with each other.

During desynchronization, sleep and wakefulness became quite erratic. Nevertheless, as both research groups noticed, sleep length was still linked to body temperature. Let me describe these findings a little more clearly, starting with those of Czeisler and coworkers[34]. In those subjects with desynchrony, there were sometimes sleep–wake cycles of extraordinary duration, of up to 50 hours wakefulness between consecutive sleep periods, even though body temperature still cycled around 24–25 hours. Typically though, the pattern consisted of regular appearances of shorter sleep, interrupted by longer sleep. Remember, the bedtimes and waking-up times were entirely self-chosen. When these sleep lengths were compared with the body temperature rhythm, it was clear that short sleeps usually began at or just after the temperature cycle trough—findings similar to those of Åkerstedt and Gillberg.

Figure 6.4 is taken from the report by Czeisler and colleagues, and shows the remarkably close relationship between sleep length and body temperature—still very apparent in desynchronized subjects. The average sleep lengths from sleep onset are shown as a column under the point of the temperature cycle at which sleep began. Rather than describe the horizontal axis of the graph in terms of physical time, which means little for this type of experiment, the circadian 'phase' is given. It consists of 360 degrees, and is equivalent to a 24-hour day—roughly, 1 hour of the day equals 15 degrees. The zero degree point is the time of the temperature trough, and 180 degrees,

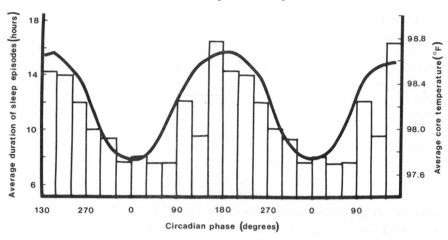

Fig. 6.4 The close association between sleep length and the point on the temperature rhythm at which sleep begins—from the 'time-free' isolation experiment of Czeisler *et al.*[34]. The circadian cycle is shown in degrees (360 degrees per 'day'), and the columns show sleep lengths. Sleep onset at the time of the temperature trough led to a short sleep of about 8 hours, whilst sleep beginning at the temperature peak led to a long sleep of around 14 hours. See text for details. (Reproduced with the permission of the American Association for the Advancement of Science)

the time of the peak. So, when the subject's chosen bedtime was near the temperature cycle minimum, at zero degrees, the average sleep length was 7.8 hours. On the other hand, sleep at the 180-degree point averaged 14.4 hours.

The association between the body temperature curve and sleep length continued to hold even when the chosen bedtime followed 20 hours of wakefulness. Bedtimes (and presumably a time of heightened sleepiness) were not entirely random, however, as the most popular time for bed was still around the temperature trough. Last, but not least, 86 per cent of all awakenings occurred on the rising phase of the temperature rhythm—findings also supporting the sleep 'terminator' idea. That is, largely irrespective of bedtime, sleep ends at a certain point on the upturn of the circadian rhythm of body temperature, even when this rhythm is free running.

For me, the sleep terminator idea also seems to be a very plausible explanation of Zulley's findings, although both he and Czeisler are more cautious about such an interpretation—the timing of sleep onset in relation to the circadian temperature rhythm may still be the real key. Zulley and colleagues ran 20 subjects in their experiment[33], half of whom became desynchronized. For those remaining synchronized, sleep usually began about 1.3 hours before the temperature trough, and lasted for around 8.3 hours. On the other hand, in desynchronized subjects there was a much wider range of possibilities for sleep onset. Nevertheless, just like Czeisler's findings, the length of sleep was still related to when during the temperature cycle sleep began. Zulley's group found that for both their synchronized and desynchronized subjects there was a consistency in the waking-up time—it occurred about 6 hours into the body temperature rise, after the trough.

There is much still to learn about the circadian timing of sleep, especially about the waking-up time in relation to the upturn of the temperature curve. We know little about the circadian temperature rhythm in natural short sleepers, or in people who have adapted to less sleep, as none of those studies measured body temperature in sufficient detail. The same applies to the extended-sleep experiments in the previous section. But of course, from the 'oversleeping' that occurred in these three circadian rhythm studies[32-34], it seems that oversleep continues as far as the termination point on the temperature curve. This implies that in normal circumstances most of us wake up about 2 hours before the real termination point, as:

1. We seem naturally to be able to oversleep by around 2 hours (see Section 6.4).
2. Åkerstedt and Gillberg have shown that sleep length from the normal sleep onset time to the temperature termination point is about 10 hours.

Maybe the terminator could be considered as a final backstop to optional sleep, in case we overshoot our usual waking-up time?

I mentioned earlier that optional sleep should have the potential to increase and shorten with seasonal changes in daily light and darkness (Section 6.3). If the circadian temperature rise has an important role in terminating sleep, then appropriate seasonal changes might be found in the circadian temperature rhythm (this might not be the only reason for such seasonal changes, of course). For example, during the winter the morning upturn of the curve may be later to allow a longer optional sleep. Unfortunately, we have little information to go by—for two main reasons. First, few people have ever looked at seasonal variations in the circadian rhythm of human body temperature. Second, as we in the Western world with our artificial lighting etc. are no longer slaves to daylight and darkness, any potential changes of this nature in body temperature may be hidden.

One investigation on Eskimos showed a 2.5-hour seasonal shift in the peak times of their circadian temperature curves during wakefulness[36], but there was no information about the temperatures during sleep, or to what extent these people used electric lights, etc. We have carried out a limited study at out own laboratory, not on Eskimos, but on students at Loughborough[37]. It had several shortcomings, however, as I will explain. Twelve men and 14 women measured their oral temperatures about every hour throughout the waking day, from morning arising until sleep. This continued for 3-week periods during December, March, and June. It was not possible to measure

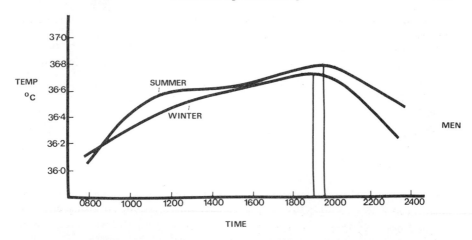

Fig. 6.5 Changes in daytime oral temperature from winter to summer in young men. Vertical lines indicate the peak times. Note the steeper morning rise for summer. See text for details. (From Horne and Coyne[36])

their temperatures during sleep, and another drawback was that subjects were unable to sleep for as long as they wanted because all of them had daytime jobs or lectures to go to. So their bedtimes and waking-up times remained constant throughout the entire study. Nevertheless, we gathered a large amount of temperature data.

As women usually have a slightly higher body temperature than men, we separated the findings into sexes. Despite the drawbacks to the study, we found distinct seasonal changes with several aspects of waking body temperature. To avoid complications, I will just compare December ('Winter') with June ('Summer'). The findings for March fell roughly mid-way. Both sexes showed very similar results, and only those for men will be shown here (Fig. 6.5). I have identified the circadian peak times by vertical lines to the time axis of the graph. It can be seen that the difference in these times going from winter to summer is a delay of just over an hour. But of greater interest were the morning temperature rises. During the winter, body temperature rose slowly but steadily from waking to its peak, almost in a straight line. On the other hand, in the summer temperature rose much more steeply during the first 2 hours after waking, and then levelled off into a shallow rise until the peak. So, if the temperature terminator idea for sleep holds, with waking not triggered until a certain body temperature point is reached, then the rapid rise of temperature early in the morning during summer suggests that if subjects were allowed to sleep on, then extended sleep would end sooner during the summer than the winter. The temperature decline after the peak time also changed with the seasons, and was steeper during the winter.

6.7 Abnormalities in the timing of sleep

The importance of a circadian 'pacemaker' in the regulation of sleep is illustrated by the variety of problems that can occur in the timing of sleep under
more everyday circumstances. The commonest of these are associated with
shiftwork and 'jet lag'. Sleep is both distorted and shortened by shiftwork,
especially by nightshifts. The picture is confused by the increased incidence
of napping, and by the fact that few shiftworkers ever have sufficient time to
adapt fully to their schedules. Also, on days off, shiftworkers usually return
to their normal sleep–wake habits. This is a very complex area, and as there
are good and recent reviews on the topic[38, 39] I shall not dwell on it.

Two abnormalities in the timing of sleep that are less confounded by other
factors, and clearly illustrate the influence of circadian rhythms, are the
'delayed sleep phase syndrome', and sleep changes in the elderly. The former
condition is a relatively new discovery, identified by the late Dr Elliot
Weitzman, together with colleagues, at the Sleep–Wake Disorders Centre at
Montefiore Hospital, New York[40]. Over a period of several years of assessing
and treating large numbers of insomniacs, it became obvious to these investigators that some patients had certain interesting symptoms in common.
Typically, there is a chronic inability to fall asleep until around 4–5 a.m., and
then to sleep quite well. But as many sufferers have to get up only a few hours
later for work, the sleep they get falls short of what I would see to be near to a
core sleep requirement that they might adapt to. Consequently, they are very
sleepy in the day. For most sufferers, this state of affairs has usually been
going on for years, and is generally quite unresponsive to sleeping tablets.
Often, these people are viewed by their doctors as anxious or even neurotic
insomniacs, despite the common finding that there is little sign of anxiety
outside their understandable worry about sleep.

Weitzman and colleagues found that the cause lay with the circadian
rhythm of sleep. Aberrantly, the mechanism regulating sleep onset seems to
have stuck. The investigators already knew that in order to shift sleep to a
different time of the day, it is much better to extend the circadian day rather
than reduce it. So, for example, it is far easier to adapt to sleeping on a
27-hour 'day' than a 21-hour 'day'. Or, to put this another way, it is easier to
overcome jet lag when flying from east to west (e.g. from the UK to the USA)
than vice versa. In the former, the day has been extended by several hours,
whereas in the latter it has been reduced. For sufferers from the delayed sleep
phase syndrome, going to bed earlier in an attempt to cure the problem in
effect shortens their day.

What they should be doing, reasoned Weitzman, is to arrive at an earlier
bedtime the other way, by lengthening the day. They must go to bed later and
later each day, continuing over a series of days, from the small hours of the
morning, through the morning and afternoon to the early evening, to end up

at, say 11 p.m. Ideally, believed Weitzman, this should be a 27-hour day, maintained for 6 days. So, for example, if sleep onset were usually 5 a.m., then the successive bedtimes would be: 8 a.m., 11 a.m., 2 p.m., 5 p.m., 8 p.m., and ceasing at 11 p.m. Thereafter, bedtime remains at 11 p.m. Patients usually have no difficulty in going to sleep at these later times during the treatment. Then, remarkably, sleep onset usually stays at 11 p.m. For most of Weitzman's sufferers the cure was dramatic. I should add that they are allowed to sleep for up to 8 hours at a time during the treatment days.

Circadian rhythms age, and many sleep researchers consider that the circadian regulation of sleep weakens somehow in the elderly, to produce both obvious and subtle changes in sleeping and waking habits. Sustained sleep at night becomes difficult in the elderly, and so does sustained wakefulness during the daytime, with naps becoming common. Typically, naps occur after lunch, and again around late afternoon. Of course, such naps are also promoted by physical infirmity, loneliness, and boredom. However, there are tremendous differences between old people in the amount of sleep taken per 24 hours, and in how it is taken. Some require much less sleep than when they were young, but others much more. If daytime naps are taken every day, as is often the case with the elderly, then these naps become part of the total daily sleep requirement, and in general terms such naps can be subtracted from what used to be for them a full night's sleep. That is, these naps are 'replacement' naps (see Section 6.4). In many elderly people, naps can add up to 2 hours a day, and if their total daily sleep requirement is, say, 7 hours a day, then this may leave only 5 hours to be taken at night.

Around mid evening, typically 9–10 p.m., elderly people tend to feel sleepy again, owing to the inability to stay awake for very long. Rather than take another nap, for say half an hour, and then be more able to stay up until midnight or beyond, they usually go to bed. Because of sleepiness, sleep comes easily then. But around 3–4 a.m. they tend to wake up, as the full sleep quota has been taken. They may well be quite alert and refreshed, but might not realize this, as 'this is the time one is supposed to be asleep'. Consequently, many believe that they have not had enough sleep, and then worry about not getting back to sleep. Twelve hours may be spent in bed overnight in an attempt to achieve the 'proper amount of sleep'. Lying awake in the small hours of the morning can be a lonely experience, and getting up into a cold house will increase the fuel bills. For one reason or another then, they may resort to sleeping tablets. The metabolism of these drugs by the body is much slower in the elderly, as the organs principally involved in their elimination, the liver and kidneys, become less efficient with age. Consequently, there are more likely to be residual 'hangover' effects of the drug the next day, which will increase daytime sleepiness, promote further napping, and reduce the sleep need the next night–necessitating more sleeping tablets, and so the vicious circle may go on.

One solution, as I have just mentioned, is for the elderly person to try and get into the habit of taking another nap at 10 p.m. (for about half an hour), rather than go to bed, and then stay up for 2 or 3 more hours. Although more time has now been lost from the night-time sleep requirement, a new bedtime at around 1 a.m. followed by 4.5 hours of sleep leads to an acceptable waking-up time.

6.8 Insomnia

If people can adapt to having less sleep, as was shown in Section 6.3, then how is it that 'insomnia' is one of the commonest complaints taken to the general practitioner? One factor is that most of us are brought up to believe that we all 'need a good 8 hours sleep a night', and this notion is being continually promoted by popular articles in newspapers and magazines. Physicians tend to endorse the idea, and 'how are you sleeping', must be one of the first questions asked of most patients. Manufacturers of sleeping tablets exploit the belief further, and it is not surprising that sleeping tablets are one of the commonest forms of prescription taken away by the patient.

Insomnia is one of the few disorders where diagnosis lies with the patient and not with the physician, since outside the EEG laboratory the real extent of the insomnia is impossible to determine. Quite reasonably, physicians view insomnia not to be a serious complaint, and as sleeping tablets are apparently now quite safe drugs many physicians see no harm in prescribing hypnotics. Irrespective of the contentious debate about whether these drugs are good for us in the long term, which I shall avoid, I consider that physicians who unreservedly give out these prescriptions are unwittingly 'rewarding' the insomniac's beliefs about the seriousness of the condition.

I have already described in some detail how the evidence from sleep deprivation research strongly indicates that sleep loss is not as harmful as is commonly thought. But many insomniacs believe that they get too little sleep, and that their health will suffer as a consequence. The key sign of disturbed or insufficient sleep is whether excessive daytime sleepiness is present. However, for the majority of insomniacs this seems not to be the case, as most are in fact getting enough sleep. Although insomniacs may report feeling 'tired' throughout the day, it may not be sleepiness but lethargy and disinterest due to depression. This is why sleep researchers specializing in sleep disorders (see Section 1.1) are careful to distinguish between 'sleepiness' (due to insufficient or disturbed sleep) and this 'tiredness'.

About 10 years ago, the US Institute of Medicine, a division of the prestigious National Academy of Sciences, was asked by President Carter to review the safety, usefulness, and the prescribing practices of hypnotic drugs. Their report[41] contained a survey of the current research on the sleeping habits of insomniacs. It turned out that, without the aid of medication, most insomniacs obtain about 6 hours sleep a night, and few take longer than 20–30 minutes to go to sleep, or have more than 20–30 minutes of wakefulness within the sleeping period. But even more interesting, the report also concluded that when taking sleeping tablets, most sufferers obtain:

1. Less than a 15-minute reduction in getting to sleep.
2. Less than a 15-minute reduction in wakefulness during the night.
3. An increase in sleep length of no more than 30–40 minutes.

Also, the report doubted whether such effects could be sustained to this extent beyond a few weeks of therapy.

So why is insomnia so distressing to the insomniac? There are many reasons, and many books and papers on the subject. Let me just take one type of insomnia as an example—that associated with a difficulty in getting to sleep, so-called 'sleep onset insomnia'. Sufferers tend to overestimate the time it takes to go to sleep by as much as threefold, not as an intended exaggeration but as a genuine belief. An estimated 1.5 hours of tossing and turning in bed may well be only half an hour. The more one worries whilst lying in bed, the slower time seems to pass. Such concerns are further compounded by worrying about 'not getting enough sleep' and anxiety about health. One reason for a greater peace of mind after taking hypnotics is not just through an improvement to sleep, but because most modern hypnotics are also tranquillizers, and reduce the accompanying anxiety.

Since anxiety seems to make the time spent awake pass more slowly, its removal creates a more accurate perception of time. Hence, the apparent time the insomniac believes it takes to go to sleep may decrease dramatically—more than can be accounted for by the genuine reduction in sleep onset achieved by the drug. This can cause the sufferer to attribute greater soporific properties to the drug than really exist. Because the perception of time may be distorted without the drug, but more reliable with it, simply using the patient's own assessment of sleep quality and quantity before and during drug treatment may not give truly reliable results compared with more objective assessments using all-night recording techniques. On the other hand, it could well be argued that it is the patients' own feelings that should be of greater concern to the physician, not such impersonal assessments. This is another controversial issue, and my book has plenty of these already. Let me extract myself from this one by giving some practical advice to the poor sleeper.

The advice concerns the improvement of sleep 'hygiene' by non-drug methods, and is recommended by many sleep disorders centres. Whilst the advantage of hypnotics is that they have an immediate effect, repeated use reduces this. On the other hand, improving sleep hygiene requires more of an effort, takes several days, maybe a few weeks, but the result is usually long lasting, more rewarding, and there are no side effects. So, I will go on to the first point of advice: it concerns daytime naps, which tend to be much more frequent in insomniacs. Although naps are inevitable in the elderly, for the young to middle-aged insomniac they must be avoided, as napping reduces sleepiness at bedtime and creates more difficulties in going to sleep at this time. Naps also further impair the insomniac's circadian sleep–wake rhythm, which in many cases is already 'weakened'. I must emphasize that for the good sleeper daytime naps may be of great benefit, and any impairment to sleep onset at night is usually minor.

The second tip for the insomniac is always to wake up at the same time every morning, using an alarm clock. This helps retrain the circadian rhythm. Weekend 'sleep-ins' are forbidden. Thirdly, going to bed at night must be avoided until sleepiness occurs, irrespective of how late this may be. If, having gone to bed, sleep does not come within a few minutes, then sufferers must get up, leave the bedroom, and do something distracting to occupy their attention. A return to bed should not be contemplated until sleepiness returns. It is important to associate the bed with sleep, and not with distressing wakefulness. Last but not least, various relaxation techniques can also be of help.

6.9 Stage 2 sleep—optional sleep?

So far, this book has made little mention of stage 2 sleep. In young adults, about 50 per cent of a normal night's sleep consists of stage 2, with SWS and REM sleep making up most of the remaining sleep. Whilst stage 2 is more prevalent in the latter part of the night, nevertheless the first three sleep cycles, core sleep, contain about 2 hours of stage 2. Should this initial stage 2 sleep be included as core sleep? Not really—as will now be seen.

From the findings of total sleep deprivation (see Tables 2.1 and 2.3) stage 2 seems to be a very dispensable sleep, as most of it is not reclaimed afterwards. I have emphasized in this book that core sleep centres on the delta EEG activity (SWS), occurring mostly in the first two sleep cycles, and to some extent in the third cycle. The accompanying REM sleep within these three cycles is also part of core sleep.

The 90-minute cycling of REM and non-REM sleep is one of the prominent characteristics of sleep (Figure 1.2). The entire night's REM sleep is not condensed into one long episode of around 100 minutes, or all the SWS into another similar block. For reasons we do not really understand, nature has produced this cyclicity in sleep, spreading out REM sleep, SWS, and the other sleep stages into separate episodes. There seems to be a maximum SWS level that each SWS episode can contain, with the first one being near to its maximum capacity (i.e. it is 'saturated'). The next episode, in the second sleep cycle, is less saturated, and the third episode may almost be empty. This is illustrated in Fig. 5.3, based on Feinberg's work[7]. Extra amounts of SWS, following sleep deprivation for example, can be fitted into these episodes, increasingly with successive SWS episodes as these are less saturated. If necessary, new SWS episodes can be created in later cycles. Even with huge demands for SWS, after many days of sleep deprivation, SWS is still not gathered as one large mass at the beginning of recovery sleep, but is spread out in portions from sleep onset.

If SWS reflects cerebral restitution, then perhaps only a certain amount of this restitution can be achieved at any one time, and periods of testing and rest are necessary before the next episode of restitution can be performed. When a complex repair or overhaul of an intricate machine is carried out, it is often wise to do this in stages, allowing rest pauses and testing. I see such rest pauses to be equivalent to stage 2 sleep, whereas the testing might be done in REM sleep, as will be seen in Chapter 8.

Fig. 6.1 is a simple diagram illustrating the progress of core and optional sleep over the sleep period. To be more accurate, I could have represented core sleep as a series of episodes during the first part of sleep, broken by periods of stage 2 sleep, and not just as a continuous block. But of more importance, Fig. 6.1 does show both core and optional sleep mechanisms to be present at sleep onset, even though it is core sleep that exerts the most influence at the beginning of sleep. I am proposing that stage 2 sleep is a manifestation of optional sleep, present throughout sleep, but obscured by core sleep at the beginning of the night. In a sense, stage 2 sleep is a 'coat-hanger' of sleep, on which can be hung the more essential SWS and some of REM sleep. These 'rest pauses' of stage 2 sleep during the first few sleep cycles might well prevent any repair process from fouling up.

When the restitutive processes of SWS are complete, stage 2 maintains sleep, with the aid of REM sleep. To my mind, stage 2 sleep is a central part of the drive mechanism of optional sleep, maintaining sleep until the wake-up point. Optional REM sleep, at this time, may well continue to test circuits, etc., although it probably has other roles, and these are discussed in some detail in Chapter 8.

Two prominent EEG characteristics of stage 2 sleep are 'spindles' and 'K complexes'. The former, sometimes also called 'sigma activity', consists of bursts of 12–14 Hz waves (Fig. 1.1), lasting for about 0.5–1 second at a time. Interestingly, but inexplicably, women seem to show more spindles than men[42]. In men, spindles appear about two to five times a minute over the night throughout non-REM sleep (except for stage 1 sleep). Spindles are absent from REM sleep, but are particularly obvious in stage 2 sleep, where their occurrence is about double that of SWS[42]. In young adults, the incidence of spindles within sleep increases with successive sleep cycles, but in healthy elderly subjects sleep spindles are generally less apparent, and there is no increasing trend over the night[43]. Some sleep researchers believe that delta waves inhibit spindles, but recent work strongly indicates that this is not so[43].

Sleep spindles are found in those mammals with a well-developed cerebral cortex, for example cats and monkeys, where there is the equivalent of stage 2 sleep (as well as SWS). Studies on the cat[44] suggest that spindles damp down irrelevant input from the senses and preserve the continuity of sleep. This seems also to be the case with humans[45], where it is thought that the increasing number of spindles over the night somehow compensates for the diminishing 'need' for sleep as sleep progresses. The lack of this spindle increase over the night in the elderly may be connected with the greater number of awakenings and disturbance to the latter part of their sleep.

The other notable characteristic of stage 2 sleep, the K complex, can also be seen in Fig. 1.1. Frequently the two phenomena coalesce, and appear as a combined waveform. Usually, K complexes appear spontaneously, with a frequency of about one per minute[46]. But often they are caused by a noise or other stimulus. Typically, the louder or more personally significant the noise, the larger is the K complex[47]. Such findings indicate that some processing of external stimuli by the cerebrum does go on during stage 2 sleep. Not surprisingly, several sleep researchers now view K complexes as extremely large evoked responses[48] (see Section 2.21); however, this is a controversial point. Like spindles, K complexes may well act to reduce or block out unwanted environmental stimuli, to prevent sleep disturbance[46], and help maintain the integrity of sleep.

6.10 Conclusions about core and optional sleep

Descriptions of core and optional sleep are given at the beginning of this chapter. By now, I hope that the reader can see that the splitting up of sleep in this way gives quite a different perspective to sleep than the popular division of REM versus non-REM sleep. The core–optional view can also be applied to the sleep of other mammals, and this forms the basis for the next chapter. One of the first points I raised in favour of the concept of core and optional sleep related to feeding and drinking. For most of us the daily intake of food and water is more than the real physiological requirement, so why not the same for sleep? Also, the opportunities to eat and drink are ever present, and there is much social facilitation here.

The more substantial points I have made in this chapter in relation to the core–optional hypothesis for sleep in humans are summarized as follows:

1. During recovery sleep after sleep deprivation, only about 30 per cent of lost sleep needs to be returned, which is made up of most, if not all, of the lost stage 4 sleep and about half of the lost REM sleep (Section 2.7). This, I argue, constitutes the return of core sleep only.
2. Natural short sleepers seem to have wholly or partly lost the usual latter part of sleep (optional sleep). Their sleep is very similar in structure and in

SWS content to the first few sleep cycles of age-related normal length sleepers (Section 6.2). That is, short sleepers retain their core sleep.

3. Following limited sleep deprivation, long sleepers absorb the extra demand for SWS into a recovery sleep which is of their normal length, whereas short sleepers have to extend their recovery sleep to fit in this SWS demand (Section 2.19). In my view, the sleep of long sleepers contains much optional sleep, and has some capacity to absorb an increased demand for core sleep.

4. Normal 7–8-hour sleepers can adapt quite successfully to 1.5–2 hours less sleep daily—that is down to about 5.5–6 hours of sleep. This is accomplished at the expense of the latter part of sleep (i.e. optional sleep) (Section 6.3).

5. Sleep can be extended easily by about 2 hours through oversleep and daytime naps, although no long-term studies have been done here. This extended sleep has the characteristics of optional sleep. If sleep is extended beyond 2 hours then there is wakefulness (see below), and further sleep becomes fitful. Some core sleep returns as a bicircadian rhythm of SWS coupled with a demand created for SWS by the interim wakefulness and REM sleep (Section 6.4).

6. There is a sleep terminator, or backstop to *uninterrupted* optional sleep, related to a critical point on the circadian temperature rise, that is reached after about 2 hours of oversleep (Section 6.6).

7. Sleep in time-free environments also shows how (optional) sleep can expand and contract, and further demonstrates that the waking-up point is linked to the circadian temperature rise (Section 6.6).

Sleepiness can similarly be subdivided into core and optional components (Section 2.14). Optional sleepiness rather than core sleepiness would mostly prevail when, for example, sleep was reduced to 5.5–hours per night in 7–8 hours a night sleepers. However, after several days this optional sleepiness diminishes, leading to what seems to be full adaptation to sleep reduction. But it is difficult to reduce sleep much further, say down to about 4.5–5 hours of sleep a day, which I have suggested is the limit to core sleep. So there is a 'fluid' region, say between 4.5 and 5.5 hours of sleep, falling between the two limits. It may well take up some extra SWS pressure owing to extended wakefulness. For example, given the positive relationship between SWS and the length of prior wakefulness, a reduction in daily sleep from 8 to 5 hours would necessitate about a 20 per cent increase in SWS.

I am not advocating that we should cut down our sleep to, say, 6 hours a day, only that it can be done. The idea of an extra 2 hours of wakefulness each day may seem appealing, as more work might be done. But my own research indicates that all that tends to happen is that more of the daytime is 'wasted', and the usual day's work is just spread out to fill the time available—one of the so-called 'Parkinson's Laws'[49]. Optional sleep is not to be viewed as wasted time, as for many people this is a period for comfort and relaxation, which may be unavailable to them during wakefulness. My advice then, is if one is happy and enjoys wakefulness, then by all means take some more, but if wakefulness brings stress, and life is a struggle, then maintain your sleep. Taking less sleep because of pressure of work is fine for a few nights, but it is not a good idea in the long term, as valuable hours of daily relaxation have been lost.

Most short sleepers seem on the whole to be healthy individuals, but it is important to distinguish whether they are 'contented' short sleepers, or have been forced into this style by various pressures of waking life. The same applies to long sleepers, as some may retreat to the oblivion of sleep as a form of escape. Whilst there has been some work on the mental health and psychological differences between long and short sleepers (Section 6.2), there has been very little research into their physical health and lifespan. In 1965, a detailed general health survey was carried out on 2222 men and 2491 women aged between 30 and 69 years living in Alameda County, California. Among the numerous questions asked of the responders was sleep length, although, these lengths could not be verified. A 9-year follow-up of the mortality rates of these people ensued[50], and over this period 210 men and 159 women died. For both groups combined, 78 per cent had slept 7 to 8 hours per night, 16 per cent 6 hours or less, and 7 per cent 9 hours or more. It turned out that long and short sleepers had a 30 per cent greater risk of dying than the 7–8 hour sleeper, and this just reached statistical significance. No particular cause of death stood out for the long and short sleepers, and most died from the usual causes—cancer, heart disease, and stroke.

In the original health survey, information about various risk factors was also obtained. Of course, the most powerful one for everyone, long, short, and normal sleepers alike, was age. This was followed by, in decreasing order of importance, general health, how many 'social networks' the individual was involved with (the fewer, the greater was the risk), sex, smoking, alcohol consumption, physical inactivity, and finally sleep length. Sleep length seemed to be a reasonably 'pure' factor, as related risks had been accounted for statistically. So, for example, increased smoking and alcohol consumption were not the cause of a higher mortality in short sleepers, (it could be reasoned that increased wakefulness allows more smoking and drinking).

The original survey also asked subjects to rate themselves for 'trouble in sleeping' on a scale of: 'often', 'sometimes', 'never'. The interrelationship of this variable with short and long sleep was not straightforward. Certainly, the incidence of 'often' in both male and female short sleepers was twice that for the 7–8-hour sleepers, but so was the incidence of 'never'! We cannot assume that the underlying causes of 'trouble in sleeping' were the same for both long and short sleepers. The investigators cautioned against jumping to the conclusion that long or short sleep was the reason for death, as sleep length may well have been just another symptom of deeper causes—stress for example. Finally, it is not known by how much the sleep lengths of these long and short sleepers were natural or forced by circumstances, or to what extent the long and short sleepers led contented versus unpressured lifestyles.

References

1. Webb, W.B. and Agnew, H.W. (1970). Sleep stage characteristics of long and short sleepers. *Science*, **168**, 146–147.
2. Webb, W.B. and Friel, J. (1971). Sleep stage and personality characteristics of 'natural' long and short sleepers. *Science*, **171**, 587–588.
3. Hartmann, E. (1973). *The Functions of Sleep*. Yale University Press, New Haven.
4. Benoit, O., Foret, J., Bouard, G., Merle, B., Landau, J. and Marc, M.E. (1980). Habitual sleep length and patterns of recovery sleep after 24 hour and 36 hour sleep deprivation. *Electroencephalography and Clinical Neurophysiology*, **50**, 477–485.
5. Oswald, I. and Adam, K. (1980). The man who had not slept for ten years. *British Medical Journal*, **281**, 1684–1685.
6. Jones, H.S. and Oswald, I. (1968). Two cases of healthy insomnia. *Electroencephalography and Clincal Neurophysiology*, **24**, 378–380.
7. Feinberg, I. (1974). Changes in sleep cycle pattern with age. *Journal of Psychiatric Research*, **10**, 283–306.
8. Stuss, D. and Broughton, R. (1978). Extreme short sleep: personality profiles and a case study of sleep requirement. *Waking and Sleeping*, **2**, 101–105.
9. Meddis, R., Pearson, A.J.D. and Langford, G. (1973). An extreme case of healthy insomnia. *Electroencephalography and Clinical Neurophysiology*, **35**, 213–214.
10. Fischer-Perroudon, C., Mouret, J. and Jouvet, M. (1974). Sur un cas d'agrypnie (4 mois sans sommeil) au cours d'une maladie de morvan. Effet favorable du 5-Hydroxytryptophane. *Electroencephalography and Clinical Neurophysiology*, **36**, 1–18.
11. Keys, A., Brozek, J., Henschel, A., Mickelsen, O. and Taylor, H.L. (1950). *The Biology of Human Starvation*. University of Minnesota Press, Minneapolis.
12. Husband, R.W. (1935). The comparative value of continuous versus interrupted sleep. *Journal of Experimental Psychology*, **18**, 792–796.
13. Johnson, L.C. and Macleod, W.L. (1973). Sleep and awake behaviour during gradual sleep reduction. *Perceptual and Motor Skills*, **36**, 87–97.
14. Mullaney, D.J., Johnson, L.C., Naitoh, P., Friedmann, J.K. and Globus, G.G. (1977). Sleep during and after gradual sleep reduction. *Psychophysiology*, **14**, 237–244.
15. Friedmann, J.K., Globus, G.G., Huntley, A., Mullaney, D.J., Naitoh, P. and Johnson, L.C. (1977). Performance and mood during and after gradual sleep reduction. *Psychophysiology*, **14**, 245–250.
16. Webb, W.B. and Agnew, H.W. (1974). The effects of a chronic limitation of

sleep length. *Psychophysiology*, **11**, 265–274.

17. Carskadon, M.A. and Dement, W.C. (1981). Cumulative effects of sleep restriction on daytime sleepiness. *Psychophysiology*, **18**, 107–113.

18. Horne, J.A. and Wilkinson, S. (1985). Chronic sleep reduction: daytime vigilance performance and EEG measures of sleepiness, with particular reference to practice effects. *Psychophysiology*, **22**, 69–78.

19. Evans, F.J., Cook, M.R., Cohen, H.D., Orne, E.C., and Orne, M.T. (1977). Appetitive and replacement naps: EEG and behaviour. *Science*, **197**, 687–689.

20. Dinges, D.F., Orne, M.T., Orne, E.C. and Evans, F.J. (1981). Behavioural patterns in habitual nappers. *Sleep Research*, **10**, 163.

21. Aserinsky, E. (1969). The maximal capacity for sleep: Rapid eye movement density as an index of sleep satiety. *Biological Psychiatry*, **1**, 147–159.

22. Aserinsky, E. (1973). Relationship of rapid eye movement density to the prior accumulation of sleep and wakefulness. *Psychophysiology*, **10**, 545–558.

23. Verdone, P. (1968). Sleep satiation: extended sleep in normal subjects. *Electroencephalography and Clinical Neurophysiology*, **24**, 417–423.

24. Feinberg, I., Fein, G. and Floyd, T.C. (1980). EEG patterns during and following extended sleep in young adults. *Electroencephalography and Clinical Neurophysiology*, **50**, 467–476.

25. Feinberg, I., Fein, G. and Floyd, T.C. (1982). Computer detected patterns of electroencephalographic delta activity during and after extended sleep. *Science*, **215**, 1131–1133.

26. Roth, B., Nevsimalova, S. and Rechtschaffen, A. (1972). Hypersomnia with 'sleep drunkenness'. *Archives of General Psychiatry*, **26**, 456–462.

27. Gagnon, P., De Koninck, J. and Broughton, R. (1985). Reappearance of EEG slow waves in extended sleep with delayed bedtime. *Sleep*, **8**, 118–128.

28. Webb, W.B. and Agnew, H.W. (1975). Are we chronically sleep deprived? *Bulletin of the Psychonomic Society*, **6**, 47–48.

29. Taub, J.M. (1981). Behavioural and psychobiological effects of ad-libitum extended-delayed sleep. In: Karacan I., (ed.) *Psychophysiological Aspects of Sleep*, pp. 10–25.

30. Webb, W.B. (1978). The spontaneous ending of sleep. *Perceptual and Motor Skills*, **46**, 984–986.

31. Kleitman, N. (1963). *Waking and Sleeping*. University of Chicago Press, Chicago.

32. Åkerstedt, T. and Gillberg, M. (1981). The circadian variation of experimentally displaced sleep. *Sleep*, **4**, 159–169.

33. Zulley, J., Wever, R. and Aschoff, J. (1981). The dependence of onset and duration of sleep on the circadian rhythm of rectal temperature. *Pflugers Archives*, **391**, 314–318.

34. Czeisler, C.A., Weitzman, E.D., Moore-Ede, M.C., Zimmerman, J.C. and Knauer, R. (1980). Human sleep: its duration and organisation depend on its circadian phase. *Science*, **210**, 1264–1267.

35. Åkerstedt, T. and Gillberg, M. (1986). A dose-response study of sleep loss and spontaneous sleep termination. *Psychophysiology* **23**, 293–297.

36. Simpson, H.W. and Bonien, J.G. (1973). *Biological Aspects of Circadian Rhythms*. Plenum, London.

37. Horne, J.A. and Coyne, I. (1975). Seasonal changes in the circadian variation of oral temperature during wakefulness. *Experientia*, **31**, 1296-1297.
38. Åkerstedt, T. (1985). Adjustments of physiological circadian rhythms and the sleep–wake cycle to shiftwork. In Folkard, S. and Monk, T.H. (ed.) *Hours of Work*. John Wiley, Chichester. pp. 185-198.
39. Kogi, K. (1985). Introduction to the problems of shiftwork. In: Folkard, S. and Monk, T.H. (ed.) *Hours of Work*. John Wiley, Chichester. pp. 165-184.
40. Weitzman, E.D., Czeisler, C.A., Coleman, R.M., Spielman, A.J., Zimmerman, J. and Dement, W. (1981). Delayed sleep phase syndrome. *Archives of General Psychiatry*, **38**, 737-746.
41. Institute of Medicine (1979). *Sleeping Pills, Insomnia, and Medical Practice*. 1OM-79-04. National Academy of Sciences, Washington.
42. Gaillard, J.-M. and Blois, R. (1981). Spindle density in sleep of normal subjects. *Sleep*, **4**, 385-391.
43. Guazzelli, M., Feinberg, I., Aminoff, M., Fein, G., Floyd, T.C. and Maggini, C. (1986). Sleep spindles in normal elderly: comparisons with young adult patterns and relation to nocturnal awakening, cognitive function and brain atrophy. *Electroencephalography and Clinical Neurophysiology*, **63**, 526-539.
44. Bowersox, S.S., Kaitin, K.I. and Dement, W.C. (1985). EEG spindle activity as a function of age: relationship to sleep continuity. *Brain Research*, **334**, 303-308.
45. Silverstein, L.D. and Levy, C.M. (1976). The stability of the sigma sleep spindle. *Electroencephalography and Clinical Neurophysiology*, **40**, 666-670.
46. Halasz, P., Pal, I. and Rajna, P. (1985). K-complex formation of the EEG in sleep. A survey and new examinations. *Acta Physiologica Hungaria*, **65**, 3-35.
47. Oswald, I., Taylor, A.M. and Treisman, M. (1960). Discriminative responses to stimulation during human sleep. *Brain*, **83**, 440-453.
48. Ujszaszi, J. and Halasz, P. (1986). Late component variants of single auditory evoked responses during non-REM sleep stage 2 in man. *Electroencephalography and Clinical Neurophysiology*, **64**, 260-268.
49. Parkinson, C.N. (1958). *Parkinson's Law or The Pursuit of Progress*. John Murray, London.
50. Wingard, D.L. and Berkman, L.F. (1983). Mortality risk associated with sleeping patterns among adults. *Sleep*, **6**, 102-107.

7. Sleep in other mammals

So far this book has concentrated on humans, but the sleep of other mammals also has a lot to add to our understanding of sleep and its function, and I shall now broaden out to other species. I will keep as my central themes: (1) a component of sleep (core sleep) is essential, for what I cannot be sure, but it may well centre on cerebral restitution, (2) sleep in mammals living in dangerous circumstances is down to core levels, whereas safe sleepers have additional sleep (optional sleep) that occupies unproductive hours and conserves energy, (3) for various reasons, the energy conservation value of sleep increases the smaller the mammal.

7.1 Dolphins

The most advanced group of mammals below humans and other apes are the *Cetacea*—the whales and dolphins. It is in only recent years that the sleep of some members of this group has been studied, and, from what we know so far, their sleep patterns are probably the most fascinating of all mammals. Let me start with one type of dolphin which, despite living in perilous circumstances, still appears to sleep, even though this jeopardizes its safety further. Presumably, what sleep it obtains (core sleep) must be vital to survival.

The blind, Indus dolphin (*Platanista indi*) appears to sleep for only seconds at a time, but many times a day. Professor Georg Pilleri, from the University of Berne, has made a detailed study of this extraordinary animal which lives in the muddy and turbid waters of the Indus estuary[1]. It swims on its side and has lost the use of its eyes, although it has a very efficient sonar system. Incredibly, it never stops swimming, seemingly because of the dangerous environment it lives in, especially during the monsoon when the Indus floods, sweeping along uprooted trees and other debris. The animal has to be very alert, avoiding not only these rapidly moving objects, but also being dashed against the rocks below. Consequently, cessation of swimming for more than a brief time would result in it being swept along by the currents, and injury.

The intrigued Pilleri put two captured animals in a large aquarium, and studied them for over 7 years. With the aid of underwater microphones, he found that these dolphins perpetually swam and almost continually emitted sonar and other sounds, except for very brief periods ranging from 4 to 60 seconds, which he attributed to 'microsleeps'. Unfortunately, because of

218

their perpetual movement, sleep EEGs could not be recorded. During the numerous microsleeps, found throughout the day and night, swimming slowed down but did not cease. When added up they came to about 7 hours per 24, which Pilleri considered to be equivalent to the average sleep length for many other mammals.

Now it could be contested that this animal may be able to swim and emit sounds during its sleep, and without any proof from EEGs of sleep occurring, further discussion perhaps ought to be curtailed. But it is unlikely that such complex manouvering and navigation could be done during sleep, even if this dolphin's brain was 'half-asleep'—an extraordinary phenomenon I will cover shortly. Assuming that the microsleeps are truly this animal's sleep, then if sleep did not serve some crucial role in such an advanced mammal it is difficult to imagine why any sleep should be kept, and not evolved out as in the case of its eyes—these are atrophied and almost functionless as they are of no use in muddy water.

Like all dolphins it has a highly developed cerebrum, and I believe that this is why the animal still needs to sleep—for cerebral restitution. What sleep it takes would presumably be core sleep, and in the circumstances I doubt whether it has any optional sleep. Nevertheless, 7 hours of core sleep a day seems a lot. However, because of the nature of the environment this animal has to maintain a high level of awareness of its surroundings (see Section 5.5), higher than for most mammals living in more static circumstances. This might well add to cerebral 'wear and tear' during wakefulness, leading to more cerebral restitution in sleep.

Recordings of the electrical activity of the sleeping brain in two species of dolphin living in the Black Sea, the bottlenose dolphin (*Tursiops truncatus*), and porpoise (*Phocoena phocoena*), have recently been made by Dr Lev Mukhametov and colleagues at the Institute of Evoluntary Morphology and Ecology of Animals, in Moscow[2]. This pioneering work required many years of development, and in all, 30 animals in captivity in an aquarium were investigated. Sleep was recorded from freely moving animals in the water, via long zero-buoyancy cables. All animals showed the same extraordinary sleep pattern. For them the term, 'to be half asleep' can be taken quite literally. They sleep with one cerebral hemisphere at a time, the other remaining awake. Both species sleep mostly at night, with sleep typically lasting for about 12 hours. The sleep period starts with one hemisphere sleeping for about 2 hours and the other remaining awake. This is followed by around one hour of wakefulness in both hemispheres, and then 2 hours of sleep in the other hemisphere, with the first hemisphere remaining awake.

Such a pattern, which continues throughout the night, is seen in Fig. 7.1, showing sleep and wakefulness in both hemispheres over 24 hours. For both hemispheres sleep consists of two types: (1) high amplitude delta activity, apparently identical to our stage 4 sleep, which occupies about 30 per cent of

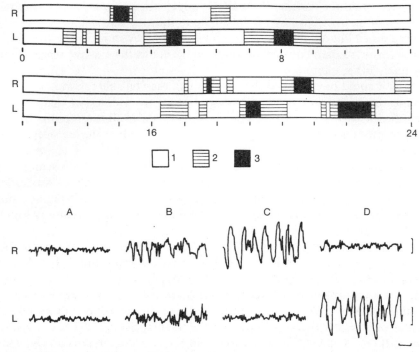

Fig. 7.1 Sleep in a bottlenose dolphin.

Upper—Progress of wakefulness (1), 'intermediate' (2) and 'deep' (3) forms of sleep in right and left hemispheres over 24 hours. Sleep usually occurs only in one hemisphere at a time with the other remaining awake. This alternates throughout the night. See text for details.

Lower—EEG patterns in the right (R) and left (L) hemispheres: (A) high frequency activity of alert wakefulness in both hemispheres. (B) low amplitude delta activity of 'intermediate' sleep in the right hemisphere, and to some extent in the left hemisphere; (C) high amplitude delta waves of 'deep' sleep in the right hemisphere only; (D) in the left hemisphere only. (From Mukhametov[2]. Reproduced by permission of Springer-Verlag NY Inc.)

sleep in these animals, and (2) a lower amplitude delta and theta activity, also containing sleep spindles, seemingly of intermediate depth, and probably equivalent to the borderline between our stages 2 and 3 sleep. Occasionally this latter sleep occurs in both hemispheres at once, but as can be seen in Fig. 7.1 the 'deep' sleep only appears in one hemisphere at a time. Interestingly, some of Mukhametov's dolphins generally showed more sleep in the right hemisphere compared with the left, and others vice versa.

Mukhametov found no signs of REM sleep in any of the dolphins he studied. There was an absence of rapid eye movements, no loss of tone in the neck muscles, no increase in brain temperature that often accompanies REM sleep in other mammals, no hippocampal theta activity or PGO spikes (see Section 8.10 for a description of these latter characteristics of REM sleep). Such an absence of REM sleep, if it can be confirmed, is of considerable importance as it indicates that, for these animals at least, REM sleep is not a crucial form of sleep. Whilst Mukhametov is convinced about these animals having no REM sleep, he is cautious about whether REM sleep could be so dispensable in other mammals. For example, REM sleep might serve a vital function in mammals, but in the case of the dolphin this may have been taken over by other unknown mechanisms.

Several possibilities have crossed my mind as to why this animal has no REM sleep. For example, REM sleep usually causes a generalized paralysis (see Chapter 8), which would impair the animal's need to keep swimming (see below). Another reason relates to dreaming. Assuming that dreaming usually accompanies REM sleep in the intact brain of advanced mammals, then a state whereby one hemisphere was awake and the other was dreaming could well present considerable problems with reality confused with fantasy. But I suspect that perhaps I am being too anthropomorphic.

Mukhametov also noticed in his dolphins that during sleep one eye remains open, with the open eye changing from side to side over the night. However, the open eye is unrelated to the hemisphere that happens to be awake at the time. Whether or not this open eye is vigilant is another matter that is unresolved (the optic nerve in the dolphin is unlike that of other advanced mammals, as all the information from one eye goes to the opposite hemisphere). In dolphins, the main connecting pathway linking the two cerebral hemispheres, the corpus callosum, is poorly developed. Although this could be a reason why the two hemispheres sleep independently, Mukhametov disagrees with such a view by pointing out that: (1) the 'half' sleep in the dolphin is also to be found in regions below the hemispheres, and for example can be seen in the thalamus; (2) other mammals with a poorly developed corpus callosum, like the opossum, have normal 'bilateral' sleep in the two hemispheres; (3) when this pathway is severed in mammals with a fully developed corpus callosum, they still carry on with 'bilateral' sleep.

Mukhametov and colleagues[3] were further able to sleep deprive one hemisphere at a time in the dolphin, by awakening the animal each time the hemisphere selected for deprivation went to sleep. The other hemisphere was allowed to sleep normally. The non-deprived hemisphere did not attempt to sleep longer in some form of compensation. However, on recovery the deprived hemisphere took extra sleep mostly in the form of high amplitude delta activity, the 'deep' sleep shown in Fig. 7.1, in the same way seen in humans after sleep deprivation. I strongly suspect that this animal's delta activity, like ours, is also core sleep. I do not know to what extent its 'intermediate' sleep may be core or optional. It should be remembered though that, because these animals were sleeping in the confined, safe environment of an aquarium, they may have been extending their sleep beyond normal limits with this 'intermediate' sleep, in a similar manner to humans (Section 6.4).

These Russian workers have also looked at the sleep of another group of marine mammals, three species of seal—the Caspian, harp, and northern fur seals. The first two showed no signs of 'half' sleep, but it was present to some extent in the fur seal. This animal had REM sleep as well as a lighter non-REM sleep, with both these sleep states appearing in the two hemispheres together. However, the 'deeper' sleep, containing much delta activity, only occurred in one hemisphere at a time, with the other hemisphere having either 'intermediate' sleep or wakefulness.

Why do these members of the dolphin family and the fur seal have such peculiar sleep? Mukhametov emphasized that marine mammals face the problem of sleeping in the water combined with a need to swim to the surface in order to breathe. This seems to have been solved in different ways. Seals (which, by the way, will sleep on land rather than in water if given the choice) show prolonged breath holding and physical immobility during sleep, lasting about 15–30 minutes (depending on the depth below water), with brief arousals for swimming to the surface to breathe. In this way both hemispheres may sleep at once, with one or both hemispheres waking in order to enable a swim to the surface. Dolphins cannot hold their breath like seals, and have to swim frequently to the surface to breathe. The evolution of the dolphins' 'half' sleep may therefore have been a necessary adaptation so that breathing could be maintained somehow by the waking hemisphere—perhaps allowing frequent swimming to the surface.

Dolphins have another peculiar problem with breathing during sleep. Mukhametov has shown that if 'deep' sleep is induced in both hemispheres simultaneously, by the use of drugs, then the animal ceases breathing entirely. Again, it avoids this problem with 'half' sleep. Such an obstacle does not seem to be present in the fur seal, as induction of this 'deep sleep' in both hemispheres does not impair breathing.

There are indications that at least another member of the whale family also has 'half' sleep. A short report[4] on the brain activity in both hemispheres during sleep in a single, captive North Pacific pilot whale (*Globicephala scammoni*), found delta activity in one hemisphere and wakefulness in the other. However, the authors were cautious about their findings, as the animal died shortly afterwards.

This remarkable development of sleep in such advanced mammals again demonstrates that sleep must serve an essential purpose. Otherwise, why should the further adaptation of sleep occur when sleep is so hazardous to breathing, and may leave the animal exposed to other dangers? It is difficult to understand how, as some might suggest, the function of sleep in this animal is wholly for occupying unproductive hours, when one side or other of its brain remains awake throughout the night. Why would Nature go to all the bother of this 'half' sleep if at least some sleep was not vital? The dolphin's cerebrum is nearly at the level of complexity as that of the human, and it is fair to assume that without sleep the dolphin's cerebrum would suffer in the same way as does ours.

On a final note, many species of bird spend a portion (but not all) of sleep with one eye open and the other closed, and this has led to speculation about whether they might also have 'half' sleep. Indeed, this now seems to be so, at least in the glaucous winged gull (*Larus glaucescens*). Very recent and remarkable work by Drs Charles Amlaner, Nigel Ball, and colleagues, now at the Zoology Department at the University of Arkansas[5], has shown that about 17 per cent of sleep in these birds is of this type, with the remainder being normal bilateral sleep.

7.2 Laboratory vs natural habitats

A major problem encountered when monitoring the sleep of animals in confinement, out of their natural habitat, is that they have little to occupy their time. Food is supplied, and there is no need to forage. Movement is restricted by a cage. So any predator or other danger they might normally encounter is absent, and they do not have to remain alert. We know that humans in similar circumstances will take more (optional) sleep (Section 6.4) and, apparently, so do farm animals living in a stall (see below).

Taking Mukhametov's dolphins for example, which had to be kept in a small aquarium, it is likely that they slept for longer than usual, presumably by taking more of the 'intermediate' sleep. On the other hand, it could be argued that they may have been distressed by the confinement and by the techniques used for monitoring brain activity. This may have resulted in sleep disturbance and reduced sleep. Mukhametov acknowledged this latter possibility, but claimed that it was not likely as his animals had several weeks to adapt to the apparatus. However, he did recognize the greater problem of confinement. So we still do not know to what extent this recorded sleep was truly natural. In theory, Mukhametov as well as other researchers interested in animal sleep should measure sleep in the animals' natural state, using, for example, small radio transmitters attached to the head ('radiotelemetry'). Whilst this has been done in some terrestrial animals, it can be extremely difficult in practice—particularly so with dolphins, as not only do transmitters have a limited range underwater, but the animals move rapidly in a territory of hundreds of square miles.

From the few studies that have looked at sleep in mammals vulnerable to predators, in both safe and dangerous environments, sleep is indeed longer when under safety, especially in farm animals. Here, there is more drowsiness—a finding carefully explored by Dr Yves Ruckebusch of the National Vetinary School in Tolouse. From extensive monitoring of farm animals, sleep in the field was found to be shorter than in the stable. Ruckebusch referred[6] to this extra sleep as 'luxury sleep', which 'exceeds the apparent physiological requirement' (p. 152). His luxury sleep is very similar in concept to my optional sleep, and predates me by several years. This luxury sleep, though, really refers to extensions of normal sleep, whereas my optional sleep also includes the latter part of normal sleep. But of course, we are dealing with different animals. He is concerned with timid farm mammals, where sleep may have already been near to a core minimum with little room for any reduction. I, on the other hand, have been relating mainly to humans, where reduction is possible.

Until now I have been describing changes in sleep length in individual animals, and am not referring to various species that are habitually 'short' and 'long' sleepers, like the deer versus the cat—a topic that I shall be coming to. However, even these long and short sleepers seem to have the capacity to extend sleep further, or, in the case of predators, reduce it. A good example of the latter comes from the renowned work on the sleep of the domestic cat, by Professor Pierluigi Parmeggiani and colleagues at the University of Bologna. His primary field of interest has been thermoregulation during sleep, especially in REM sleep (see Chapter 8). It is Parmeggiani who must take much of the credit for the idea of dividing sleep into the two types that I call core and optional sleep, which he refers to, as 'obligate' and 'facultative' sleep. Because of his other interests, Parmeggiani has only given his idea cursory attention since his conception of it in 1970[7]. His perspective mostly applies to REM sleep[7]. I use my two terms rather than his, as mine are simpler to refer to, and encompass both REM and non-REM sleep.

During the course of experiments on thermoregulation, Parmeggiani and his coworker Dr Carlos Rabini[7] studied cats sleeping in cold environments. As the environmental temperature fell, sleep became shorter and more inter-rupted, which is not surprising. But the interesting finding related to REM sleep, which was particularly prone to be lost, seemingly to be replaced by wakefulness. However, when the cats were allowed recovery sleep at a normal temperature, missing REM sleep was only reclaimed when its loss exceeded about 60 per cent of the usual daily levels. This apparently dis-pensable 60 per cent was described by Parmeggiani as 'facultative sleep', with the remaining 40 per cent being an 'obligate quota'—reclaimed when lost. Such percentages are very similar to those found for recovery sleep in humans after sleep deprivation (Chapter 2). We only reclaim around 30–50 per cent of lost REM sleep. Parmeggiani believed that the reduction of REM sleep in the cold was due to a failure the cat has with thermoregulation during this type of sleep, leaving the animal very vulnerable to unwanted body heat losses. Such problems are not present in non-REM sleep, and therefore relatively more of this sleep can occur in the cold. By the way, the state of thermoregulation during REM sleep is itself a matter for debate, which is covered in Sections 8.11 and 8.12.

7.3 Statistical analyses of mammalian sleep

Several sleep investigators have collated data on the characteristics of sleep in a variety of mammalian species, especially sleep length, and the amount of

REM and non-REM sleep. Through the use of various complex techniques of statistical correlation, these amounts have been compared with other variables that fall under the two headings:

'Constitution'—for example, body weight or metabolic rate (metabolic rate is proportional to body weight raised to the power of 0.75—see Sections 2.2 and 7.4), brain weight, lifespan, gestation time, etc.
'Sleep safety'—for example, the threat of predation, and how physically safe the sleeping animal is—does it sleep in a tree or burrow?

Over the last decade, three such analyses have been performed, by different people, using up to 53 mammalian species each time. Although such findings have shed some light on our understanding of sleep, the outcome has not been so clear as many had hoped. The problems have been threefold. First, there is the validity of the actual sleep data used, as of necessity most of this information has come from laboratory studies. So there may be some doubt about whether the sleep that was recorded is typical of what would be expected from the animal free in its natural surroundings, not only able to forage and move around, but also perhaps under threat from predators. Second, there has been a difficulty with the types of mammals put into the statistical 'melting pot'. For example, there may be too much bias towards one group of animals (e.g. rodents), causing distortions. Third, there has been debate about the statistical analyses themselves, and whether these have been 'correctly' interpreted, even though there may not be any agreed-upon correct interpretation.

Bearing such points in mind, let me go through these findings, starting with the earliest and most substantive of the three analyses, carried out in the early 1970s at the University of Chicago Sleep Laboratory by Drs Harold Zepelin and Allan Rechtschaffen[8]. They based their results on the sleep of 53 mammalian species. Simple observations of animals sleeping in the wild tended to be excluded by the authors as being unreliable. They looked for objectivity in the data to be used, and in most cases this was based on EEG measurements. In many respects this reasoning is sound, but it meant that most of the data they used came from laboratory investigations. The aspects of sleep used by Zepelin and Rechtschaffen were: total sleep, amounts of non-REM and REM sleep, percentage of REM sleep, and time between successive periods of REM sleep ('sleep cycle' length). These were compared with constitutional variables such as lifespan, metabolic rate, and brain weight.

One dilemma encountered by Zepelin and Rechtschaffen was what to do with 'drowsiness', found extensively in ruminants. Was this to be classified as sleep or wakefulness? During drowsiness these animals usually stand still and chew the cud. Their eyes slowly open and close, and the head may droop. In some mammals such as humans, drowsiness only occupies a few minutes of the day and poses no problems, whereas for the cat and cow drowsiness occupies several hours a day. The not-ideal solution, somewhat reluctantly applied by Zepelin and Rechtschaffen (p. 245), was based on the expediency that drowsiness is halfway between sleep and wakefulness. So they added half of drowsiness time to the sleep quota, and half to wakefulness. Amusingly, 'to be half asleep' takes on another interpretation here, contrasting with that of the dolphin!

The species used in Zepelin and Rechtschaffen's analysis covered 12 orders and 33 families, ranging in body size from the elephant and giraffe to the mouse and little brown bat, and varying in level of evolutionary advancement from the insectivores (such as the tenrec and hedgehog) to the apes (the human and chimpanzee). These species contrast with each other in many other respects, such as food habits, safety, climate, and whether they hibernate. Although such factors could not be considered by the investigators, I must emphasize that Zepelin and Rechstchaffen fully appreciated these finer points, and treated with considerable caution both their statistical analyses and conclusions.

The statistic used by the authors was 'Pearson's correlation coefficient'. For readers not familiar with this method, correlations are typically performed between two variables, and give an index of the extent to which one variable relates to the other. Of course, this does not imply that one causes the other, as both may be the result of a deeper cause. Correlation coefficients have a plus or minus sign and a number that indicates the strength. Values range from minus one (100 per cent negative correlation—both factors change in completely the opposite direction), through zero (no correlation), to plus one (100 per cent positive correlation—both change in completely the same direction). If a correlation is squared and multiplied by 100, then the 'shared variance' is obtained, and describes how much of one variable can be predicted from the other. For example, a correlation of 0.5 gives 25 per cent shared variance—that is only one-quarter of the value of one factor can be explained by the other, leaving three-quarters still to be accounted for. The correlation scale is exponential, as, for example, to double the shared variance to 50 per cent the correlation only has to rise to 0.7, and to triple this variance to 75 per cent the correlation rises to 0.87, etc.

The most apparent outcome from Zepelin and Rechtschaffen's findings was a + 0.64 correlation between sleep length and metabolic rate (i.e. the smaller the mammal, the longer it slept). This suggested to the authors that sleep may have the function of enforcing rest and saving energy. But as there were inconsistencies, with a few small mammals sleeping little, and some large ones sleeping a lot, the investigators were only tentative in their proposal that metabolic rate helped determine sleep length. Shared variance only came to 41 per cent, and both variables may simply be the result of some other common cause. This latter point may particularly apply to another noticeable finding, that sleep length was correlated negatively (– 0.52) with lifespan (i.e. the longer the sleep, the shorter the life), as the most likely explanation is that both lifespan and sleep length independently depend on metabolic rate. Remember also that this latter correlation is across species, and does not apply to individuals within a species—e.g. short sleepers amongst humans do not live longer.

Although brain weight also correlated negatively (-0.71) with sleep length, the underlying factor was again almost certainly metabolic rate—increasing metabolism comes with a smaller body size, and therefore there is a smaller brain. Interestingly though, and for reasons that were not clear, brain weight correlated very highly with sleep cycle length ($+0.92$). Nothing of great interest was found for REM sleep. Whenever relatively high correlations were found, these were by virtue of the relationship between REM sleep and total sleep length—longer sleep means more REM sleep.

The second set of statistical analyses on sleep was by Drs Truett Allison and Domenic Cicchetti, from the Veterans Administration Hospital in West Haven, Connecticut[9]. This appeared 2 years after that of Zepelin and Rechtschaffen, and concentrated upon the effects of safety on sleep, as this was not covered previously. Allison and Cicchetti obtained data suited to their needs from 39 species of mammal, many being from the same sources used by Zepelin and Rechtschaffen. Three aspects of safety were adopted: (1) the degree to which an animal was preyed upon, (2) safety of the sleeping place, for example whether the animal slept in a burrow, up a tree, or was exposed, (3) 'overall danger', an amalgam of categories (1) and (2).

Constitutional variables similar to those used by Zepelin and Rechts-chaffen were also taken, for example body weight (not metabolic rate, note), brain weight, and lifespan. Only two aspects of sleep were employed: the amounts of REM and non-REM sleep. Total sleep time was not reported on, as Allison and Cicchetti claimed that non-REM sleep was so highly corre-lated with total sleep time (82 per cent shared variance) that a further corre-lation using total sleep would not add any more to the findings.

Correlations coefficients between all the constitutional variables and both REM and non-REM sleep turned out always to be negative. For example, between non-REM sleep and (1) lifespan, (2) body weight, and (3) brain weight, the respective correlation coefficients were -0.38, -0.71, and -0.68. The authors of course emphasized that such correlations by them-selves do not reveal true relationships, nor do they show which variables are particularly important in accounting for sleep differences between mammals. To improve matters, Allison and Cicchetti carried out more sophisticated calculations using 'factor analysis'. I shall not go into detail about this tech-nique, except to say that it enables one to look at a matrix of correlations between many variables from different 'angles', and extract any key factors running through the matrix. Correlation coefficients as such are not produced by this technique, but something similar called 'loadings', which also range from – 1 to + 1. For simplicity, let us consider correlation coefficients and loadings to be the same.

Two fairly powerful underlying factors emerged:

1. *Body size* influenced non-REM sleep more (– 0.63 loading) than REM sleep (– 0.40 loading)—larger size means less of both types of sleep.
2. *Overall danger* influenced REM sleep (– 0.69 loading) more than non-REM sleep (– 0.48 loading)—more danger leads to less of both types of sleep.

Of course, body size and overall danger are not entirely independent of each other. For example, not only do larger mammals have less non-REM sleep, but there is also some influence of danger, as it is more difficult for them to use safe refuges such as trees or holes.

This relationship between body weight and non-REM sleep endorsed Zepelin and Rechtschaffen's findings of an association between sleep length and metabolic rate. Remember, total sleep is mostly made up of non-REM sleep, and metabolic rate depends on body size.

Allison and Cicchetti remind us that even though two powerful factors had been identified, other variables influencing sleep still need to be found. They also recognized that by including large herbivores in their analyses, as they did, there may have been a substantial improvement of the correlation between non-REM sleep and body size across mammals in general. High amounts of total sleep are a particular disadvantage to large herbivores as they have to spend much time in eating (see Section 7.9). In fact, a later analysis by Meddis, which I am coming to, concluded that herbivores had such a powerful effect on the statistics that these animals were the real cause of the overall relationship between body weight and non-REM/total sleep length. But this issue must not detract from Allison and Cicchetti's major finding of the strong inhibition that 'overall danger' has on REM sleep, even though the majority of the variance is still unaccounted for. Why danger diminishes REM sleep more than non-REM sleep was a puzzle to the investigators. In my view, though, this further suggests that part of REM sleep is dispensable, with the 'lost' REM sleep being part of optional sleep.

The third and most recent statistical analysis of mammalian sleep was carried out by Dr Ray Meddis[10], my colleague at Loughborough University. He used a total of 65 species. Most of the sleep data came from sources common to the two previous analyses, with the addition of some new findings. He adopted most of the variables used before, with some more, including:

Encephalization—an estimate of how advanced the cerebrum is.
Grazing—whether or not the mammal is a herbivore.
Brain maturity at birth—animals born relatively mature (i.e. precocial) have

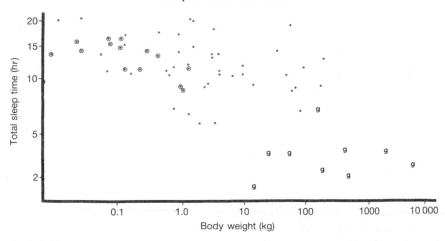

Fig. 7.2 Plot of body weight against total sleep time for 65 species of mammal. (g = grazer, * = non-grazer, ⊛ = rodent). Values have been converted to logarithms to straighten any potential trends, and to compress the otherwise massive scale for body weight. The apparent fall in sleep length with increasing body weight is lost when grazers and non-grazers are treated separately. See text for details. (Reproduced by permission of Ray Meddis)

more developed brains than those born immature and in a helpless (altricial) condition.

Meddis's results were both interesting and disappointing, as some of the apparently clearer findings from the previous analyses now become clouded, especially the relationship between total sleep length and body weight. This now dropped to a correlation of – 0.61 (37 per cent shared variance). As non-REM sleep showed a similar outcome to total sleep time in this and in most other respects, I will be dealing with total sleep time alone. The variable that had the greatest effect on total sleep time was grazing, with the correlation between the two being – 0.79 (62 per cent shared variance). In fact, when the grazing animals are taken out from the correlation between body weight and total sleep time, the correlation fell to – 0.1—next to nothing. It seems that the significant correlation between body weight and sleep length is an artefact produced by including grazing animals! This can be seen in Fig. 7.2 showing total sleep time plotted against body weight for all the species Meddis used. Grazing animals are identified by 'g', and the remainder by '*'. For interest, I have also identified the rodents, by ⊛. When grazers and non-grazers are combined, a fall in sleep length with increasing body weight is apparent, but within each of these two groups the trend is minor—likewise for the rodents.

Meddis produced another surprising outcome, this time for REM sleep. Whilst overall danger correlated negatively with REM sleep (– 0.66), supporting Allison and Cicchetti's finding, an apparently better predictor of REM sleep turned out to be brain maturity at birth, correlating − 0.73 (55 per cent shared variance) with REM sleep. That is the greater this maturity and precociousness of the animal at birth, the less is the REM sleep in the adult.

Such a correlation might seem odd, as we are considering REM sleep in the adult, not at birth. But from the work of Jouvet-Mounier and colleagues[11], which I will be describing in Section 8.3, we know that the sleep of neonatal mammals born in an advanced state contains less REM sleep than does the sleep of a more immature neonate. Consequently, as the amount of REM sleep within sleep declines as mammals get older, those with less REM sleep to start with, at birth, may well have less later. Although this might well explain Meddis's findings, I must emphasize that he provides other possible interpretations that the curious reader should read[10].

Meddis found that the correlation between overall danger and brain maturity at birth is almost negligible (+ 0.1), indicating that the correlation REM sleep has with overall danger is independent of its relationship with brain maturity. If both these variables are combined (overall danger and brain maturity at birth), then a far better correlation is now produced with REM sleep than by either variable alone. This came to an impressive + 0.94, accounting for 88 per cent of the shared variance.

After seeing a draft of Meddis's paper, Zepelin had the opportunity to comment on it, to which Meddis replied. The exchange between the two makes interesting reading[12]. As one might expect, Zepelin homed in on the issue of grazers, and accused Meddis of being rather arbitrary in deciding which mammals are to be classified this way. Whilst Meddis viewed grazers to be hoofed (ungulate) mammals like the horse, deer, goat, elephant, sheep, and cow, Zepelin on the other hand argued that, for example, the gorilla, rabbit, guinea pig, and beaver ought to be included as well, because they also graze. Zepelin's definition therefore contains a wider variety of animals. I think that the issue is best resolved if I substitute the term 'ungulate' for 'grazer' in Meddis's analyses. Then his conclusion still stands—that one group of mammals seems to be distorting the high correlation between body weight and total sleep time across all the mammals. If the ungulates are removed from the analysis the correlation falls profoundly.

Zepelin and Meddis also debated about other biases in the types of mammals used, and the levels correlations have to achieve before reaching statistical significance. Again, I will not go into details, except to mention that Meddis stressed that, in order to try and understand what factors really influence sleep, we should look for relatively high values of shared variance, and not waste too much time on correlations of, say, under 0.4.

In some respects we are now back where we started, as the net outcome of the analyses by Zepelin and Rechtschaffen, Allison and Cicchetti, and

Meddis is that we are still unclear about what factors influence total sleep length, although we do have more insight into REM sleep. It is easy for me to be wise after the event, and the comments I am about to make are not meant to be critical of these analyses. The hypotheses and constitutional variables used were reasonable to begin with. I am just going to illustrate how complex the factors that influence sleep must be, and that we should only consider those analyses as starting points. Besides, even the largest sample was limited to only 65 species, whereas ideally hundreds would be necessary as a good sample—after all, there are around 37 000 species of living mammals.

Influences on sleep length will vary from species to species, and it is unlikely that one or even a few such factors will be prominent throughout all mammals. Even amongst the rodents there is a wide variety of ecological niches, ranging from tree-dwelling seed eaters living in cold climates to desert-living insect eaters dwelling in burrows. Body size also varies substantially in the rodents—from the mouse to the beaver for example. There is even a problem over what is the 'true' body weight of some of these animals. For example, hibernators can easily double their weight from spring to autumn, due to large fat deposits and growth of hair. For correlations between body weight and sleep length, body weight without fat and fur (lean body mass) would be more appropriate.

A key factor that is difficult to measure, but must have a crucial role to play in determining sleep length, relates to what other demands there are on the animal's time, for example how long has to be spent looking for food and in eating? The type of food is important, and grazer versus non-grazer is only one dimension. 'Non-grazer' includes carnivores, fruit eaters, seed eaters, etc., and covers foods of varying energy and protein contents. A carnivore can eat in a few minutes sufficient to last it for a day or longer, but the food of a grazer is of such low nutritional value that the animal has to spend much of the day eating in order to survive. On the other hand, there is another contrast in the time it takes these two groups of animals to look for food. The grazer, surrounded by grass, may use up only minutes during the day in this pursuit, whereas the carnivore can spend all day this way, without success. Any potential for sleep must depend on how much spare time remains after the demands of feeding and foraging.

It might be argued that the total time spent looking for food and in eating comes to the same figure for both groups of animal, but this is a controversial point. Of course, for the laboratory-confined mammal where there is easy access to food, little or no time has to be spent in foraging. Also, the food may be in 'pellets' and nutritionally dense, with less time than would be normally spent in eating. As I have already pointed out, much of the sleep data that is available on mammals comes from assessments made in the laboratory, and may be quite unlike that in the wild, where there is likely to be less opportunity for sleep owing to different feeding and other pressures.

The sleep which I have just been describing mostly falls into my category of optional sleep. However, core sleep is also implicated. Hunting for food and stalking prey require a more advanced behaviour than does chewing grass all day. Not surprisingly, carnivores generally have a more highly developed cerebrum and greater degree of encephalization than do grazers—a topic that will be dealt with in Section 7.8. The point I want to make now is that because of this greater encephalization more cerebral recovery may be needed in sleep, and, in my view, carnivores might well need more core sleep. Of course, herbivores have to remain vigilant for predators, but the 'collective vigilance' of the herd in which they usually live allows most individual members to have a low level of awareness, except that is those members acting as sentinels on the herd's perimeter.

Other factors that are easily overlooked in correlations between constitutional variables and sleep length come under the heading of 'energy conservation during sleep'—almost certainly a crucial function of sleep in small mammals. Whilst small mammals like rodents may sleep longer than large mammals, suggesting that sleep may be conserving energy, we must not forget:

1. The extent of the fall in metabolism during sleep.
2. Whether a torpor develops.
3. Whether there is a nest and how thermally insulating it is.
4. Whether several animals huddle together when sleeping.
5. Whether the animal is nocturnal or diurnal and naturally lives in a hot or cold environment.

The importance of these points will now be discussed.

7.4 Sleep—the immobilizer and energy conserver for small mammals

I mentioned in Section 4.2 that small mammals such as rodents and insectivores do not have the capacity to show useful amounts of relaxed wakefulness. I argued that there are two causes for this. Firstly, relaxed wakefulness is an advanced form of behaviour involving 'contemplation' or the like, and this is beyond the ability of their cerebrum. Secondly, in their natural state they have little time for such relaxation, as more vital activities have to be carried out, particularly feeding, and to a lesser extent, infant rearing, sexual behaviour, and grooming. Therefore, when these essential tasks are completed, the animals need to be immobilized to prevent any wasting of energy over less fruitful activities. Saving energy in this way conserves the local food resources, and allows more individuals to flourish in the area. Another advantage of immobility, it will be remembered, is to allow mitosis and other aspects of body restitution to proceed without hindrance

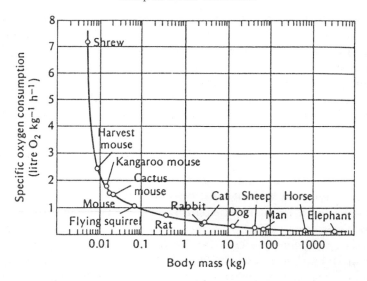

Fig. 7.3 Resting metabolic rate rises with decreasing body size. Body weight is on a logarithmic scale. (From Schmidt-Nielson[13]. Reproduced by permission of Cambridge University Press)

(Section 4.4). Sleep is the *only real* immobilizer for these animals, and as I have just outlined sleep has the further energy-saving advantages of confining the animal to the insulation of its nest, encouraging huddling, and allowing a torpor to develop. On the other hand, the well-developed cerebrum of advanced mammals allows them to sit and relax during wakefulness, and energy can be conserved this way without them having to sleep in order to be immobilized.

Fig. 7.3 shows the accelerating (exponential) rise in metabolic rate as body size gets smaller, going from the elephant to the shrew. In Section 2.2 I mentioned that the problem for small mammals is that their body surface is relatively large in relation to body volume, and as a result, much body heat can be lost to the outside[14]. To compensate, the animal has to have a higher heat production—the metabolic rate is greater, more oxygen is consumed, more energy stores are burnt up, and more food has to be eaten[14]. In real terms, small species of shrew have to eat their own body weight of food each day to survive. The mouse, somewhat larger, has to eat one-quarter of its body weight a day, and at the other extreme the elephant eats only one-twentieth of its weight. Put differently, one human body weight's worth of mice (about 5 000 mice) would have to eat 17 times more food per day than a human[15]. This is why so much of wakefulness in these small mammals has to be spent foraging for food, and when completed the next best thing for them to do is to minimize body heat loss by retiring to the nest. The laboratory

mouse is different in both these respects. No foraging is necessary, as food is
forever in easy reach, and the laboratory environment is usually quite
warm—so the need to stay in the nest and conserve body heat is not so great.
Besides, not many laboratories supply their animals with nesting material
anyway.

There is a potential problem for one of my themes—the point that, in order
to maximize energy conservation, small mammals should not waste energy in
useless physical activity, and should be immobilized (by sleep). In certain
respects it can be argued that physical activity in small mammals is far less
costly than is the case for a larger animal such as a dog (see below), and the
small mammal can, after all, waste time running around. Let me explain
further, firstly by looking at the energy cost of physical activity. Fig. 7.4
comes from the work of Dr Richard Taylor and colleagues, based at the
Zoology Department, Duke University. It shows how oxygen consumption
increases with running speed in a variety of mammals, ranging in size from a
mouse to a large dog. Resting metabolism (i.e. zero speed) is greater in the
smaller mammals, for reasons I have already explained. For all the animals,
however, there is a linear relationship between running speed and oxygen
consumption—but there are also important differences.

In the mouse, for example, the difference between its resting metabolic
rate and that of running at half of its top speed is about 1 litre of oxygen per

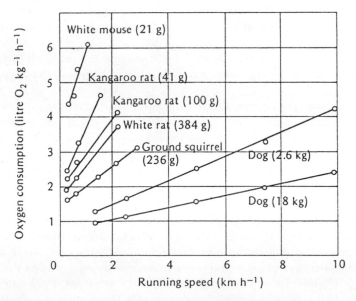

Fig. 7.4 Energy cost of running in various mammals—this rises more steeply with
increasing running speed as body size decreases. See text for details. (From Taylor et al.[16].
Reproduced by permission of Cambridge University Press)

kilogram body weight per hour, which is an increase of about 55 per cent over resting levels. On the other hand, for the larger dog also running at half of its maximum speed these values are about 0.7 and 150 per cent respectively. If one just looks at the percentage increases, then it seems that, in energy terms, the mouse is far more able to afford to run around as much as it likes—the increase is only a third of that of the dog. Taking this perspective into the realm of sleep, one could instead claim that for a small mammal the energy-saving value of immobilization (via sleep), to prevent the animal from moving about needlessly, is low when compared with that of large mammals.

But this outlook begs the real issue on two accounts. Firstly, whereas a wild mouse spends almost all of wakefulness moving around, as it is unable to sit still for very long, the reverse is generally true for the dog and other advanced mammals having relaxed wakefulness. So the total extra energy expended by the ever-active mouse during wakefulness is much greater than at first it might have seemed. Furthermore, remember, that in absolute terms the mouse still uses up more energy by being active, as the difference between running and resting was 1 litre of oxygen per kilogram body weight per hour, compared with 0.7 for the dog. Secondly, small mammals have many preda-tors, and the nest, burrow, etc, provide protection. Spending excess time for-aging or wasting time out in the open heightens the risk of being caught. The prudent mouse keeps its foraging to a minimum, and stays in the safety of its nest for as long as possible each day. For these small mammals, sleep is the mechanism that implements this confinement in the absence of relaxed wake-fulness. Nature has provided a delicate balance of pay-offs between sleep, foraging, and danger for these small mammals.

Confinement to a nest gives the opportunity to huddle, and sleep is *the* occasion for huddling in small mammals. In this respect, sleep saves even more energy. Huddling reduces the body surface area that is exposed and in effect creates a larger animal with a surface area smaller in proportion to its body size. The value of huddling in energy conservation terms is impressive, and has been well demonstrated in a classical experiment carried out around 40 years ago by Dr Oliver Pearson from Harvard University[17]. Using a calor-imeter, he measured the oxygen consumption of between one and four mice under two conditions—when huddled, and when kept apart. At an environ-mental temperature of 26°C, about 4°C cooler than thermoneutrality, oxygen consumption of four huddled mice is about half that of the four animals sleeping alone. This can be seen in Fig. 7.5—the greater the number of animals huddled together, the more is the energy saving. As the outside temperature increases to thermoneutrality and beyond, the likelihood of huddling falls, because of overheating.

Unfortunately there are few, if any, findings available on small mammals that can be used to compare metabolism during normal active, foraging wakefulness with that during the immobility of sleep. So I am unable to

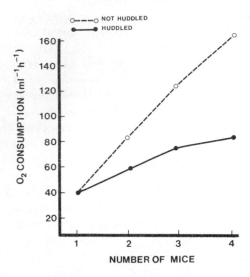

Fig. 7.5 The energy saving of huddling—oxygen consumed by mice huddling together or kept apart. This falls to half when four mice are together. (From Pearson[17]. Reproduced by permission of the Ecological Society of America)

demonstrate how much energy is really saved through sleeping rather than by being awake. Pearson measured oxygen consumption over 24-hour periods in a variety of newly captured wild rodents, but did not have the facilities to monitor their sleep. Other excellent studies of body temperature and metabolic changes during EEG monitored sleep have been carried out on small mammals; unfortunately, owing to the leads from the electrodes etc., the animals have to be confined to a small cage and movement restricted.

There have been several detailed investigations comparing metabolism during sleep with that of wakefulness in much larger mammals, particularly humans. But with these animals, sleep is no longer the only immobilizer, and wakefulness is typified more by relaxed wakefulness. Consequently, in relation to this form of wakefulness, the average fall in metabolism during sleep is relatively small—not enough to warrant sleep being described as a significant conserver of energy. In the cow and sheep, there are respective falls of 10 per cent and 13 per cent in oxygen consumption from relaxed wakefulness to sleep[18]. With humans this is around 9 per cent[19-21], which excludes the circadian rhythm in metabolism, where there is a fall to a low point during the night whether one is asleep or not. Metabolism in human sleep will be covered in more detail in Section 8.12 (also see Fig. 8.4).

7.5 More energy savings if sleep develops into a shallow torpor

During food shortages or a fall in the environmental temperature, the energy saving of sleep can become exceedingly high in a small mammal if sleep develops into a shallow torpor ('aestivation'). One popular school of thought believes that sleep, shallow torpor, and hibernation (deep torpor) are all on the same continuum. The main advocates of this theory come from two closely associated Californian research groups, one at Stanford University led by Dr Craig Heller in association with Dr Steve Glotzbach, and the other at Santa Cruz led by Drs Ralph Berger and Jim Walker. Heller and colleagues have pointed out[22] that at an environmental temperature of 0°C a small mammal weighing 100 grams can, through lowering its body temperature by 2°C during sleep (which is a typical body temperature drop for sleep in such a mammal), survive for 5 days without food. This is 1 day longer than if it remained awake but inactive. If sleep now develops into a shallow torpor and body temperature drops by 10°C then the same animal can remain alive for 7 days. But by hibernating, with a body temperature fall of about 33°C, and regulating this at around 7°C, the animal can survive for 65 days.

In the laboratory there have been practical problems with measuring oxygen consumption in small mammals sleeping and entering a shallow torpor, especially if they are going to sleep within a mass of nesting material. But recording body temperature and brain activity present less difficulties. Under the circumstances of sleep and torpor, body temperature changes also provide a good guide to metabolic rate.

The two Californian groups have carried out pioneering experiments demonstrating how sleep can lead to a shallow torpor, and in some animals on to hibernation. Shallow torpor is common amongst small mammals, and is clearly associated with sleep. But hibernation is rarer, even though it is entered via sleep. One well-known investigation into shallow torpor by these groups[23] was carried out on the round-tailed ground squirrel (*Citellus tereti-caudus*). Four animals were each monitored continuously for 10–26 days, with recordings made of the EEG and brain temperature (an index of body temperature).

Shallow torpor was induced by food deprivation, although water was freely available. These animals are naturally day-active, sleeping by night. In the daytime they remained fairly active despite the lack of food. Daytime brain temperature ranged between 34°C and 37°C, but during night-time sleep it fell to about 32°C. The four animals began to show periods of shallow torpor respectively after 2, 3, 5, and 19 days of food deprivation. Usually, shallow torpor occurred during sleep, and was typified by a fall in brain temperature of about 1°C every 40–50 minutes, eventually to stabilize at

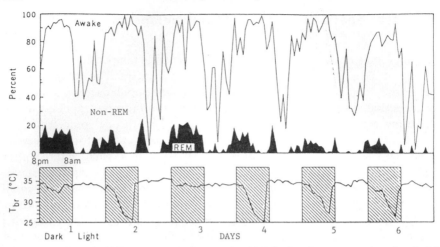

Fig. 7.6 Sleep and shallow torpor in a ground squirrel—hourly percentages of wakefulness, REM sleep, and non-REM sleep over 6 days and nights in *Citellus tereticaudus*, deprived of food. Falls in brain temperature (Tbr) during sleep on nights 2, 4, 5, and 6 show that a shallow torpor had developed. REM sleep also fell on these nights. See text for details. (From Walker *et al.*[23]. Reproduced by permission of the American Association for the Advancement of Science)

around 27°C for 1–4 hours. This would then return to waking levels over another hour. The whole period of shallow torpor, from beginning to end, lasted about 10 hours. Similar periods then usually followed at 24 to 48-hour intervals, and the sequence of events can be seen in Fig. 7.6, which covers 6 days of recording in one animal. Brain temperature changes are shown on the lower graph.

It can be seen that for this particular animal there was no shallow torpor on the first and third nights, but for the other nights brain temperature fell and the torpor developed. The upper graphs give the sleep and waking patterns. Note how wakefulness still occupies most of the daytime, even when shallow torpor happened at night. During nights occupied by sleep alone, rather than by sleep and torpor, sleep occupied much (82 per cent) of the night, with about 17 per cent of this sleep being REM sleep and the rest non-REM sleep. In nights of torpor, total sleep increased to about 92 per cent of the time and mostly consisted of non-REM sleep, as REM sleep fell to about 5 per cent. The EEG activity of non-REM sleep during shallow torpor was similar to that of normal sleep, but the amplitude was lower.

At 26°C, the lowest brain temperature recorded, REM sleep completely disappeared, and the investigators considered that this was due to the inability of REM sleep to regulate brain (and body) temperature at such a low level. Interestingly, compensatory REM 'rebounds' did not occur when brain temperature rose back to normal levels. In my opinion, this apparently lost REM sleep would mostly have been optional REM sleep. The indication that thermoregulation is impaired during REM sleep was clearly shown in another study by Glotzbach and Heller[24], and I will cover this phenomenon in more detail in Sections 8.11 and 8.12.

The Californian groups emphasized that *body temperature is still carefully regulated during non-REM sleep and shallow torpor*—that is, it is controlled not only in its descent into shallow torpor, but also within this torpor and during its ascent back to waking levels. Therefore, this torpor must not be confused with the type of torpor that reptiles enter during their sleep. In reptilian torpor, body temperature falls uncontrollably and is at the mercy of the prevailing environmental temperature. There is no control of this fall by thermoregulation, as reptiles cannot thermoregulate. On waking, reptiles are very sluggish and warm up slowly with the increasing temperature of the day, assisted by some heat production by body muscles gradually becoming more active.

Berger and Walker[25] have proposed that in mammals non-REM sleep evolved hand in hand with warm-bloodedness (homeothermy), so that body temperature and metabolism could be regulated at a lower level during sleep for the purposes of *conserving energy*. However, I suspect that whilst this proposal may well be applicable to the sleep of small mammals it may not be so relevant to non-REM sleep in larger mammals, where neither metabolism nor body temperature fall by very much (see Section 8.12). Part of Berger and Walker's case concerns their view that non-REM sleep is only found in mammals and birds—the homeothermic animals. These researchers support earlier views that non-REM sleep is absent in reptiles, amphibians, etc., with what sleep these poikilothermic animals have being apparently a form of REM sleep.

So, REM sleep is supposed to be the 'primitive archisleep', which in birds and mammals is a remnant of the reptilian state of inactivity or sleep. As reptiles are 'cold blooded', then we might expect thermoregulation during REM sleep in homeothermic animals to revert to this reptilian mode. I shall come to this intriguing idea in more detail in Chapter 8, although I should say at this point that I believe this outlook to be very debatable. Whilst REM sleep might indeed in some senses be 'primitive', I consider that this form of sleep is not a throwback to the reptilian era, but is a special development for the mammalian and avian fetus, continuing into adulthood in a diminished form.

Berger and Walker consider that non-REM sleep is not to be found in reptiles, and there is debate around this topic as well. It is a particularly difficult issue to resolve. Non-REM sleep as we know it in mammals is generated in the cerebrum, but reptiles, etc., have so little cerebrum that its electrical activity is overwhelmed by those of other brain regions. Even though 'less advanced' mammals such as rodents have a poorly developed cerebrum, it is still considerably larger than that of reptiles. However, in the mammalian brain there are still some electrical signs of non-REM sleep below the level of the cerebrum, and in particular, there is what is known as the 'limbic spike'. Recently, Dr Krystina Hartse with Dr Allan Rechtschaffen at the Chicago University Sleep Laboratory looked to see whether signs of this activity could be found in sleeping reptiles[26]. Not only were these limbic spikes found, but drugs that alter this spike activity in mammals seemed to have the same effect on the reptilian limbic spikes. Such findings suggest that reptiles could well have some form of non-REM sleep.

But to be fair to Berger and Walker the question of whether non-REM sleep is present in reptiles is not crucial to their argument that this form of sleep evolved to regulate body temperature and metabolism for energy conservation. Even if it is present in reptiles, there is no reason why it could not have evolved different functions in mammals, including the production of shallow torpor in small mammals.

Mammalian shallow torpor, unlike the deep torpor of hibernation, has a circadian rhythm and is normally confined to the usual sleep episodes, with the animal awake for the rest of the day. Sometimes, though, a shallow torpor can continue uninterrupted for much longer, even for days. Remember, shallow torpor is typically brought about by food restriction, and in animals living in a cold climate it is more likely to occur in the autumn and spring, giving way to hibernation in the winter. On the other hand, in desert-living animals like the round-tailed ground squirrel, whose sleep and torpor I have just described, food restriction is more likely in the arid summer months, and can lead to the hibernation-like state of 'aestivation'.

A good example of the seasonal development of hibernation in an alpine mammal is found in the golden-mantled ground squirrel (*Citellus lateralis*), again studied by the two California groups[27]. Typically, these animals enter hibernation through sleep and shallow torpor. Sometimes there are brief periods of wakefulness during the initial entry into hibernation, delaying full hibernation. Usually though, when the animal decides to hibernate, the process occurs fairly quickly after sleep onset, with sleep first giving way to shallow torpor and a disappearance of REM sleep. In a matter of hours, brain temperature falls to about 10°C, the EEG becomes flat, without any sign of non-REM sleep, and hibernation sets in.

Rather than hibernate during the winter, some mammals living in cold climates have developed the ability to go into a particularly prolonged sleep-cum-shallow-torpor called 'seasonal sleep', where brain temperature remains very close to normal levels. The animals are quite easily aroused, and it is fairly clear that they are just asleep. Seasonal sleep can be found in the bear, some species of chipmunk, and probably the badger, skunk, and racoon[28]. Grizzly bears will spend 3 months of the winter like this in their lair, when females will also give birth and suckle young. Much fat is built up over the summer, which is used as the food reserve. Not surprisingly, 25 per cent of the

bears' body weight can be lost during these times. But because of
and near normal body temperature during seasonal sleep, it is unl
they are really conserving much energy in this way. Such a mamm
sion of sleep is clearly a special and almost unique adaption of sleep. I suspect
that, at least for the bear, an advanced mammal with a well-developed cerebrum, seasonal sleep is another albeit extreme example of optional sleep
designed to overcome the monotony of the winter darkness.

7.6 Night- versus day-sleeping mammals

Within any climate, environmental temperatures are invariably colder by
night and warmer by day. This can influence the energy-saving value of sleep,
depending on whether the mammal sleeps by day or by night. Interestingly,
nocturnally active mammals usually have a lower body temperature and
metabolic rate than similar-sized day-active counterparts[29]. Diurnally active
mammals tend to regulate their body temperatures at around 40°C, whereas
nocturnal mammals fall into two categories. One has a more 'primitive' type
of temperature regulation, where body temperature is kept at around 30°C,
and is typified by many of the insectivores. The second, found in many nocturnal marsupials, has a more advanced thermoregulation, where body
temperature is kept at about 35°C. During non-torpor sleep, most members
of these three groups of mammals maintain their body temperatures near to
waking levels.

The consequences of being a diurnal or nocturnal sleeper for the energy
conservation value of sleep seem to be quite important, although it is a matter
that has not received much attention. There are several lines of exploration
that could be developed to illustrate this importance, and here is one. If an
animal is active by day, maintaining a relatively high body temperature, then
it risks overheating during the day. So it is more likely to have a thinner fur or
coat than any nocturnal counterpart. The likelihood is also greater that this
mammal will need to retire to the insulation of a nest when it sleeps, because it
has a higher body temperature, thinner coat, and sleeps at the colder time of
day. From the perspective of energy conservation during sleep, the nocturnal
mammal, therefore, has several advantages. Its heat loss during sleep is
relatively smaller because the animal maintains a lower body temperature, it
sleeps at a warmer time of the day, and it has a thicker coat. Such factors
would further allow it to survive and sleep in cooler ecological niches not
occupied by diurnal mammals. It may even forgo having to sleep in a nest
every day, which would allow it a greater home range for foraging, as it could
now sleep in any appropriately safe spot.

Whilst I may have over-generalized in this line of thinking, nevertheless it
again highlights the complexity of the issues surrounding the energy conservation benefits of mammalian sleep.

7.7 Food, feeding behaviour, and cerebral development

The evolution of the mammals tended to produce animals with increasing body size, and certain other developments were able to take advantage of this, particularly the advancement of the cerebral cortex. I have already described how this advancement brings the ability to display relaxed wakefulness (Section 4.2), and that for mammals like the ungulates, carnivores, and primates, sleep is no longer *the* immobiliser. However, if sleep provides cerebral restitution, then an advanced cerebrum may require more of this restitution during sleep, and therefore a greater need for core sleep (see later). But, as I will be suggesting, there may well be differences in the amounts of core sleep required between many of the ungulates on the one hand, and carnivores and primates on the other. Although both have an advanced cerebrum, that of the ungulates seems to be not so well developed—a factor probably associated with different food habits and feeding styles.

Let me now cover these points in a little more depth. A large body size means a lower metabolic rate (Fig. 7.3), and so less energy (food) is required in proportion to body weight. This allows two contrasting courses for the evolutionary development of larger mammals to occur. One builds on the general principle that, as relatively less food is necessary, larger mammals need not devote so much of the day actually eating, but could spend more time in hunting and foraging. Therefore, they can have a more extensive home territory, and risk (or lose) more time in looking for foods that are nutritionally rich, especially meat. The alternative evolutionary course is for larger mammals to take advantage of foods of very low nutritional value, particularly grass. But so much grass has to be eaten that they must spend most of the day in feeding, and cannot risk a lot of time in looking for food in case too much actual feeding time is lost and the animal starves.

The first course of evolution is typified by the carnivores and the primates, and the second by the herbivorous ungulates such as antelope and cattle. However, if animals in this second group become very large, like the elephant, then they can have the best of both worlds, up to a point. Their great size requires relatively very little food per kilogram of body weight, and although they are herbivores they do not have to spend almost all of the day eating, but can risk time in foraging for more choice vegetation.

Grazing on grass is a monotonous and mundane behaviour that contrasts with the awareness and guile that hunting or foraging for food requires. Grazers are surrounded by their food from dawn to dusk, and daily life mostly consists of routine behaviour that is repetitive and stereotyped. They move around relatively little, and do not experience a constantly changing scene. Consequently, there is little new stimulation or varied bombardment of the cerebrum by sensory information. Although they have to be on the look-out for predators, these grazers are usually within a herd. Whilst an

individual animal's awareness may be low, when this is added
awareness levels of other herd members the 'collective awareness'
is high.

The grazing ungulate, then, typically has a cerebrum that
advanced as that of the carnivore (reflected in EQ differences-
section), and in this respect might well have less need for cerebral restitution
during sleep than does the carnivore. The life of the carnivore contains much
more variety, as this creature usually has to move over a wide and less
familiar territory to seek out, stalk, and catch its prey. The less predictable is
the source of food, the more flexible and adaptable the behaviour needs to
be, and the greater the demand on the cerebrum. In my view this would point
to a potentially greater need for cerebral restitution during the sleep of carnivores, and hence more core sleep.

When carnivores eat they usually gorge themselves, not knowing when
exactly the next meal will come. Because meat is nutritionally rich, taking
many hours to be digested, such a meal can sustain them for several days.
There may be little else to do for the next day, except to sleep (probably
extended optional sleep), 'contemplate', and indulge in more leisurely
pursuits such as playing with cubs (remember, an advanced cerebrum also
indicates a long learning period in infancy, and much playing). There is often
plenty of relaxed wakefulness. When I watch wildlife films on wolves, foxes,
jackals, hyenas, lions, bears, etc., I cannot help but be impressed by how
much time these animals may spend sitting or lying relaxed and just watching
what is going on around them.

Grazing ungulates do not sleep for more than a few hours in every 24, but
have much drowsiness instead, particularly during the night. One reason, of
course, is that they are particularly vulnerable when asleep, and drowsiness
allows better vigilance compared with sleep. However, for those that also
chew the cud, there is another reason. Rumination takes up a lot of time and
can only be done during wakefulness or drowsiness, not in sleep. In fact, for
these animals most of drowsiness is occupied by rumination.

To come to my main point, I suspect that the need for core sleep in
ungulates is lower than that of carnivores owing to a poorer cerebral advancement, or rather lower 'encephalization'. I first mentioned this term in Section
7.3, when referring to Meddis's work. Although he found that encephalization was a poor predictor of the sleep parameters he used (e.g. REM and
non-REM sleep), he did not view sleep in terms of core and optional sleep,
and neither would have most other investigators of mammalian sleep.
So at the moment I do not have proof of whether, for example, carnivores and primates really do have more core sleep than do most grazing
ungulates.

7.8 Encephalization

One of the pioneers in the study of encephalization in mammals is Dr Harry Jerison from the University of California at Los Angeles. His classic book, *The Evolution of the Brain and Intelligence*[30] devotes much time to the comparative sizes of mammalian brains. He termed the ratio of actual brain weight to expected brain weight, as the 'encephalization quotient' (EQ), which mostly relates to the size of the cerebrum. Mammals with an EQ below 1.0 have a brain (i.e. cerebrum) that is smaller than would be expected from their body weight, while an EQ above 1.0 indicates a larger than expected brain. Consequently, an EQ of 2.0 means a brain twice the size expected, and an EQ of 0.5 half the size. For most mammals the usual EQ range is between 0.5 and 1.5. Scores above 1.5 can be regarded as 'high', and, as will be seen, there are many mammals with even greater values apart from ourselves.

A selection of EQs from a variety of mammals is shown in Table 7.1 taken from Eisenberg (see below), with the range going from 0.5 for the European hedgehog, an insectivore, to 7.5 for humans. Most rodents have values around 1 or just under, although tree-living varieties, particularly squirrels, that have to move in three dimensions, leaping from branch to branch, have a higher EQ—of around 1.4. Carnivores usually have values well above 1 with, for example, the fox having an EQ of 1.9, and the tiger 1.4. The elephant comes out at about 1.9, and primates excluding humans range between 1.6 for the more primitive lemur, to about 2.5 for the chimpanzee and 3.4 for the capuchin monkey. Dolphins can have remarkably high values of up to 4.9. Ungulates, on the other hand, tend to have EQs under 1.

Jerison pointed out that a low EQ (under 1) means that the mammal has a repertoire of stereotyped behaviour 'preprogrammed' into fixed routines, that can be very complex. Also, the brain has a reduced memory capacity to store and retrieve information, and the ability to learn is limited. Although such animals have most of their senses functioning adequately, only one or two of these senses will be developed to any sophisticated degree. In the case of insectivores these are usually smell and hearing. But for very high EQ mammals like monkeys, such sophistications may be present with several senses, that is vision, smell, touch, and hearing. Jerison also found that low EQ mammals were more likely to be nocturnal, and have poor vision. High EQ mammals on the other hand were more likely to be diurnal, with a very well-developed visual system that usually included stereoscopic depth perception and colour vision.

Dr John Eisenberg, from the Smithsonian Institute in Washington DC, has made further use of EQ assessments in the study of the evolution and advancement of mammalian behaviour. His views are to be found in his stimulating book, *The Mammalian Radiations*[31], which is an analysis of trends in evolution, adaptation, and behaviour. In it he develops some of

Table 7.1 Encephalization Quotients — from a selection of mammals taken from Eisenberg[31]. Figures rounded up. (c = about.) See text

Mammalian group	Animal	EQ
Marsupials	Opossum (*Didelphis*)	c0.5
	Greater kangaroo (*Macropus*)	0.5
Insectivores	Hedgehog (*Erinaceus*)	0.5
	Shrew (*Sorex*)	0.5
	European mole (*Talpa*)	c0.8
Edentates	Long-nosed armadillo (*Dasypus*)	c0.6
	Giant ant-eater (*Myrmecophaga*)	0.8
Bats	Flying fox (*Pteropus*)	0.9
	Vampire bat (*Desmodus*)	1.2
	Little brown bat (*Myotis*)	0.6
Rabbits	Hare (*Lepus*)	0.5
Rodents	Tree squirrel (*Sciurus*)	1.4
	House mouse (*Mus*)	0.8
	Rat (*Rattus*)	0.8
	Porcupine (*Hystrix*)	0.9
	Guinea pig (*Cavia*)	0.9
Ungulates	Zebra (*Equus*)	1.7
	Donkey (*Equus*)	1.0
	Rhinoceros (*Diceros*)	0.5
	Warthog (*Phacochoerus*)	0.6
	Camel (*Camelus*)	1.0
	Sheep (*Ovis*)	0.5
	Thomson's gazelle (*Gazella*)	0.9
	Giraffe (*Giraffa*)	0.4
	Elk (*Cervus*)	0.9
	Reindeer (*Rangifer*)	0.9
	Goat (*Capra*)	1.1
Elephants	Indian elephant (*Elephas*)	1.6
Carnivores	Fox (*Vulpes*)	1.9
	Weasel (*Mustella*)	1.9
	Badger (*Meles*)	0.9
	Tiger (*Panthera*)	1.4
	Leopard (*Leopardus*)	1.5
	Racoon (*Procyon*)	1.4
Dolphins	Bottle-nose dolphin (*Tursiops*)	3.2
	Porpoise (*Phocoena*)	4.9
Primates	Lemur (*Lemur*)	1.6
	Slow loris (*Nycticebus*)	2.3
	Spider monkey (*Ateles*)	2.6
	Capuchin (*Cebus*)	3.4
	Macaque (*Macaca*)	2.3
	Gibbon (*Hylobates*)	3.1
	Gorilla (*Gorilla*)	c1.6
	Chimpanzee (*Pan*)	c2.5
	Man (*Homo*)	c7.5

Jerison's ideas further. For Eisenberg, a high EQ is not only associated with more versatility in behaviour, but a longer development period in infancy to allow much learning from the parents. In this respect, it is perhaps surprising to note that Eisenberg found no relationship between EQ values and the amount of helplessness or maturity at birth ('precociality'). Even within orders of mammals such as the rodents, carnivores, and primates, there was no such association. As might be expected, a long infancy and dependency on the parent means that fewer litters are produced over time, and/or fewer infants per litter. A high EQ is also associated with a longer lifespan, which makes sense as so much time and effort has been invested in the animal's infancy. I must emphasize that there is only an association between EQ levels and all these phenomena, as we cannot be sure about causations.

As I have already mentioned, hunting behaviour requires a high EQ, as locating, stalking, and capturing prey need adaptability and cunning. In the case of prey that also have a high EQ, Eisenberg points out that there is usually active offensive behaviour, such as counter-attacking, or complex fleeing manouvres. This contrasts with the passive protective responses of low EQ animals, like rolling up into a ball as in the case of the hedgehog. Moving in three dimensions is also related to a high EQ, which is found in tree-dwelling mammals that jump from branch to branch. Hence the relatively high EQ of the squirrel compared with other rodents, and an important reason for the higher EQ of monkeys. A similar principle applies to mammals that jump obstacles and manoeuvre on land at high speed, and is a likely reason why the horse and zebra have higher EQs (at 1.7) than the donkey (around 1.1) or cow (about 0.8). Although gazelles and antelope can run and leap at high speeds, they are more limited in their manoeuvrability, and this may be associated with their relatively lower EQs of around 1. Marine mammals move in three dimensions and have high EQs, although there are many other contributory factors here. Finally, Eisenberg has shown that a high EQ is also found in mammals having a rich but dispersed source of food, which brings us back to the carnivores, and contrasting with the poor but ubiquitous food and low EQs of the grazing ungulates.

Why am I describing EQ and behaviour to such lengths?—because across mammals, any need for cerebral restitution during sleep, and for core sleep, would in my view, increase with higher EQs. Therefore, increasing amounts of core sleep will accompany the more advanced forms of behaviour, as outlined by both Jerison and Eisenberg:

- High learning ability.
- Sophisticated development of three or more senses.
- Widespread food source.
- Hunting behaviour.
- Active avoidance of predators.
- Long infancy.

7.9 Conclusions so far

We still have much to understand about mammalian sleep, and although many studies have been carried out on a variety of mammals most of these animals have been confined to the laboratory setting, away from their natural state, where sleep is subjected to many pressures alien to the laboratory. However, there are great practical problems in monitoring the sleep of mammals in the wild, and I am not being critical of the laboratory investigations. Nowadays though, with the new technological advancements in microelectronics (e.g. radiotelemetry and lightweight videocameras), more openings are available to make measurements outside the laboratory.

Statistical analyses of the amounts of REM and non-REM sleep across mammals, and how these might be associated with certain constitutional and environmental variables such as body weight, precociality at birth, being an ungulate, encephalization, and danger, have produced equivocal findings. One clear outcome is that there is less REM sleep in those mammals living in dangerous environments, suggesting that at least some of REM sleep is dispensable. However, the equivocal outcomes from the other findings are not surprising when we consider some further factors I have described that could influence sleep. These interact with each other in often subtle ways, changing from one group of mammals to another.

For example, if the animal is small (having a high metabolic rate and food requirement), with a low EQ and little relaxed wakefulness (which is a good description of most rodents), then the function of sleep is more likely to be towards energy conservation, and the facilitation of increased body restitution through physical immobility (Section 4.4). Although there may be some cerebral restitution, this would be less than in the case of a large mammal with a high EQ, where sleep has a low energy conservation value, but may be particularly helpful in occupying unproductive hours. No doubt Nature has moulded sleep into optimal amounts to fit the requirements of each species. Fig. 7.7 a, b, and c illustrate in a simple way some of the changes to sleep function that I believe have occurred during mammalian evolution.

Whilst the REM/non-REM division of sleep makes sense from certain perspectives, we have probably become too hardened in seeing sleep only in this way. Why should either of these sleep states be an essential feature of sleep, to be related to various constitutional variables? Instead, I have argued in favour of dividing sleep into core and optional sleep, as I consider this to make more sense from the functional viewpoint. But few other people see sleep in this way. The marker I have used to identify core sleep is EEG delta activity, but unfortunately, for the majority of mammals for whom EEG findings are available, the information is not detailed enough for me to establish how much of their sleep could be core sleep. So, I have based my case for core and optional sleep on the numerous findings from human studies, and have extended it to other mammals.

To summarize briefly the main topics I have covered in relation to the value of sleep as an energy conserver, this not only depends on body size and the ability to display relaxed wakefulness, but on other critical variables such as whether sleep confines the animal to the insulation of a nest, encourages huddling, can develop into a shallow torpor, or occurs during the warmer daytime or cooler night-time.

In the case of many small mammals, sleep is relatively safe, as they are usually confined to a burrow or other secure place. But it becomes more hazardous with increasing body size, particularly for the ungulates, where sleep length tends to be short, and presumably near to a core amount. As these mammals have a lower EQ (particularly the grazing ungulates) than, for example, the carnivores and primates, their need for core sleep could well be lower. Nevertheless, despite the great danger of sleep for certain ungulates, some sleep still seems to be essential and it has not been evolved out.

An excellent example of this last point is the giraffe. It sleeps for a total of about 2 hours a night, and like any other mammal has to lie down if it wants to obtain anything better than drowsiness or very light sleep. This ungainly animal's problem is not so much in lying down, but in getting up, as this takes about 15 seconds—a long time if there is danger around. Although no EEG records have been made of its sleep, detailed visual observations have been taken[32]. Between three and eight times a night the giraffe lies down on its haunches for periods of about 3–75 minutes. For the rest of the night, whilst standing, it usually supports itself against a tree. Most of its lying is spent awake chewing cud, with the neck vertical. We do not know much about drowsiness in the giraffe, but part of this lying develops into sleep, with the neck becoming 'S' shaped, a cessation of chewing, and the eyes unfocused but open. These periods are probably non-REM sleep, with each lasting about 5–30 minutes, and are followed by 1–10 minutes of what seems to be REM sleep. Here, the neck and head sag further to lie upon the animal's flank in a 'sleeping swan' position, with the eyes closed. Remember that during REM sleep in other mammals the muscles of the head and neck lose their tonus. In the giraffe this would cause a collapse of the neck, and probably is the reason why the neck is rested in the way I have described.

All mammals have to sleep. Extensive observations on many species failed to find any non-sleepers (readers interested in this information should consult the excellent comprehensive and recent review of all the studies so far conducted on mammals and other animals, written by Drs Scott Campbell and Irene Tobler[33]). Very strong evidence favouring sleep having an essential life-preserving purpose, at least in the more cerebrally advanced mammals, comes from the dolphins. The blind Indus dolphin risks its life if sleep lasts for more than a few minutes, and it has developed multiple 'microsleeps' as a solution. In the bottle-nosed dolphin, normal sleep impairs its breathing, so it has become adapted to sleeping with one hemisphere at a time. Why would such complex changes occur to sleep if some sleep was not essential? This must be a powerful argument against those people who dismiss sleep purely as a 'non-behaviour'[34] or as a near-redundant instinct[35].

The evolutionary advancement of the mammals tended to bring an

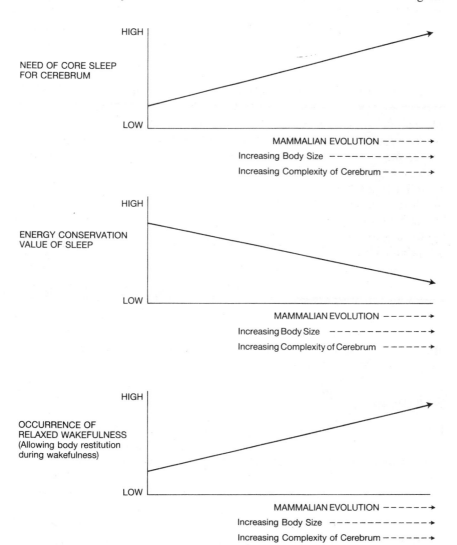

Fig. 7.7 Simplified graphs summarizing the key points discussed in Chapter 7—showing how various aspects of sleep function will change with mammalian evolution. Note that evolution tends to bring increases in body size and in the complexity of the cerebrum.

increased body size, with a relative reduction in metabolism and food need. Less time could be spent in feeding and more time in other pursuits. Or, more time could be used in eating foods of a low nutritional value, as is the case with grazing ungulates. Concomitant with this advancement came further developments of the cerebrum. EQ rose, at least for the carnivores and primates, but less so for most of the grazing ungulates, as their stereotyped feeding behaviour does not require such cerebral development. Compared with the ungulates, the carnivores and primates have greater use of their more sophisticated cerebrum, perhaps a greater need for cerebral restitution during sleep, and therefore a greater need for core sleep (Fig. 7.7).

Ungulates have large amounts of relaxed wakefulness, but also much drowsiness, and many sleep researchers have commented on this. It will be remembered that Zepelin and Rechtschaffen (Section 7.3) wrestled with the problem of how to classify this state—was it sleep or wakefulness? The compromise was to call half of it sleep and half wakefulness. In Ruckebusch's[36] pioneering work on drowsiness in ungulates (in domesticated animals though) he found that for every 24-hour day, sheep spent about 4 hours in drowsiness and 4 hours asleep. For cows these figures were 7.5 hours and 4 hours respectively, and for the horse 2 hours and 3 hours. Why do these animals, like the giraffe, bother to sleep at all, when they could simply extend drowsiness by a few extra hours? The reason is, I believe, that some sleep is essential—probably for the cerebrum.

Carnivores and primates usually have much less drowsiness, and sleep for much longer than do the ungulates. Drowsiness in the ungulates may well substitute for optional sleep by occupying time and allowing greater vigilance. Another reason for so much drowsiness in ruminants is that sleep prevents rumination, whereas drowsiness allows it to continue. This does not apply to the horse, of course, which is not a ruminant, but is still a short sleeper, seemingly for reasons of sleep safety.

7.10 Infancy

I have just described how certain functions of sleep, such as energy conservation, cerebral restitution, and any need for body restitution, will change with mammalian evolution, especially in relation to increasing body size and increasing complexity of the cerebrum. However, this particularly applies to adult animals. On the other hand, mammalian infants have a lot more in common with each other. They are all fairly helpless, have rapid body and brain growth, and relatively high rates of learning. To these ends, it is likely that sleep may have a much more common function across the infants of mammals than across the respective adults. For example, in the typical infant, sleep may well play a more dominant role in cerebral restitution, as there is so much novelty in the sensory bombardment of the cerebrum, and many new neural networks are developing—so there would be greater amounts of core sleep. Optional sleep may also be longer, but not necessarily to conserve energy, or to occupy 'unproductive hours', but to serve a role unique to the infant—providing the mother with respite and allowing her to carry out other essential activities such as obtaining food.

Therefore, within any species, sleep would change its function in subtle ways from infancy to adulthood. However, and this is my final theme for this chapter, humans may be different in this respect, as the function of our sleep may not change so much from infancy to adulthood as it does for most other mammals. My case concerns the evolutionary process by which humans seem to have evolved from our ape ancestors—neoteny—the retention of fetal- or infant-like characteristics into adulthood (with sexual development brought forward to allow the organism to reproduce without having to become the typical adult). In simpler terms, many aspects of our infancy do not really end with childhood, but continue to adulthood and old age[37, 38].

In many respects, the human adult resembles the human baby far more than does the typical infant ape or monkey resemble its adult form. Let me start off with the head, for example; the extensive alteration in the chimpanzee face from infancy to adulthood can be seen in Fig. 7.8. Also, the

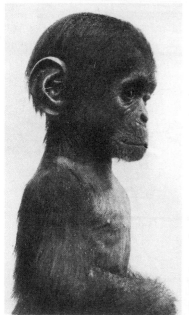
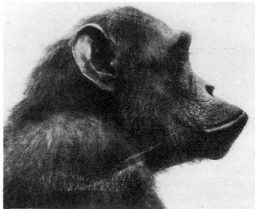

Fig. 7.8 The infant ape bears a much greater resemblance to we humans than does the adult—baby and adult chimpanzee. See text for details. (From Naef[39]. Reproduced by permission of Springer-Verlag NY Inc.)

likeness of the infant chimp to the human adult is striking, and contrasts
dramatically with the adult chimpanzee, which looks so unlike us.

So many of our adult features resemble those of the fetal or infant ape[37, 38].
Apart from our relatively high brain weight, the absence of brow ridges, the
angle the head makes with the spinal column (to give an erect head), the
presence of a forehead and flatness of the face, all to be seen in Fig. 7.8,
the shape of the human adult brain and the proportions of the lobes of the
cerebral hemispheres also resemble those of the infant monkey much more
than those of the adult animal[37]. There are aspects of human adult behaviour
that are infant like. I do not mean what could be commonly called 'childish-
ness' and 'immaturity', but the retention into adulthood of a high degree of
learning ability, curiosity, exploration, and playfulness. We take these for
granted, but they are not to be found to this extent in other adult mammals.
Leaving the brain and behaviour, and going downwards to the rest of the

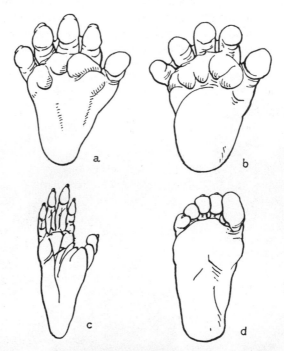

Fig. 7.9 Feet—another example of similarities between the human adult and fetal monkey:
(a) fetal macaque monkey, (b) fetal human, (c) adult macaque, (d) adult human. The human
adult foot bears a much greater resemblance to that of the fetal monkey than to that of the
adult animal, especially in relation to the positions of the big toe, and the width of the foot in
proportion to its length. Also, the similarity between the adult and the fetal foot is much
greater in the human than in the macaque. (From de Beer[37]. Reproduced by permission of
Oxford University Press.)

body, there are numerous other examples[36, 37] of the similarity between the human adult and infant or fetal ape. There is our hairlessness, the position of the human vagina, and even our feet, especially the position of the big toe. Fig. 7.9 compares the feet of the adult macaque monkey and adult human with those of their fetal forms. The odd one out is that of the adult monkey. The adult human foot resembles those of both the fetuses, and changes less from its fetal state than does that of the adult animal. (The macaque is not an ape, of course—I could not locate such pictures for apes, but I am assured that the same principles apply to the feet of the baby and adult chimpanzee.)

A similar concept could apply to the function of human sleep—perhaps it is 'infant' like (excepting of course, the notion that sleep gives the mother some respite). I readily admit that this is a speculative idea, particularly as we cannot be sure of what the functions of sleep are in the human adult, let alone in the human infant, where less research has been done. However, the point that I am trying to illustrate is that if, for the typical mammal, the function of sleep does alter from infancy to adulthood, then doubt can be cast upon whether this also applies to the same extent in humans. That is, for the most part, the functions of human sleep, particularly in relation to the cerebrum, may not change substantially from infancy to adulthood.

References

1. Pilleri, G. (1979). The blind Indus dolphin, *Platanista indi. Endeavour*, **3**, 48–56.
2. Mukhametov, L.M. (1984). Sleep in marine mammals. In: Borbély, A.A. and Valatx, J.L. (ed.) *Sleep Mechanisms*. Springer, Munich. pp. 227–238.
3. Supin, A.Y., Mukhametov, L.M., Ladygina, T.F., Popov, V.V., Mass, A.M. and Polyakova, I.G. (1978). *Electrophysiological Study of Dolphins Brain*. Nauka, Moscow.
4. Serafetinides, E.A., Shurley, J.T. and Brooks, R.E. (1972). Electroencephalogram of the pilot whale *Globicephalia scammoni*, in wakefulness and sleep: laterality aspects. *International Journal of Psychobiology*, **2**, 129–135.
5. Ball, N.J., Amlaner, C.J., Shaffery, J.P. and Opp, M.R. (1987). Asynchronous eye closure and hemispheric quiet sleep of birds. In: Koella, W.P. (ed.) *Sleep 1986*. Gustav Fischer Verlag, Stuttgart. (in press).
6. Ruckebusch, Y. (1977). Sleep and the environment. In: Koella, W.P. (ed.) *Sleep 1976* Karger, Basel. pp. 152–169.
7. Parmeggiani, P.L. and Rabini, C. (1970). Sleep and environmental temperature. *Archives of Italian Biology*, **108**, 369–387.
8. Zepelin, H. and Rechtschaffen, A. (1974). Mammalian sleep, longevity, and energy metabolism. *Brain and Behavioural Evolution*, **10**, 425–470.
9. Allison, T. and Cicchetti, D.V. (1976). Sleep in mammals: ecological and constitutional correlates. *Science*, **194**, 732–734.
10. Meddis, R. (1983). The evolution of sleep. In: Mayes, A. (ed.) *Sleep Mechanisms and Functions*. Van Nostrand Reinhold, London. pp. 57–106.

11. Jouvet-Mounier, D., Astic, L. and Lacote, D. (1970). Ontogenesis of the states of sleep in the rat, cat and guinea-pig during the first post-natal month. *Developmental Psychobiology*, **2**, 391–399.

12. Zepelin, H. (1983). Note by Harold Zepelin. In: Mayes, A. (ed.) *Sleep Mechanisms and Functions*. Van Nostrand Reinhold, London. p. 93.

13. Schmidt-Nielsen, K. (1983). *Animal Physiology*. University Press, Cambridge.

14. Kleiber, M. (1961). *The Fire of Life: An Introduction to Animal Energetics*. John Wiley & Son, New York.

15. Haldane, J.B.S. (1965). On being the right size. In: Shapley, J., Rapport, B. and Wright, T. (ed.) *The New Treasury of Science*. Harper Row, New York. pp. 474–478.

16. Taylor, C.R., Schmidt-Nielsen, K. and Raab, J.L. (1970). Scaling of energetic cost of running to body size in mammals. *American Journal of Physiology*, **219**, 1104–1107.

17. Pearson, O.P. (1947). The rate of metabolism of some small mammals. *Ecology*, **28**, 127–145.

18. Toutain, P-L. and Webster, A.J. (1975). Equilibre energetique au cours du sommeil chez les ruminants. *Comptes Rendus Academie des Sciences (Paris)*, **281**, 1605–1608.

19. Haskell, E.H., Palca, J.W., Walker, J.M., Berger, R.J. and Heller, H.C. (1981). Metabolism and thermoregulation during stages of sleep in humans exposed to heat and cold. *Journal of Applied Physiology*, **51**, 948–954.

20. Shapiro, C.M., Goll, C.C., Cohen, G.R. and Oswald, I. (1984). Heat production during sleep. *Journal of Applied Physiology*, **56**, 671–677.

21. Haskell, E.H., Palca, J.W., Walker, J.M., Berger, R.J. and Heller, H.C. (1981). The effects of high and low ambient temperatures on human sleep stages. *Electroencephalography and Clinical Neurophysiology*, **51**, 494–501.

22. Heller, H.C., Walker, J.M., Florant, G.L., Glotzbach, S.F. and Berger, R.J. (1978). Sleep and hibernation: electrophysiological and thermoregulatory homologies. In: Wang, L. and Hudson, J.W. (ed.) *Strategies in Cold: Natural Thermogenesis and Torpidity*, Academic Press, New York. pp. 225–265.

23. Walker, J.M., Garber, A., Berger, R.J. and Heller, H.C. (1979). Sleep and estivation (shallow torpor): continuous process of energy conservation. *Science*, **204**, 1098–1100.

24. Glotzbach, S.F. and Heller, H.C. (1976). Central regulation of body temperature during sleep. *Science*, **194**, 537–539.

25. Walker, J.M. and Berger, R.J. (1980). Sleep as an adaptation for energy conservation functionally related to hibernation and shallow torpor. *Progress in Brain Research*, **53**, 255–278.

26. Hartse, K.M. and Rechtschaffen, A. (1980). The effect of amphetamine, nembutal, alpha-methyl-tyrosine, and parachlorophenylalanine on sleep-related spike activity of the tortoise, *Geochelone carbonaria*, and on the cat ventral hippocampus spike. *Brain, Behaviour and Evolution*, **21**, 199–222.

27. Walker, J.M., Glotzbach, S.F., Berger, R.J. and Heller, H.C. (1977). Sleep and hibernation in ground squirrels (*Citellus* spp.): electrophysiological observations. *American Journal of Physiology*, **233**, R213–R221.

28. Hudson, J.W. and Bartholomew, G.A. (1964). Terrestrial animals in dry heat:

estivators. In: Dill, D.B. Adolph, E.F. and Wilbur, C.G. (ed.) *Handbook of Physiology: Adaptation to the Environment—Vol. 4*. Springer-Verlag, Berlin. pp. 541–550.

29. Crompton, A.W., Taylor, C.R. and Jagger, J.A. (1978). Evolution of homeothermy in mammals. *Nature*, **272**, 333–336.

30. Jerison, H.J. (1973). *The Evolution of The Brain and Intelligence*. Academic Press, New York.

31. Eisenberg, J.E. (1981). *The Mammalian Radiations*. Athlone Press, London.

32. Kristal, M.B. and Noonan, M. (1979). Note on sleep in captive giraffes (*Giraffa camelopardalis reticulata*). *South African Journal of Zoology*, **14**, 108.

33. Campbell, S.S. and Tobler, I. (1984). Animal sleep: a review of sleep duration across phylogeny. *Neuroscience and Biobehavioural Reviews*, **8**, 269–300.

34. Webb, W.B. (1975). *Sleep the Gentle Tyrant*. Prentice-Hall, New Jersey.

35. Meddis, R. (1977). *The Sleep Instinct*. Routledge and Keegan Paul, London.

36. Ruckebusch, Y. (1972). The relevance of drowsiness in the circadian cycle of farm animals. *Animal Behaviour*, **20**, 637–643.

37. de Beer, G. (1958). *Embryos and Ancestors*. University Press, Oxford.

38. Gould, S.J. (1977). *Ontogeny and Phylogeny*. University Press, Harvard.

39. Naef, A. (1926). Uber die Urformen der Anthropomorphen und die Stammesgeschichte des Menschenschadals. *Naturwiss*, **14**, 445–452.

8. REM sleep

8.1 Perspectives on dreaming

One is led to suspect that the activity of the extra-ocular musculature and the lids might be peculiarly sensitive indicators of CNS changes associated with the sleep–wakefulness cycle. The disproportionately large cortical areas involved with eye movements, the well-defined secondary vestibular pathways to the extra-ocular nuclei, and the low innervation ratio of the eye muscles point to at least a quantitative basis for their reflection of general CNS activity[1].

So began the circumspect opening paragraph of the classic paper by Aserinsky and Kleitman, published in 1955, that first described in detail the link between dreaming and rapid eye movements. These investigators briefly mentioned such a link earlier, in 1953, in a short paper concerned with the association between body movements and eye movements during sleep[2]. Then, they reported that out of 27 awakenings of sleeping subjects showing rapid eye movements, 20 occasions produced accounts of dreaming involving visual imagery, whereas out of 23 awakenings when there were no eye movements, only 4 led to claims of dreaming. Aserinsky was at the time a graduate student in Kleitman's laboratory, and he moved off to Jefferson Medical College in Philadelphia as soon as his thesis was completed. There, he was unable to devote much time to sleep research, and 14 years were to elapse before his next major contribution on rapid eye movements appeared (Section 6.4).

Aserinsky and Kleitman[1] reported that periods of rapid eye movements and dreaming first appear after about 3 hours of sleep, last for about 20 minutes, and return at about 2-hour intervals. However, this information was rather vague and not quite correct. Another of Kleitman's graduate students, William Dement, took up the challenge, and looked much more closely at rapid eye movements and dreaming. Like Aserinsky, he measured eye movements from electrodes around the eyes. There is a small potential difference between the retina and cornea, picked up by these electrodes, and eye movements can be registered easily. With Kleitman, Dement carried out a remarkably detailed and thorough investigation, reported in their famous paper of 1957, 'Cyclic variations in EEG during sleep and their relation to eye movements, body motility, and dreaming'[3]. Emphasis was given to the regular occurrence of REM sleep throughout sleep, at approximately 70–90-minute intervals, and to the characteristics of the rapid eye movement bursts.

But, as Kleitman later pointed out in his book[4], the discovery in his laboratory of an association between eye movements and dreaming was not altogether new. For example, in 1892 G.T. Ladd, a professor of mental and moral philosophy at Yale University, reported through pure introspection about his own sleep that during deep dreamless sleep his eyes were stationary, but during dreaming sleep he was 'inclined also to believe that, in somewhat vivid visual dreams, the eyeballs move gently in their sockets, taking various positions . . .' How he came up with these ideas is a mystery. As Kleitman noted, neither Ladd nor his associates actually watched the eyes of sleepers. This would have been a simple task as the rapid eye movements of REM sleep can be easily seen under the eyelids. Such observations were not made until 1930, when a Dr E. Jacobson, having noticed that waking people move their eyes when trying to recollect some visual event, also observed eye movements during dreaming. Later, in a popular book, '*You Can Sleep Well—The ABC's of Restful Sleep for the Average Person*', published in 1938[5] he suggested 'watch the sleeper whose eyes move under his closed lids . . . awaken him . . . you are likely to find that . . . he had seen something in a dream'.

Dreaming is not solely associated with REM sleep, and occurs to some extent in non-REM sleep. Conversely, REM sleep sometimes appears without dreaming. In another study[6] Dement and Kleitman woke up nine subjects a total of 191 times from REM sleep, and collected reports of dreaming on 152 occasions (80 per cent). Out of 160 awakenings of these same subjects from non-REM sleep, only 11 reports of dreaming were obtained (7 per cent).

By the end of the 1950s Kleitman had reached 65 years of age and was obliged to retire shortly after these discoveries, and his laboratory had to close down. However, the phoenix was reborn, as by this time Allan Rechtschaffen had arrived at Chicago University, and was establishing his own laboratory. One of his first graduate students was David Foulkes, whose area of interest happened to be dreaming. But in contrast with the findings of Dement and Kleitman[6], Foulkes[7] reported dream-like mental activity in 74 per cent of awakenings from non-REM sleep, against 88 per cent for REM sleep. The disagreement between these two studies over the incidence of 'dreaming' in non-REM sleep appears to lie in what is meant by 'dreaming'. In non-REM sleep, dreaming is less 'visual' and involves more thinking and remembering, whereas real dreaming is more bizarre, emotional, and vivid. Nowadays, to avoid this confusion, the typical mental activity of non-REM sleep is usually called 'thinking' or 'mentation', compared with the true dreaming of REM sleep. Even so, some dreaming is still to be found in non-REM sleep.

Other interesting mental states exist in sleep outside REM sleep, particularly the less bizarre visual imagery experienced by many people during drowsiness and light sleep. 'Hypnagogic' is the term used for the imagery at sleep onset, whereas 'hypnapompic' imagery occurs around awakening. Although having different names, both seem to be the same phenomenon, and are derived from the Greek '*hypnos*' (sleep), '*agogos*' (leads), and '*apophysis*' (outgrowth). Some conscious control can be exerted here, and a few people can maintain these pleasant states for many minutes. The more abnormal mental experiences in sleep include sleepwalking, and the alarming 'night terror'. It must be remembered, as I mentioned in Section 5.10, that they occur in SWS, not in REM sleep. Sleep talking is quite common, specially among children, and is usually associated with stage 2 sleep.

The ability for most people to recall their dreams on awakening in the morning is very limited, as the memory for dreaming is very short lived. Recall is best if one wakes or is awoken from a dream. Many studies have shown how the memory rapidly fades. For example waking someone up 5 minutes into non-REM sleep after the end of a REM period only produces fragmented accounts of the dream, and by about 10 minutes into non-REM sleep there is little or no recall[8]. It is generally thought that the reason why some people are good recollectors of their dreams in the morning is that they wake up periodically during the night from their dreams. If they go over the dream during this brief wakefulness, then it can recounted again later. Absence of any knowledge of dreaming may simply be a sign of good and undisturbed sleep.

Aristotle, in his *Parva Naturalia*, gave an insightful account of how dreams are formed, after dismissing the current view of the time that they are 'sent by the gods'. Dreams, he surmised, were mostly based on residual images left in the mind from various events previously seen or thought about. These presented themselves:

With even greater impression . . . like little eddies which are being formed in rivers . . . often remaining like what they were when they first started, but often, too, broken into other forms by collisions . . . If one violently disturbs these residuary movements they become confused . . . this may occur particularly in people who are atrabilious, or feverish, or intoxicated. (p. 460).

Returning to present day research, it is clear that not only do dreams include some of the previous day's happenings, but during dreaming, sounds and other non-arousing stimuli from outside the sleeper can also be incorporated. In a further study[9] from Kleitman's laboratory, a variety of stimuli were given to subjects in REM sleep: noise tones, light shining into the face, and the most effective—spraying water onto the skin. On 33 occasions when the spray did not wake the subject, 14 of the dream narratives included falling water. But when this water spray was given in non-REM sleep there were no reports of 'thinking about water'. A fortuitous outcome was that an alarm bell, really meant to wake up the subjects, found its way into about 10 per cent of dreams when it failed to wake them up. Usually it appeared as the ringing of a doorbell or telephone.

Events in dreams seem to run their full course in the same time it would take to visualize the experiences in wakefulness. There is little evidence to support the idea that dreams are all over in a 'flash', or are substantially compressed in time. This latter notion was challenged as early as 1897 by a Dr J. Clavière[10] who took as one example the famous dream by a fellow Frenchman, Maury, who was awoken by a board falling on his neck. Maury recounted a long story of events in his dream that ended in him being guillotined, that is, when the board fell. Therefore, Maury argued, the whole dream must have been constructed the instant the board fell, but Clavière doubted the accuracy of the account.

Whether or not dreams run at normal time was a topic also investigated in Dement and Kleitman's second study[6]. Subjects were woken up either 5 or 15 minutes into a period of REM sleep, and had to say for how long they thought that the dream had been going. The reports were compared with the EEG assessments of the REM sleep, and it was found that the subjects were correct for about 75 per cent of the occasions. Interestingly though, if subjects were woken at the end of 30–60 minutes of REM sleep, their accounts were no longer than those from 15 minutes of REM sleep. They only remembered the last part of the dream, and apparently the first part was forgotten. Often during REM sleep there are small arousals and body movements, first noted by Aserinsky and Kleitman[2]. These, claimed Dement and Kleitman[6], fragment sleep so that memory of material prior to the arousal is lost.

Dreams are mostly visual in character, and this is not surprising when one considers that vision is our dominant sense. Some people appear to dream in colour, and others not. One of the most plausible reasons for these differences between people was given by Kleitman in his simple maxim—'One dreams as one thinks'. Several studies have been conducted in answer to the obvious question of 'what do blind people dream about?'. It is fairly clear that for people born blind, or who lose their sight before the age of 5 years, dreaming is mostly auditory, and to some extent tactile. A famous study[11] carried out by Berger and colleagues (the same Ralph Berger who now works on thermoregulation during sleep—Section 7.5) in 1961 looked at eye movements during REM sleep in the blind. He found that for those blind since birth there were no rapid eye movements during REM sleep, whereas for those who became blind later such eye movements were present, but varied according to the length of blindness.

REM sleep is prolific in the newborn. In fact, in humans it seems to be at its height in the fetus, at about 6 months gestation. At this age the fetus may be having around 15 hours REM sleep a day. The intriguing but apparently unanswerable question is whether any form of dreaming is going on at this time? Clearly, any dreaming here is not going to be as we know it, particularly as the cerebrum is only partly developed. However, as will be seen in Section 8.3, with or without dreaming, REM sleep may be playing a crucial role in cerebral development.

As far as we know, REM sleep is found in most other mammals. There seem to be few exceptions apart from the dolphin and perhaps other whales. The primitive egg-laying mammals such as the spiny anteater (*Tachyglossus*) seem to be the only other category of REM-less mammal. Whilst it cannot be established whether other mammals dream during REM sleep, there is no justification for claiming that humans are unique in this respect. There are some signs that at least in the more advanced mammals there may be dreaming. Many dog owners can testify to the periodic yelping, growling and excitement of their sleeping pets, which is best explained by 'dreaming'.

The contents of dreams and what they mean have been a focus of countless writings since writing began. The most substantive report of how the ancient cultures viewed and interpreted their dreams, especially the Greeks and Romans, comes from the five volumes of *'Oneirocritica'*, written by Artemidorus in the second century AD. Over 3000 dream accounts were given, with the translation of numerous dream symbols (e.g. the right hand = father, son or friend; left hand = mother, wife or mistress; foot = slave; a dolphin in water = good omen; out of water = bad omen). Artemidorus wisely insisted that dreams be interpreted in relation to each dreamer, their customs, and where they live. This is why dream interpretation was so difficult, and could only be left to a few informed individuals. Even Sigmund Freud was impressed by these writings, and often referred to Artemidorus.

Whether or not dreams can be interpreted is a topic beyond my comprehension, and often beyond the understanding of many people who write about the meaning of dreams. Sometimes, it can be difficult to say who is fantasizing more, the dreamer or the dream 'interpreter'. Aristotle noted again in *Parva Naturalia* that:

The most skillful interpreter of dreams is he who has the faculty of observing resemblances. Anyone may interpret dreams which are vivid and plain. But . . . dreams are analogous to forms reflected in water . . . if the motion in the water is great, the reflection has no resemblance to the original. Skilful is he who could rapidly discern . . . the rapid and distorted fragments . . . for internal movements effaces the clearness of dreams. (p. 464).

Viewing dreams as portents of the future has been another popular approach for dream 'interpreters'. Again, the sceptical Aristotle has some comments to make here, as 'most prophetic dreams are . . . mere coincidences'. But he points out that dreams can set one's mind up to change behaviour and bring about a foreseen event—'for as when we are engaged on any course of action, or have performed certain actions . . . the dream movement has had a way paved for it, which in turn should prove a starting point for action to be performed'. (*Parva Naturalia*, p. 462).

I do not want to dismiss entirely the principle of dream interpretation, as in certain circumstances dreams can be of help in understanding the pressures confronting patients with severe mental problems, and to some extent Freud may be correct in saying that dreams are the 'royal road to the unconscious'. But to endorse Artemidorus' point, it is crucial to know the patient before any 'interpretation' can begin, and I see little evidence in support of a notion for universal symbols in dream imagery common among humans. So for example, 'dream dictionaries' and schemes for 'dream analyses by mail', where there is no rapport between the dreamer and interpreter, must be treated with the greatest of suspicion. Freud's views on the interpretation of dreams are highly contentious, of course, particularly because of their great sexual bias. Because of this, several of his notable early followers went off to create their own schemes of dream interpretation. Today's state of the art of dream interpretation is still best summed up by the disheartened Freud in his '*New Introductory Lectures on Psychoanalysis*'[12] published in 1933:

But if you ask how much of dream interpretation has been accepted by outsiders—by the many psychiatrists and psychotherapists who warm their pot of soup at our fire (incidentally without being very grateful for our hospitality), by what are described as educated people, who are in the habit of assimilating the more striking findings of science, by the literary men and by the public at large—the reply gives little cause for satisfaction (p. 8).

Dream interpretation is one matter, but the role of dreams is another, and Freud could be right in his view that dreams were 'wish fulfilments to provide a substitute way for discharging repressed emotions or unconscious wishes.' These feelings are probably not as sexually oriented as Freud suggested, but are much more diverse, like most modern psychoanalists believe. Nevertheless, Freud had a remarkable insight into dreaming. In particular, he saw that at least two types of mental activity seem to be going on, which he described as the 'manifest' and 'latent' content of the dream. The latter is an expression of basic biological drives (which for Freud were mainly sexual). However, these may be too emotive for the sleeper to handle, and this is where a form of censor comes in, to moderate the offending parts and to produce the 'manifest' dream. Freud explained several mechanisms by which the manifest dream was produced, such as 'condensation'—the clustering of several meanings into an image, and 'displacement'—the shifting of emotionally painful experiences onto a more benign image.

What impressed Freud, and many others including myself, is how remarkably elaborate dreams are for most people, and he noted 'we have found evidence in the dream, thoughts of a highly complex intellectual function, operating with almost the whole resources of the mental apparatus'. The process becomes even more awesome when one considers how it is almost impossible for most people to produce such colourful and complex scenarios within their waking imagination that could continue for half an hour or so.

Freud also regarded the dream as the 'guardian of sleep', and in this respect so did his contemporary, Dr Carl Jung[13] who, like Freud, also considered that dreams had a compensatory function. Through their content and release of emotions, Jung proposed that 'dreams contribute to the self-regulation of the psyche'. For Jung, though, dreams were the expression of the:

collective unconscious—that lies at a deeper level and is further removed from consciousness than the personal unconscious—in the dream the psyche speaks in images and gives expression to instincts which derive from the most primitive levels of nature.

Interestingly, present day research shows that one of the more noticeable effects of REM sleep deprivation seems to be to heighten various 'basic' drives during wakefulness, although this is more apparent in animals than in humans (see Sections 8.6 and 8.7). Whether or not REM sleep deprivation is the same as dream deprivation is, of course, another matter.

One of the more recent reviews on the less psychoanalytical side of dreaming is to be found in the book *Sleep and Dreaming* by Dr David Cohen, a leader in this field, from the University of Texas[14]. Cohen points out that dreaming may not simply be the reflection of one's anxieties, but a process for solving emotional or intellectual problems. Dreams may help organize our thoughts and sort out the day's events.

Alternatively, dreams could just be the mind's junkyard. The advent of computers has prompted the still popular idea that dreams represent the clearance of irrelevant memories from the previous day[15]. Somehow, the mind is supposed to sort through all the day's memories, storing the key material for the long term, and throwing out the irrelevant material to avoid the unwanted clutter of our memory banks. This clutter is 'discharged' by the process of dreaming, and is a reason why dreams are seldom remembered— they are not supposed to be remembered. I will come back to these 'memory consolidation' theories in the next section as mostly they are not concerned with dreaming *per se* but with REM sleep.

I am tempted to argue that if dreaming is generally confined to REM sleep, then as about half of REM sleep falls into my division of optional sleep, about half of dreaming would also seem to be non-essential and relatively dispensable. Therefore, any views that dreaming is a crucial process must be reconciled with its apparent dispensability. This would seem to pose a particular problem for the memory clearout hypothesis I have just mentioned. But there are good counter arguments. For example when sizeable portions of REM sleep are removed (Sections 2.7, 6.3) through sleep deprivation or adaptation to less sleep, potential dream loss could well be compensated by more dreaming shifting into the non-REM sleep of core sleep. Some sleep researchers, like Dr Rosalin Cartwright from the Rush-Presbyterian-St Luke's Medical Centre in Chicago, would argue further. She believes that the act of fantasizing, as in dreams, is of such importance to our mental health that if the dream outlet for fantasizing is reduced we compensate by fantasizing more during wakefulness[16].

On the other hand, many sleep researchers believe that too much attention is paid to the function of dreaming, viewing it to be of little consequence, and just a by-product of REM sleep—that is, the purpose of REM sleep is not simply to allow dreaming. One of the most parsimonious, and rather cynical accounts of dreaming that I know of has been given by Kleitman[4]:

> To those who insist that because dreams occur they must serve a particular purpose, it may be pointed out that not all processes have a teleological explanation. Vomiting, for instance, when it is elicited by some irritating matter in the stomach, serves a good purpose in evacuating the stomach and removing the irritant. The same vomiting act, when resulting from motion sickness, serves no physiological purpose. The explanation of the latter type of vomiting is that the vestibular centres of the medulla were unduly excited from the unusual motion of the body, and this excitation has spread to the neighbouring vomiting centre. This explanation is correct, but not teleological. Dreaming may be considered a crude type of cortical activity associated with a recurrent appearance of stage 1 EEG (REM sleep) in the course of a night's sleep . . . As such, dreaming sleep need not have any special function and may be quite meaningless. (p. 107).

More recently, two celebrated neurophysiologists in the field of sleep who are also psychiatrists, Drs Alan Hobson and Bob McCarley from Harvard Medical School, put forward a controversial theory also implying that dreaming was incidental to REM sleep. Their 'activation–synthesis' hypothesis[17], proposed that dreaming is the result of a near-random barrage (activation) of the cerebral cortex (where dreams occur) by neural impulses from the more primitive basal parts of the brain that initiate REM sleep. The cerebrum tries to make some sort of order out of this chaos, by releasing stored memories that are somehow weaved together into a dream (the synthesis). According to Hobson and McCarley, the distortion and bizarreness of the dream is not the result of unconscious wishes and subtle psychological factors arising from within the cerebrum, as many others such as Freud have claimed, but much more of a random and meaningless process.

The basal part of the brain that Hobson and McCarley consider to be the main REM sleep generation centre, responsible for the activation of the cerebrum, lies within the region called the pons—specifically, the 'FTG' neurones (the initials 'FTG' come from the French language version of 'the giant cells of the pontine tegmentum'). However, there is now strong doubt about whether these cells are *the* REM sleep centre, particularly as it has since been shown by two other leading neurophysiologists, Drs Dennis McGinty and Jerome Siegel from the Sepulveda Veterans Administration

Medical Center in Los Angeles[18], that FTG cells also fire in a similar way during wakefulness. In fact, this firing seems to be linked to real or attempted body movements. In response to these findings, Hobson and McCarley contend that the firing is much greater in REM sleep, and in this respect different to that of wakefulness.

Needless to say, Hobson and McCarley's theory created a considerable stir in other quarters, with one of the greatest critics being Dr Gerald Vogel, an eminent sleep researcher from Emory University, Atlanta, Georgia. Vogel pointed out[19] that Hobson and McCarley have only been able to infer that dreaming is caused by a random discharge of FTG cells to the cerebrum, and there is no real proof of this. Other research has shown that the cerebrum itself plays a crucial role in the initiation and organization of dreams. For example, the generation of REM sleep by the FTG cells falls dramatically in cats without a cerebrum. The cerebrum is not a slave to the FTG cells, but clearly, can influence them in return. Vogel further attacked the idea that the FTG cells were the generators of REM sleep, and also he considered that much of our non-REM mentation, as well as hypnagogic and hypnapompic imagery, is in fact dreaming. That is, for Vogel dreaming occurs outside REM sleep, and outside the activation of FTG cells anyway. Hobson and McCarley have now modified their theory somewhat. It still attracts much interest and has its supporters.

8.2 REM sleep—memory, homeostatic, sentinel, and motivational theories

Over the last 30 years since the 'discovery' of REM sleep there have been a variety of theories about its function, rather than that of dreaming itself. Most only give a cursory mention to the possible role of non-REM sleep, and in this respect cannot be seen as general theories for sleep function. Even more proposals have appeared about the neurophysiological mechanisms in the brain that produce REM sleep, including that of Hobson and McCarley just mentioned. Generally, though, these do not tell us what the purpose of REM sleep is, nor why such mechanisms are there in the first place.

The most prominent theories about the function of REM sleep fall under the heading of 'memory consolidation', briefly mentioned in the last section. There are variations on this theme, with the most recent proposal, dealing with forgetting rather than with remembering, by the Nobel Laureate and molecular geneticist, Dr Francis Crick, and a colleague, Dr Graham Mitchison[20]. REM sleep, they suggested, is involved in a form of cleansing operation in the cerebrum to get rid of spurious connections between neurones which inevitably arise in the myriad of neural networks during wakefulness. The authors subscribe to the idea that memories are stored through the development of new neuronal connections, which include useless memories from events happening that day. These pointless memories, that is the bad connections, must be removed in order to avoid the brain becoming cluttered up. REM sleep somehow gives the cerebrum a steady series of 'bangs' (to use the authors' terminology) to knock them out. To explain the absence of REM sleep in primitive egg-laying mammals, Crick and Mitchison point out these animals are unusual in having an exceptionally large cerebrum, with plenty of spare capacity that can absorb this clutter, and so REM sleep is not required. This presumably is also the authors' explanation for the lack of REM sleep in the dolphin (see Section 7.1), although the animal is not mentioned by them. In all, this is an intriguing theory, but so far there is little experimental evidence to support it.

Whilst on the one hand we have a famous molecular geneticist giving a neurophysiological explanation for REM sleep, a renowned neurophysiologist and sleep researcher has turned to genetics in his quest for the answer. Professor Michel Jouvet, from the Université Claude-Bernard in Lyons, points out that the various instinctual behaviours that animals are born with must be genetically coded. He proposed[21] that during REM sleep this repertoire of behaviour and its codes are somehow read through and checked within the brain. If any changes need to be made as a consequence of the animal's experience with real life, then these can be done during the 'read out', and the appropriate recoding performed. Again, there is little proof for this idea, although he has shown in experiments with less advanced mammals, where behaviour is largely governed by instincts, that REM sleep deprivation impairs the ability to modify these behaviours. However, there is at least one other explanation for such a finding, which I will be describing in the next section. Also, it is difficult to see how Jouvet's idea applies to advanced mammals such as humans, where there is so little instinctual behaviour.

Most other memory consolidation theories claim that REM sleep expedites the sorting out of the day's events, with the important memories stored in an organized way, particularly through the laying down of new neural networks and/or the formation of special memory proteins. Generally, such theories give little account of how unwanted memories are removed, apart from the idea that dreams are made up of these throw-out products[15]. That proposal[15] came out in 1965 in the wave of the new computer era, with the authors drawing the analogy that dreaming was 'systematic program clearance'. A similar notion, appearing a year later[22], drew stronger parallels with computers by proposing that, 'the two main functions of (dreaming) sleep are to destructuralise or erase data storage and to reinforce the program (character) of the organism' (p. 260).

Some of these memory consolidation theories incorporate what seems to be a psychoanalytic approach[23, 24], believing that the stored memories can somehow be integrated into the personality. Emotional or threatening experiences are particularly handled in this way and kept out of our waking consciousness. With the result that personality and emotions may even be altered or adapted during REM sleep[25].

Numerous experiments have explored the various memory consolidation theories in humans and other mammals (mostly rodents). One approach is to deprive the organism of REM sleep and see how this affects memory. Overall, the findings with humans are unimpressive, and at best any impairment to memory is small—certainly not substantial enough to show that memory consolidation is an important function of REM sleep (see Section 8.7). On the other hand, the animal findings may seem more convincing (see Section 8.6). But there is a caveat—they have been beset with problems arising from the techniques used to deprive animals of REM sleep. For many of these studies, at least some of the apparent effects of REM sleep deprivation on learning is an artefact of the experimental method, as will be seen later.

The mid 1960s was a boom time for other ideas about REM sleep, following the many reports from animal studies that this sleep seems to be an aroused state. These were interpreted in several ways, with one popular theory being the *homeostatic* hypothesis, proposed by Drs Harmon Ephron and Patricia Carrington, respectively from New York Medical College and Columbia University[26]. They saw REM sleep as a counterbalance to the progressive fall in vigilance that occurs in non-REM sleep (seen as a loss of 'cortical tonus'). This potentially dangerous state of affairs, leaving the sleeper more open to attack, is rectified by REM sleep, which stimulates and excites the cerebrum enough to restore its 'tonus'. After a while, non-REM sleep can return, and the whole cycle is repeated.

Ephron and Carrington were not very clear about the purpose of non-REM sleep, except that it brought cerebral rest 'in response to the overloading of sensory and memory systems with increasing data in waking life'. The authors pointed out that within the organism the levels of non-REM and REM sleep are carefully balanced to ensure that cortical 'tonus' stays within certain limits—that is 'cortical homeostasis' is maintained. Although Ephron and Carrington considered that REM sleep allows sleep to continue without the animal having to awake in order to restore the tonus, they make no mention of whether wakefulness can substitute for REM sleep. By the way, they were not the first to adopt the term 'homeostatic' for a theory about sleep, as Jung also used it, within a different context, for his theory of dreams. He believed that dreams were homeostatic in 'regulating the psyche'[13].

Ephron and Carrington's hypothesis was also incorporated into the *phylogenetic* or *sentinel* theory of sleep, conceived in 1966 by Dr Frederick Snyder, who was then at the National Institute of Mental Health in Maryland[27]. He believed that the general function for sleep in mammals was to conserve energy—the longer the sleep, the better in this respect. Again though, there was the problem that the sleeper was left vulnerable. But according to Snyder, REM sleep not only brought consciousness nearly up to the waking level, allowing the animal a quicker response to danger, but REM sleep also produced momentary arousals into wakefulness, allowing fleeting glimpses into the outdoor world to check for danger. Safe sleepers have less need for these brief awakenings. Certainly there is strong evidence showing that animals sleeping in a strange environment wake up a lot, and as they become more accustomed to the situation these awakenings disappear.

Why then, from Snyder's standpoint, do very safe sleepers, such as humans and members of the cat family, need to have any REM sleep at all? Here Snyder brings in the homeostatic hypothesis, saying that REM sleep prevents sleep becoming too 'deep', as even the safest sleeper may have the occasional need to wake up fairly quickly. Snyder also proposed that in many respects REM sleep is a substitute for wakefulness, to maintain sleep. This is better than the alternative, of the animal having to wake up periodically to get its 'cortical homeostasis'. Awakenings, of course, bring body movements that can attract predators, whereas REM sleep keeps the animal relatively immobile. But for Snyder there was something more subtle in REM sleep than it being simply a substitute for wakefulness. He was impressed with the findings at the time that REM sleep deprivation made animals more 'excitable' during wakefulness (see below). Snyder saw this phenomenon to be beneficial to vulnerable sleepers, as not only do they have more wakefulness in substitution for REM sleep, to give them greater surveillance, but during this wakefulness they will also be more excitable and reactive to any danger. Conversely, he claimed, REM sleep dampens down this excitability to the extent that safe sleepers, in having more REM sleep, are much calmer during wakefulness.

This dampening effect is an attractive idea, even though it may simply be a variation on Freud's view that dreams discharge inner tensions. Nevertheless, the theme has also been taken up by Vogel, whom I mentioned in the last section for his comments on the activation–synthesis hypothesis. He produced a *motivational* theory about REM sleep[28], following the accumulating evidence showing the 'excitability' produced by REM sleep deprivation. Such findings are impressive in animals, and reviews of these effects by Vogel and by others[29] show that REM sleep deprivation increases sensitivity to various stimuli, reduces fear, heightens exploration and dominance, and raises general 'drive behaviour', reflected by increased eating, grooming, sexual activity, and aggression. The brain itself shows more excitability, as not only are these animals more prone to epileptic seizures, but their evoked potentials (see Section 2.21) are larger, and they have a greater desire for their brain 'pleasure centres' to be stimulated. Most of these effects continue for as long as the REM sleep deprivation lasts, but soon disappear on recovery.

REM sleep deprivation in humans is far less dramatic, and I have already given a brief account (Section 5.9) of how subjects behave after seven nights without REM sleep. Although there are other reports of increased appetite, aggression, and sexual interest, as well as enhancement of evoked potentials, such findings are minor[28, 29]. But as Vogel points out these modest effects are from subjects who are in good mental health. He suggests that there is a 'ceiling' on the amount of excitability that can be produced by REM sleep deprivation, with these people probably already near their maximum. Consistent with this idea is the common finding that antidepressant drugs, which suppress REM sleep, do not affect drive behaviour or mood in normal people. On the other hand, in severely depressed patients REM sleep reductions produced either by waking, or by antidepressant drugs, can lift mood dramatically. For a more permanent effect though, this deprivation has to last for about 3 weeks[30].

Vogel's ideas are attractive, but there is still the question of whether REM sleep really keeps excitability and drives dampened down? There is the alternative explanation that heightened drives, etc., are an artefact of the stressful procedures of REM sleep deprivation, with REM sleep itself having no dampening effect. However, Vogel makes a strong case for the former, which he sees to be particularly appropriate to the advanced mammals. For them, he suggests that such dampening of more 'basic behaviours' by REM sleep releases the animal from its instincts, gives more flexibility to other behaviours, and allows more 'thinking for itself'. I have much support for Vogel's views, although I strongly suspect that stress artefacts from the REM deprivation procedures used in the animal studies do add to the excitability due to the loss of REM sleep (Section 8.5).

8.3 Abundance of REM sleep in early life—the ontogenetic hypothesis

The newborn human spends nearly half of sleep in REM sleep. In 1-month premature babies this rises to 67 per cent, and up to 80 per cent at 2 months prematurity[31]. In absolute terms we are talking about 8 hours of REM sleep per 24 hour day at birth, and nearly double this amount for the 2-month premature baby (that sleeps for most of the time). A similar phenomenon, of large amounts of REM sleep around birth, is found in the newborn of most mammals, and for that matter in chicks (adult birds have very little REM sleep). Nevertheless, there are differences between mammals, depending on how well developed they are at birth. Mammals born precocious, that is with their brain and physical abilities in a fairly advanced state, particularly to allow walking within minutes of birth, have relatively little REM sleep.

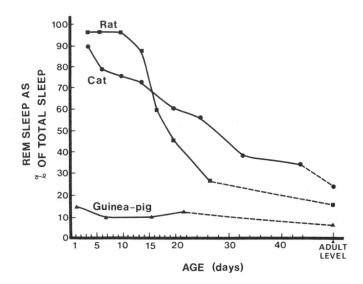

Fig. 8.1 Changes in levels of REM sleep with age—REM sleep around birth follows a 'maturity law'—as the cerebrum develops, the amount of REM sleep falls. The rat and cat are born in a helpless state, with a less-developed cerebrum than the guinea pig. The latter has much lower amounts of REM sleep at birth, although it had higher levels during gestation. (From Jouvet-Mounier et al.[32]. Reproduced by permission of John Wiley and Sons Inc.)

Typical examples are the ungulates, such as antelope, goats, cattle, etc., where it is vital for the newborn to be mobile and avoid predators.

Precocious young are also found in the guinea pig, whose levels of REM sleep from birth to adulthood are shown in Fig. 8.1. Contrast this with the kitten and rat pup, born blind, immobile, and quite helpless—described as 'altrical', and able to be protected by the mother. Here, as can be seen in Fig. 8.1, REM sleep makes up nearly 100 per cent of sleep at birth, but falls quite rapidly to about 30–40 per cent within a month. Usually, because of their poorer development at birth, gestation time is relatively shorter. Nevertheless, the 'maturity law' for REM sleep still holds, with the amount of REM sleep at birth declining as the degree of brain development increases. Precocious—altrical is really a dimension from one extreme to the other, as most mammals, especially primates, lie somewhere between. Humans are more altrical than most primates.

The impressive levels of REM sleep in early mammalian life led three investigators, Drs Howard Roffwarg, Joseph Muzio, and William Dement, to come together from their different establishments to propose, 20 years ago, what they refer to as the *ontogenetic* hypothesis for the function of REM sleep[33]. For them, the most important function of REM sleep lies with the early development of the cerebrum. The decline in REM sleep in later life is because this function has mostly been fulfilled. Although Roffwarg and colleagues concentrated mainly on humans, their theory also applied to other mammals. They felt it was most unlikely that the human fetus experiences what we understand as dreams, because the visual system is so poorly organized at that time. This is not to say that dreams do not occur in some simple way, but that we should concentrate on the non-dreaming aspects of REM sleep, especially the excited state of the cerebrum during this sleep. Roffwarg's group saw two possible lines of reasoning, one, the 'passive' theory that large quantities of REM sleep were due to a lack of some restraining influence in the cerebrum, and the other, the 'active' theory, that the developing cerebrum needed REM sleep, which was generated for this purpose.

They provided several powerful arguments in favour of the active theory. For example, experiments on the cat showed that REM sleep falls when the cerebrum is removed. If the cerebrum were inhibiting REM sleep then the opposite should happen. Roffwarg and colleagues proposed that the growing cerebrum needed stimulation in order to develop properly, and this is what REM sleep was doing. They were impressed by findings from other studies outside sleep research, showing that lack of stimulation for the cerebrum leads to various impairments in its function. Obviously, the best way of providing stimulation is for the senses to bombard the cerebrum with information, which happens after birth when the senses begin to work fully. But within the dark and muffled confines of the uterus there is little stimulation, and of course most of the senses are not sufficiently developed to receive information anyway. So, for the ontogenetic hypothesis, REM sleep is an internally generated form of substitute stimulation, which to a lesser extent is also necessary after birth.

According to these authors, there are two possibilities why REM sleep is retained in the adult, and both could be happening. Firstly, that the cerebrum needs more stimulation than is obtained during wakefulness. Secondly, and to quote them, that 'the REM process serves to maintain the central nervous system in a state of physiological readiness so that it may react swiftly to the exigencies of the real world' (p. 618). This latter idea is very similar to parts of the homeostatic and sentinel hypotheses already mentioned.

Recent work on human babies, by Drs Victor Denenberg and Evelyn Thoman, from the University of Connecticut, has tried to test out the ontogenetic hypothesis[34]. The investigators reasoned that if REM sleep is an internal form of stimulation substituting for that of wakefulness, then the two should be inversely related. Therefore, the more time that is spent in wakefulness the less would be spent in REM sleep, and vice versa. However, they needed to establish that any such relationship was not simply an artefact of sleep length, as obviously the more one sleeps the less one can be awake.

This was done statistically, whereby the influence of non-REM sleep was neutralized. Following detailed observations of 2 to 5-week-old babies at home, the data showed a high negative correlation of – 0.82 between REM sleep and wakefulness, that is the greater the wakefulness the less the REM sleep.

Denenberg and Thoman subdivided wakefulness into 'waking active' (eyes open and physical movement), 'quiet alert' (eyes alert and scanning, with little physical movement), 'fuss or cry', and 'drowsy'. Interestingly, the behaviour that showed the greatest negative correlation with REM sleep was 'quiet alert'. As they pointed out, other work outside the field of sleep has shown that babies can only attend to new features in the environment (with the accompanying sensory stimulation of the cerebrum) when in this state, and not during 'waking active'.

How do the other theories about REM sleep explain the large amounts of this sleep in the fetus and newborn? Most give this topic only a cursory look as they are really directed towards older mammals, and are usually non-committal about what happens in early life. Ephron and Carrington, in their homeostatic hypothesis, seem to come out in support of the ontogenetic theory, but have little else to say apart from implying that an underdeveloped cerebrum has the problem of maintaining its 'tonus', and needs extra REM sleep for stimulation. Although Snyder's sentinel theory also appears to favour the ontogenetic hypothesis, in that REM sleep promotes cerebral organization, he is also sympathetic to the view that development of the mammalian fetus may reflect various stages in evolution. So he sees the possibility that REM sleep may be a primitive carryover from the now extinct early mammals where this sleep is supposed to have been abundant. For Snyder then, the large amounts of REM sleep in present day fetuses may be just a reflection of this 'recapitulation' of the past.

The idea that the *very early* stages in fetal development follow the evolution of the species has been a controversial theory in biology for over a hundred years, and it has its attractions. But there are many structures in the mammalian fetus that were certainly not present in its adult ancestors, for example the fetal membranes including the placenta. So Snyder's use of recapitulation to explain the abundance of REM sleep in the mammalian fetus is pure surmise. Also, from what evidence we have so far, there is little indication of REM sleep being the evolutionary primitive sleep (see Section 7.5). For example, it is absent in the most primitive living mammals—the egg-laying duck-billed platypus and echidna. Although there have been some claims that REM sleep is present in reptiles, this is far from clear, and it is fair to say that no one has yet produced any convincing evidence to this effect. Certainly, there are no findings of the common signs of REM sleep such as rapid eye movements, and a profound loss of tonus in the face and neck muscles. REM sleep has the potential to be detected in reptiles if it were present. From what we know about REM sleep in mammals, it is generated in structures below the cerebrum, which mostly can also be found in reptiles. This contrasts with non-REM sleep, which is mainly generated in the forebrain, which is poorly developed in reptiles—see Section 7.5.

Returning to the theme of how REM sleep theories explain the abundance of this sleep in early life, whilst Vogel's motivational hypothesis makes little mention of the topic, Crick and Mitchison's idea that REM sleep 'unlearns' faulty neural circuits has more to say. They propose that many wrong connections are likely to be made during cerebral development, and much REM sleep is necessary to eliminate them. Jouvet's genetic programming theory also provides good reasoning, by claiming that as fetal development is the time when instinctual behaviours are being programmed into the brain, considerable checking via REM sleep is needed.

So far, I have been discussing the high amounts of REM sleep found up to and around the time of birth. What about the dramatic fall (in both relative and absolute terms) in REM sleep in the human baby following birth from about 8 hours a day in its first week to around half this level by its first birthday? Now, some of the theories of REM sleep are less clear here. Although a general argument is that REM sleep falls because of the overall drop in total daily sleep over the first year, this total sleep is not halved as is the case for REM sleep, but only drops by about a quarter, and cannot account for all of the REM sleep decrease. The ontogenetic hypothesis has a good explanation of course—with increasing cerebral maturity there is less need for the extra stimulation provided by REM sleep, and, besides, wakefulness can substitute for REM sleep to a large extent. On the other hand, the memory consolidation theories now begin to creak a little, including that of Jouvet, as the first year of human life is a time of considerable learning, when the infant is being bombarded with new information. Surely, in order to deal with all this memory consolidation, REM sleep should be increasing not decreasing? But the consolidation theories could argue that owing to better cerebral organization and an increasing experience of life, the cerebrum becomes more efficient in handling this inflow, so that less REM sleep is necessary!

8.4 Sleep after increased learning

In juvenile or adult mammals, REM sleep appears to increase somewhat after heightened learning during the previous period of wakefulness, and this seems to bear out the consolidation theories. Interestingly, the situation is not so simple at it seems, as not only are there alternative explanations outside these theories, but in the experiments on humans there is no sign of any heightening of REM sleep. In Section 5.5 I discussed the effects that increased daytime awareness during wakefulness had on subsequent sleep. Various studies were described, that had either bombarded human subjects with novel sensory and learning experiences, via window shopping and sightseeing etc., or had made subjects learn to see their environment in a different way, through the wearing of distorting prisms or lenses. These latter experiments were specifically designed to test the memory consolidation ideas of REM sleep, with the expectation that REM sleep would be increased on the subsequent night. Whilst nothing was found for REM sleep levels with any of these studies, the 'real-world' encounters led to rises in SWS. I explained this in terms of SWS representing some form of recovery for the cerebrum. For example, the increased daytime awareness leads to raised cerebral metabolism, and more cerebral 'wear and tear'.

In the animal experiments the most common candidates for study are laboratory-bred mice or rats, and occasionally rabbits and cats. Around 25 such studies have been carried out over the last 15 years, with the type of learning experience falling into two main categories:

1. The animal is trained to perform correctly at a task, such as running through a maze, or discriminating between certain shapes. This usually involves the giving of electric shocks or other aversions when mistakes are made.
2. The animal is placed, often for many days, in what is called an 'enriched' environment containing many objects, with which the animal interacts. There is more space for the animal to move about compared with the control condition, which is an 'impoverished' environment of a small cage, usually measuring about one body length (including tail) by a half by a half. In my opinion, one should regard the term 'enriched' as poetic licence for a more natural environment, whereas the caged condition is quite unnatural. It should be remembered that whilst laboratory rats have been bred for many generations, they can still easily revert to the behaviour and lifestyle of the wild variety, as shown when they escape and live 'wild'.

According to the consolidation theories, REM sleep should be increased after both types of learning, that is there should be more REM sleep following the training days compared with non-training days (method 1), and in the enriched compared with the impoverished environment (method 2). Several excellent reviews of these animal studies have been written, particularly by Drs Michael McGrath and David Cohen from the University of Texas[35], and more recently by Dr Carlyle Smith from Trent University, Ontario, Canada[36]. As I have mentioned, the consensus is that REM sleep indeed rises after both types of learning experience. However, much of this is due to an overall increase in total sleep length, with non-REM sleep also rising. When this factor is removed, it seems that what is left is not so much any sustained rise in REM sleep, but increases in only certain portions of REM sleep within the entire sleep period. Smith refers to these as 'windows' in sleep, which tend to appear soon after sleep onset but sometimes occur up to several hours into sleep. Control animals show no changes within these windows.

However, there is another factor to consider, coming from the ideas put forward by both Snyder and Vogel (Section 8.2) that REM sleep dampens down excitability during wakefulness. The electric shocks and other 'aversive stimuli' used in the training sessions are likely themselves to raise this excitability, and so will living in an 'enriched' environment. Therefore, I suggest that more REM sleep may be required not to consolidate increased learning, but instead just to reduce this excitability. It could be contended that my argument is groundless, especially in relation to the shocks, etc., as there is usually a control animal also given an electric shock at the same time. To continue this riposte, these animals should be equally excited, and would also show a similar need for REM sleep if it were necessary for dampening excitability.

No, not so—as remember this control animal is probably doing nothing in particular at the time of its shocks. On some occasions it might be grooming or eating, and at other times walking around its cage, or even taking a short sleep. Consequently, it cannot associate any particular behaviour with being 'wrong', and it does not know what to do in order to avoid these unpleasant surprises—as far as it is concerned they come out of the 'thin air'. In such circumstances when nothing can be done to avoid the problem, animals demonstrate 'helplessness'. Excitability and arousal fall, and inactivity sets in. They go off their food, and, to be anthropomorphic, they seem to become withdrawn. Such effects have been well described, although outside the context of memory and sleep research[37]. But in the case of the experimental animal at whom the shocks are really directed, it has control over these unpleasant experiences by learning to avoid making mistakes at whatever the task has been given to it. These animals remain in a heightened state of alertness. In summary, the 'aversive stimuli' can have opposite effects on the excitability of the experimental and control animals, raising and lowering it respectively.

8.5 REM sleep deprivation in animals—background

The memory consolidation theories for REM sleep function are having increasing difficulty in handling REM sleep deprivation findings, as it is clear from both animal and human studies that even the longest periods of deprivation do not incapacitate memory, and at best only produce modest decrements. Furthermore, with the animal experiments there are other unwanted factors to be contended with outside the area of memory. These focus on problems with the methods used to deprive animals of REM sleep, and again on the increases in 'excitability' and in drive behaviour.

Let me start with the procedures. The typical animals used are, again, rats and mice, with the usual method for producing REM sleep deprivation being the 'pedestal' technique. The underlying rationale is that these animals dislike getting wet and will avoid water. Single animals are placed on a small, round pedestal located one centimetre above a bath of water deep enough to prevent them from walking away. The pedestal is only large enough to accommodate the animal's body, so its head is above the surrounding water. There the animal stays, often for days at a time. Food and drinking water are always available. During wakefulness and non-REM sleep, tonus in the neck muscles keeps the head above the water, but in REM sleep tonus is lost and the head dips in, immediately waking the animal up. This happens whenever REM sleep begins. Sometimes the animal falls into the water. The method effectively removes about 80–90 per cent of REM sleep, but because sleep is so disrupted the animal also loses some non-REM sleep.

Not only is the animal REM sleep deprived, but the technique itself is obviously stressful, and a 'stress control' is necessary. This normally consists of another animal being placed on a slightly larger platform, allowing REM sleep to occur as the head can rest on the edge and avoid dipping into the water. Nevertheless, the term 'stress control' is somewhat of a euphemism, as the stress cannot be as great as that of the experimental animal even though both are subjected to platform confinement. The experimental animal not only also loses REM sleep, but has considerably more sleep disruption, and falls into the water more often. Therefore, we do not know whether differences in behaviour between the two animals are due to REM sleep loss alone, overall sleep disruption, falling into the water, or all of these. Only infrequently is any measure of stress actually carried out on these animals, and then the usual check on stress is through weighing the adrenal glands at autopsy. Whilst these weights often rise by similar extents for both groups of animals, this is a crude measure if the deprivation only lasts for a few days (which is the typical period), as this is too short a time to allow the adrenals to enlarge noticeably. Besides, adrenal weights do not necessarily relate to the output of the stress hormone cortisol, and it will be remembered that it was for this reason that Rechtschaffen's laboratory relied mostly on the measurement of blood cortisol levels rather than on adrenal weights (Section 2.2).

To allow animals more movement whilst undergoing REM sleep deprivation, some laboratories use a 'multiple' platform technique, consisting of about five platforms above the water linked by narrow bridges permitting the animals to walk about from platform to platform. Control animals have larger platforms. Although still effective in removing REM sleep, this method is not up to the standards of the single platform in this respect, as to some extent the animals can support their heads on the bridges.

By far the majority of REM sleep deprivation experiments on rodents has been done with the single platform technique, but now there is a dry method for deprivation that is creating much interest—the 'pendulum' technique[38]. The animal is placed in a relatively large cage with a smooth flat floor. The whole assembly slowly rocks backwards and forwards, and the animal is liable to slide from one end of the cage to the other, unless it can exert some counteracting muscular effort. This can largely be achieved during non-REM sleep, and most of this sleep is retained. But as this ability is lost during REM sleep, owing to the paralysis of voluntary (skeletal) muscles, the rocking causes the animal to roll or slide about and wake up. There is a control condition of gentler rocking and less sliding, allowing most of REM sleep to be kept.

In fact the pendulum is better at removing REM sleep than either the single or multiple platform methods. For example, over a 3 day period it resulted in an 87 per cent loss of REM sleep, against 80 per cent for the single platform[38]. However, this is not without cost as the pendulum causes more sleep disturbance and a greater loss of the deeper form of non-REM sleep[38]. Weighed against this is the considerable advantage that the animal is dry (see below), is much less confined, and can move about. But of course it is obliged to be mobile—a factor that could create other problems.

One of the most interesting findings from using the pendulum method is that rats deprived of REM sleep in this way are less likely to show learning impairments than animals REM sleep deprived by the single platform—a perplexing finding especially for the investigators[38]. I strongly suspect that much of the experimental evidence from the platform experiments supporting a relationship between REM sleep and learning is simply an artefact of two other factors: (1) the stress of the procedure, and (2) the 'excitement' from the enhanced drive behaviour produced by the REM sleep deprivation itself (see next section). Therefore, perhaps the pendulum technique is either less stressful, or, the greater loss of the deeper non-REM sleep coupled with the increased sleep disturbance may be counteracting this 'excitement'. I will be developing this last idea further shortly.

There is one further point that I wish to take up concerning the platform techniques of REM sleep deprivation—the wetness. In Section 2.2, I mentioned that the main organ used by most rodents to regulate body heat loss is the tail. An unfortunate consequence of the single and multiple platforms is that because of the smallness of the platforms the animal's tail inevitably drops over the edge into the cool water and remains partly submerged—so there is a major risk of heat loss. This could be worsened as REM sleep deprivation may impair thermoregulation in small mammals (see Section 2.2). These factors must add to the stress and to any loss of learning. The control animal has the advantage in not only having its thermoregulation intact, but because it sits on a larger platform less of the tail is in the water. These potential complications for the platform methods, overcome by the dry pendulum technique, have never been systematically investigated. Body temperature measurements have been taken during platform experiments, and reported to be unchanged. But this tells us little about thermoregulation, as of course, metabolic rate (heat production) can rise to compensate for any extra heat loss, without affecting body temperature.

8.6 REM sleep deprivation, learning, and drive behaviour

The learning tasks given during REM sleep deprivation are similar to those used in the studies of increased learning on REM sleep, mentioned in Section 8.4. Most require the animal to learn to run a simple maze, or to run in a certain direction when a light or sound comes on. An 'aversive stimulus' is given (typically an electric shock) when a mistake is made, and the learning ability is judged by how many training trials are required before the animal can do the task perfectly. Such tasks have little bearing on the animals' normal behaviour, and for this reason the results may not be relevant to real life. And of course, when this learning is coupled with the problems associated with the various types of REM sleep deprivation procedures, then one might question the relevance of this field of research to the understanding of the function of REM sleep.

Nevertheless, let me briefly go through the findings on REM sleep deprivation and learning in animals. As in the last section, I shall base this on the two reviews, by McGrath and Cohen[35], and by Smith[36]. Both divide the learning into two types of task which, for reasons I will not go into, are called 'prepared' and 'unprepared'. Instead, it is not an overstatement to use the terms 'simple' and 'difficult' respectively, as I shall do here. Typically, in simple tasks, the animal has to learn (via the 'aversion') to avoid a 'forbidden zone' within a special cage, or turn right at a 'T' junction in a maze. Difficult tasks involve avoiding two or more forbidden zones, or to negotiate correctly several successive 'T' junctions.

REM sleep deprivation can be given either before or after the learning. In the former, the measure of learning is the number of trials that have to be given, or the time taken before the task can be done correctly. For experiments when the deprivation is given after the learning, animals are previously trained near to perfection, and then given either REM sleep deprivation or the control condition. A retest then follows, to see how much of the memory has been retained. The score can be the time taken to complete the task, or the number of trials necessary to do the task successfully. Smith cites 15 experiments where the deprivation precedes the training, and over 50 for the other way round[36]. The outcome can quickly be summarized for the former—doubtful. Nine involved simple tasks, and six difficult tasks. Out of those nine, six reported that REM sleep deprivation made learning significantly worse compared with control conditions. Although this may seem impressive at first glance, Smith goes on to find faults with most of them, mainly in their flawed designs (these criticisms being largely different from those of my own already mentioned). For the six difficult tasks, only one claimed any significant effect of REM sleep deprivation, and, according to Smith, most of these studies were also deficient in some way. Not surprisingly, in ending his discussion of the effects of REM sleep deprivation on subsequent learning, Smith makes the all too familiar remark, that 'more research needs to be done in this area before any conclusions can confidently be made. At the moment, the case . . . is weak' (p.163).

But he is more positive in his appraisal of the 50 or so studies that looked at REM sleep deprivation after training. Nearly all of them used simple rather than difficult learning tasks. Smith finds that about two-thirds of these studies reported that REM sleep deprivation reduces learning to a significantly greater extent than under control conditions, with the remainder reporting no such differences. He also brings in his proposal of the REM sleep 'window' I mentioned in the last section by suggesting that loss of this part of REM sleep will have the greatest repercussions for learning. However, the appearance of this window seems to vary in time, depending on various circumstances that I shall not go into.

In sum, and in relation to the memory consolidation hypothesis for REM sleep, I find the field of REM sleep deprivation and learning in animals unconvincing. This is because of: (1) what still seems to me to be equivocal results from a group of learning tasks unrealistic to the normal life of a rodent, (2) problems with the procedures, with the resultant stress, and with the possible impairment to thermoregulation which are not the same for the control animals, and (3) unwanted effects of increased drive behaviour (see below). Admittedly, this is a rather summary dismissal that neglects the various components of learning, for example whether REM sleep aids the formation of memory, or improves recall. However, I do not think that it is necessary to become involved with such details until these other issues have been resolved by the investigators themselves.

Of greater importance for me at the moment are the findings of increased drive behaviour produced by REM sleep deprivation. This excitability will distract the animal from its learning task, and could well be crucial to any learning impairment. Such increases in basic drives like eating, aggression, dominance, exploratory behaviour, grooming, etc., have been described in detail by Vogel[28], and more recently in an update by myself and Michael McGrath[29]. There is no shortage of such findings, and for example, we located 23 separate accounts. *It is still not clear, though, to what extent these behaviours are due directly to some association between REM sleep and drives (cf. Vogel), or to an artefact of the stress produced by the deprivation procedure, or to both mechanisms.* This does not really matter, though, as all I am concerned about is that the drive behaviours occur, for whatever reasons.

Studies on rats outside the field of sleep deprivation have shown that if they are given mildly stressful stimuli such as a small electric shock, pinching the tail, frustration, excessive handling, isolation, or confinement, then they become excitable and show greater drive behaviours[39]. Some of these stimuli, especially frustration at being prevented from sleeping, isolation and confinement are obviously found in the pedestal procedures of REM sleep deprivation. Remember that control animals have a larger platform and are able to sleep better, and so levels of confinement and frustration must be lower. An important finding with those stress studies is that the appearance of a drive behaviour depends on whether the appropriate target objects are present. For example, if there happens to be plenty of food around at the time of the stress then excessive eating will predominate. On the other hand if the animal is male and other males are around then aggression will occur, or if the other animals are females then sexual activity will increase. All these behaviours have been seen in REM-sleep-deprived animals when they are taken off their pedestals. Obviously, only a limited number of drive behaviours can be displayed when the animal is actually confined to a pedestal, such as increased grooming, eating, and drinking.

One reason, it seems, why stress increases drives is that the stereotyped behaviour produced by the drives helps block attention to the stress by keeping the animal occupied with something else[39]. Obviously, this stereotypy also prevents the animal from being flexible in its behaviour, and it will be less inclined to learn something new. So, if REM sleep deprivation is more stressful than a control condition, then the animal may be more concerned about reducing stress through producing stereotyped behaviours than about anything else.

As such behaviour helps the animal to reduce the impact of stress, any potential rise in the physiological responses to stress, such as growth in the adrenal glands or a larger output of cortisol, may be reduced. This could also explain the frequent claim that REM-sleep-deprived animals are no more stressed than 'stress control' animals, because the growth in the size of the adrenal glands is apparently the same for both animals (but remember, the sensitivity of adrenal growth as a measure of stress is also a debatable point—see last section). This is a small detail, though, and must not detract from my key point that REM sleep deprivation causes greater drive behaviour, for whatever reason, which is more likely to be responsible for the learning impairments, not some direct link between REM sleep and memory consolidation.

8.7 REM sleep deprivation in humans

The lack of any profound effect of REM sleep deprivation on human behaviour other than to produce sleepiness is perhaps surprising from the memory consolidation viewpoint, given our relatively enormous reliance on memory. When discussing Vogel's proposals (Section 8.2) I mentioned that there are only a few signs in humans of any increase in drive behaviour or excitability, except perhaps in the case of patients suffering from endogenous depression. Our behaviour is not governed by basic drives to the same extent as is rodent behaviour, and this might help explain the different effects of REM sleep deprivation. One crucial factor separating these human experiments from those on animals is that there is little additional stress imposed on human subjects, whereas for the rodents this is a considerable problem.

Of the two reviews on REM sleep and learning I have referred to[35,36], only that by McGrath and Cohen covers the human findings. Again they divide up the various studies according to whether simple ('prepared') or difficult ('unprepared') tasks had been given, and whether the REM sleep deprivation preceded or followed the learning. Both types of task have usually involved listening to words. With simple tasks this tends to consist of a straightforward list of about a dozen words to be remembered, whereas with difficult tasks the subject might have to remember the details of a complicated short story. Although there have not been many of these experiments, all had a control condition of an equivalent amount of non-REM sleep deprivation. Usually the deprivation of whatever type of sleep lasts for only one or two nights, as beyond this time sleep becomes very disrupted.

So, I will go onto McGrath and Cohen's conclusions for the human studies. It is clear that, given either before or after learning, REM sleep deprivation does not lead to any greater learning impairment on simple tasks, but difficult tasks are more affected. Whilst these latter findings can reach statistical significance, the effects are still relatively small, and not convincing enough to support any theory that REM sleep has a crucial role to play in the consolidation of memory. Exactly why REM sleep deprivation is more likely to affect the recall of difficult material is the matter for a debate that I shall not pursue. One would at first have to examine these experiments in more detail to see, for example, whether sleep was disrupted to the same extent by both the REM and non-REM sleep deprivation (control) conditions, as this can be very difficult to accomplish[40].

8.8 Brain protein synthesis and related findings

One common view about how long-term memories are stored in the brain is that it is done through the formation of memory proteins, following short-term storage via 'reverberating' networks of neurones. Such proteins could be produced within nerve endings or neuroglia (see Section 5.11). There have been several reports showing that protein synthesis increases within the brain during REM sleep—findings which have been used to endorse the idea that memory proteins are specifically made during REM sleep. Some of these findings are based on the remarkable technique of examining the protein content of fluid extracted from the living brain of a sleeping animal[41]. Unfortunately though, this method tells us little about what is going on inside neurones or neuroglia, which is where memory proteins are presumed to lie. Other techniques taking extracts from within brain cells (after the animal is killed during REM sleep) obtain proteins from numerous chemical pathways. So we have no idea which, if any, of these could be 'memory proteins', as opposed to those simply linked to the generalized increase in neural activity and brain metabolism during REM sleep.

It is possible to block protein synthesis by certain drugs, such as the antibiotics 'anisomycin' and 'chloramphenicol' and the toxic antitumor drug 'vincristine'. Often, the effect in animals is to impair the storage of new memories—a result seeming to confirm the view that memories are stored as proteins. Also, these drugs reduce the amount of REM sleep to a much greater extent than non-REM sleep. Often, the impaired memory is seen to be directly related to the reduced REM sleep, and here then seems to be more support for the memory consolidation theories of REM sleep. But such conclusions are all too easily jumped to and there is another explanation.

Given at therapeutic doses to treat infections, etc., these drugs can affect REM sleep in experimental animals. But in order to impair memory as well, the doses have to be higher. A variety of side effects are commonly produced, such as diarrhoea and malaise, which may seem minor to the experimenter. But examinations by a veterinary surgeon are seldom if ever done. These effects must distress the animal, and its memory is likely to be impaired simply because of this distress, as well as by any putative suppression of protein synthesis. Distress, rather than an impairment to the formation of memory proteins, could be another reason why the animal has less REM sleep. Remember, REM sleep is a fragile sleep, and is more liable to be lost than non-REM sleep when there is danger or distress. Whilst control groups of animals are used for these drug studies, they are usually given a pharmacologically inert substance such as saline. Ideally, something to produce the side effects alone should be administered.

Other investigators interested in memory proteins and REM sleep have looked at RNA turnover, where a rise usually heralds an increase in protein synthesis (see Section 4.1). The technique is first to put a radioactive label on RNA, by injecting the animal with a biochemical marker that becomes incorporated into the RNA molecule. Then, when the animal is in REM sleep it is killed and the brain immediately removed. RNA turnover is measured by assessing the number of labels on the RNA. RNA takes many forms, some of which are predominantly found within cell nuclei, and others within the surrounding cytoplasm. One of the most detailed series of studies in this area[42] looked at the RNA content of nuclei from neurones and neuroglia taken from the cerebal cortex of the rabbit. The outcome was not straightforward, as for certain large nuclei the RNA turnover was lowest in REM sleep and highest in the deeper form of non-REM sleep. On the other hand, for small nuclei there was no difference between these sleep states. Overall, these and related findings are puzzling, and of unknown meaning for both REM and non-REM sleep.

Because it is commonly thought that REM sleep serves an essential repair or memory consolidation function for the brain, more so than non-REM sleep, various events within the brain during REM sleep tend to be interpreted from this outlook. It particularly applies to the rise in neural activity found within the cerebral cortex during REM sleep, compared with the low activity and apparently more vegetative state of non-REM sleep. The high neural firing in REM sleep is seen to represent something beneficial. However, given that there is no real evidence to support this supposition, one could just as well argue that when neural firing is high, then little repair and restitution can be going on, as these latter events are best accomplished when neural activity is low. Similar arguments also apply to interpretations for the increases in the brain's blood flow, metabolism, and temperature during REM sleep, that I will describe in Section 8.11.

8.9 Conclusions so far about the functions of REM sleep

To summarize what I have covered so far on the function of REM sleep, it seems that all we have in favour of the memory consolidation theory is, at best, only weak evidence from humans and questionable findings from animals. Much of the data from animals are affected by the unwanted effects of other changes in behaviour, which are probably further enhanced by the stress of the procedures of REM sleep deprivation, especially in the case of the pedestal techniques. Even though stress control measures are taken, these do not seem to be adequate. Besides, the types of learning task adopted are usually traumatic in themselves, and have uncertain bearings on what these animals would learn naturally. Overall, REM sleep deprivation findings from animals seem to offer better support for those theories suggesting that REM sleep has something to do with reducing both drive behaviour and the general level of 'excitement' during wakefulness. Increases in REM sleep in animals following experiences of 'enriched environments' can be explained either by a need to reduce this excitement, or of course by the memory consolidation approach.

REM sleep is predominant in the fetus, suggesting that it is here where its function really lies. This is why the ontogenetic hypothesis (that REM sleep stimulates the developing cerebrum) is so attractive. REM sleep may at least partly act as a substitute for wakefulness because, as will be seen shortly, REM sleep is so alike wakefulness. This substitution may not only act to keep the sleeping brain stimulated without the mammal having to wake up, but also have the role of dampening down drive behaviours and excitement during wakefulness.

8.10 Similarities between REM sleep and wakefulness

REM sleep is accompanied by several remarkable phenomena apart from dreaming, and many are reminiscent of wakefulness. Prominent among these is the high level of neuronal firing within much of the CNS. In the cat, the similarity between the EEG of REM sleep and that of alert wakefulness can be seen in Fig. 8.2, and is the main reason why REM sleep has also been called 'paradoxical' sleep—the animal is asleep, but the EEG indicates wakefulness. Most mammals are like the cat in this respect, with REM sleep remarkably like alert wakefulness. The main exceptions are humans and other higher primates, where the EEG of REM sleep bears a greater similarity with stage 1 sleep. This can be seen in Fig. 1.1, and is why human REM sleep was once called 'stage 1-REM' sleep.

Because of the alertness of the cerebrum during REM sleep, animals have the potential to move about actively and even run around at this time. To a more modest extent the same probably applies to humans. The reason why animals and humans remain so still in REM sleep relates to a 'locomotor centre' within the pons, a region lying near the FTG neurones that I mentioned in connection with Hobson and McCarley's theory (Section 8.1). This centre produces a general paralysis in nearly all voluntary muscles, particularly those of the limbs and trunk, and prevents all but small movements and twitches. The paralysis lifts when REM sleep ends. Sometimes though, as many people have occasionally experienced on suddenly awakening from REM sleep, and especially from a nightmare, the paralysis remains for a short while. The term 'postural atonia' (no tone in postural [voluntary] muscles) is commonly used to describe this paralysis. However, most postural muscles do retain their background resting tonus—it is their ability to contract that is blocked. But there is one exception—the muscles of the face and neck, where the background tonus is also largely lost. This is the reason why electrodes are placed here (usually on the chin in the case of humans), as a further guide to the presence of REM sleep (see Section 1.3).

If the locomotor centre is destroyed, then the voluntary muscles are freed from their paralysis and the animal will move around during REM sleep. This was shown in pioneering work on the cat during the early 1960s carried out by Jouvet (whose 'genetic programming' hypothesis I introduced in Section 8.2). More recently, further work in this area has been carried out, again on the cat, by another leading sleep neurophysiologist, Dr Adrian Morrison from the School of Vetinary Medicine at the University of

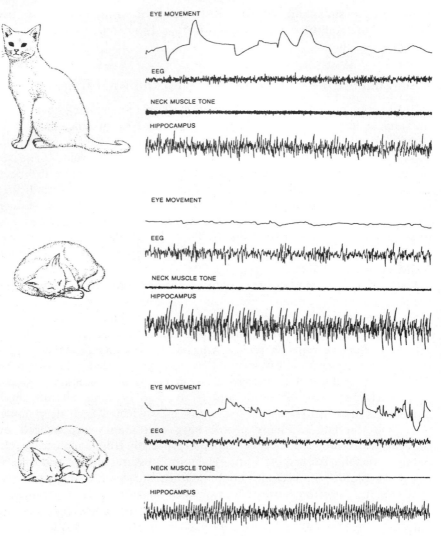

Fig. 8.2 States of alertness in the cat—wakefulness (upper), non-REM sleep (middle), and REM sleep (lower). During wakefulness the eyes and head move in response to visual stimulation, the EEG contains low amplitude high frequency waves, and the neck muscles have a relatively high tonus. The hippocampus produces much theta activity (see text). In non-REM sleep there are no eye movements, the EEG is of high amplitude and low frequency, neck muscle tone is lower, and there is no hippocampal theta. REM sleep is very similar to wakefulness, as can be seen in the EEG, eye movements, and the re-occurrence of hippocampal theta. However, neck muscle tone is lost (see text). (From Morrison[43]. Reproduced by permission of W H Freeman & Co.)

Pennsylvania. He incapacitated various parts of the locomotor centre, with the result that when REM sleep began, the non-paralysed animal typically raised its head and appeared to look around as though something was attracting its attention. The head may turn rapidly, seemingly following an imaginary moving object, and the animal often paws the air as if trying to catch something. Although the eyes are partly open, it is unlikely that anything is seen as the pupils are very constricted, letting little light through. Also, cats have a second eyelid, a nictitating membrane, which in wakefulness is only visible when the animal blinks. However, in the non-paralysed REM sleep this membrane remains half over the eye, partly obscuring the pupil. Further evidence that such a cat does not really see anything, was shown by Morrison when he placed an anaesthetized rat on the floor in front of the cat—it was ignored.

Nevertheless, the cat may well get up and appear to walk purposefully towards something, or even run around in an excited state. Often this develops into attacking behaviour, still directed towards an imaginary object, and involves anger, drawn claws, and hissing. After a few minutes the animal may lie back down, but if REM sleep continues mobility will usually return, coming and going like this until the REM sleep episode is over. Interestingly, the animals can be awakened without difficulty during these movements, and will cease what they were doing. After no more than a second or so of mild confusion they are able to attend to whatever woke them up. This rapid transformation is quite remarkable, and I have witnessed all these events myself at Morrison's laboratory. We will never know whether these animals are acting out their dreams, but it certainly looks like it. This 'window on the sleeping brain', to use Morrison's words[43] is providing considerable insight into the underlying workings of REM sleep. But he is cautious about his findings, and reminds us that these fascinating activities during REM sleep are the product of a damaged brain. It is possible, therefore, that an intact brain might not have such a potential to produce searching and aggressive behaviours during REM sleep, and that the surgical procedures could be stimulating this mobility as well as removing the paralysis.

Another strong sign of the similarity between REM sleep and wakefulness relates to a 7 Hz EEG activity in the theta range of frequencies (see Section 1.3), found in an evolutionarily old part of the cerebrum called the hippocampus. Hence this activity is called 'hippocampal theta'. As can be seen in Fig. 8.2, it is found in wakefulness, is absent from non-REM sleep, but re-appears in REM sleep. The meaning of this activity for behaviour is not fully understood, but it is thought to be associated with the redirecting and alerting of attention to new stimuli. Humans also demonstrate hippocampal theta, although it cannot usually be seen on the standard EEG, and electrodes have to be placed within the brain for this purpose.

Although neural firing rates in many parts of the brain are high during both wakefulness and REM sleep, during REM sleep the firing pattern can be broken down into two components—the 'tonic' background activity that is continuous throughout REM sleep, and the 'phasic' activity of superimposed periodic bursts of firing lasting a few seconds at a time. It is this phasic activity that coincides with the more obvious signs of REM sleep, especially the rapid eye movements themselves (see Fig. 8.2). These are not continuous (Section 1.2), and in fact for much of REM sleep the eyes are still. The ears also have their equivalent of eye movement bursts, with minute muscles of the middle ear that regulate the tension of the eardrum and ear ossicles, showing similar surges of activity, called 'MIMAs' (middle ear muscle activity).

Behind the phasic neural activity, rapid eye movement bursts, and MIMAs is another phasic electrical event that seems to be closely linked to the source of all these activities—the ponto-geniculo-occipital (PGO) spikes. These are very large electrical discharges (spikes) arising from 'burst cells' in the pons and rising to parts of the visual system, especially the geniculate body (a relay station between the eyes and rest of the brain) and the occipital area of the cerebral cortex. The burst cells are different from the FTG cells mentioned in Section 8.1. There is a complex and debatable relationship between these two groups of cells, as well as with other brain mechanisms underlying the control of REM sleep. I shall not go into this topic. PGO spikes were thought to be the key feature of REM sleep, which were unique to this sleep, distinguishing it from both non-REM sleep and wakefulness.

However, it is now known that this is not the case, as has been recently shown for example by Morrison and a colleague, Dr Robert Bowker[44]. They noticed that although EEG recordings of sleeping animals in a normal quiet environment produced the classical picture of PGO spikes only appearing in REM sleep, when the animal's cage was tapped during non-REM sleep, PGO spikes re-appeared. Further work showed, surprisingly, that the spikes could easily be produced in REM or non-REM sleep, simply by sounds or by touching the sleeping animal. So, argued Morrison, PGO spikes seem to be some sort of general alerting response, and if we were to look more carefully they would probably to be found in wakefulness as well.

Stimulated by these findings, Bowker and Morrison widened their interest to look at what researchers outside the field of sleep call 'eye movement potentials', found during wakefulness but occurring in identical parts of the brain to where PGO spikes appear during sleep. These potentials were orginally thought to depend on the lighting level in the cat's environment, as they had not been noticed in awake cats in the dark and were therefore presumed to be quite distinct from PGO spikes. It turns out however, that the methods used in the experiments may have been confusing matters, and centre around the fact that, to keep the animals calm, recordings are usually

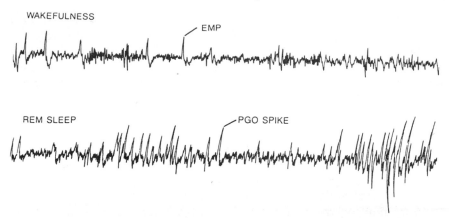

WAKEFULNESS

EMP

REM SLEEP   PGO SPIKE

Fig. 8.3 Eye movement potentials (EMPs) are the same as PGO spikes—electrical activity in the visual cortex of the cat during wakefulness and REM sleep. EMPs can be seen during wakefulness, and appear to be identical to the ponto-geniculo-occipital (PGO) spikes found during REM sleep. These apparently one-and-the-same phenomena appear to be alerting responses. See text for details. (Recordings provided by Adrian Morrison)

done in quiet and dimly lit rooms. Not surprisingly, awake cats become bored as there is nothing to attract their interest. Hence, there were no eye movement potentials. But if, as Bowker discovered, the animals are aroused by the smell of fish for example, then they look around for the source of the smell and eye movement potentials readily appear. Careful examination of these potentials now shows them to be identical to PGO spikes! The similarity between these two phenomena can be seen in Fig. 8.3. To summarize, Morrison proposes that PGO spikes and eye movement potentials are simply part of a generalized alerting response that can be produced during waking, REM, and non-REM sleep. However, in REM sleep PGO spikes can also arise spontaneously, without any stimulation.

In further work, Morrison has shown that, in addition to the locomotor centre that inhibits muscular contraction, there is another region in the brain stem that he refers to as a 'locomotor generator', giving the animal the impulse to move. Normally, in REM sleep this is switched off. If, instead, during REM sleep the animal is to be mobile, not only has it to be free of the paralysis produced by the locomotor centre, but metaphorically speaking it also has to be given a 'push' to start from the locomotor generator. The interaction between these two mechanisms is subtle. During REM sleep, particularly when the phasic activities such as rapid eye movements, MIMAs, and PGO spikes occur, both the locomotor mechanisms are involved—that is, one is activated to produce the paralysis and the other is inactivated to ensure no push start. Interestingly, Morrison points out that this situation can also occur during aroused wakefulness. For example, most of us have experienced a moment of hesitation, even physical weakness, when an unpleasant surprise comes along. An extreme example is to see a car suddenly bearing down on you when crossing the road, causing you to go 'weak at the knees', or become 'petrified by fear'. The disorder 'cataplexy' may be an abnormal and extreme example of this response, when sudden but normal heightening of the emotions, as in laughing or crying, trigger exaggerated levels of weakness to the point of physical collapse. Sometimes sleep, commonly REM sleep, is also brought on as well, and when this happens the condition is called 'narcolepsy'.

According to Morrison, normal REM sleep seems to be a type of exaggerated alertness whereby an immobilized animal experiences a large number of what could be described as 'surprises', generated from within the brain and not from the environment (as sensory input into the brain is largely cut off at this time). These are mostly reflected in the phasic (PGO) activity of REM sleep, and this behaviour is remarkably like what is known in wakefulness as 'orienting responses'. We all experience such responses throughout the day, whenever something unexpected attracts our attention—for example a knock on the door causing us to 'prick up our ears', a sudden movement at the edge of our field of view causing the head to turn and look at it, or a sudden and strange smell that makes us sniff. Orienting responses are automatic, and occur before one really knows what is going on. They do not necessarily cause fright, but are simply a mechanism for producing a total switch of attention to the new event so that one can become fully aware of it.

Accompanying these orienting responses are momentary physiological changes, especially to the heart and cardiovascular system. For example, the heart beat at first slows down and then quickens, blood flow to the skin momentarily increases, and blood-pressure falls then rises. Breathing is also affected, often very noticeably by 'catching one's breath'. There are degrees of these changes, depending on the level of the surprise, with the greatest effects coming from frights. Not only might we be 'petrified with fear', but for a second or so the heart rate drops dramatically to give the feeling of 'missing a beat'. Fortunately, we encounter few such alarms during a normal day, unlike the many quickly forgotten orienting responses, all of which produce the small changes in physiology. In REM sleep, it is unlikely that the phasic events, or what seem to be orienting responses, cause much of a surprise to the sleeper, otherwise waking would occur. Nevertheless, there are certainly measurable short-lived changes to many physiological systems during these phasic episodes of REM sleep, happening to a much greater extent than in non-REM sleep[45].

A recent carefully conducted study on humans has clearly shown this with heart rate during REM sleep[46]. Obvious heart rate slowing associated with bursts of eye movement activity typically started about 3 seconds before the eye movement activity began. The authors reported that this slowing was very similar to that found by other investigators for awake subjects suddenly attending to new stimuli and showing orienting responses. What exactly the stimuli could be during REM sleep is a mystery, and it is not known how or if they are related to an event 'seen' during dreaming.

To summarize this section, it seems that during REM sleep the firing of the FTG cells, the appearance of hippocampal theta activity, and the well-known phasic events of REM sleep such as PGO spikes, rapid eye movements, MIMAs, and heart rate slowing, are just like orienting responses of wakefulness. That is, REM sleep is very similar to alert wakefulness. We might even begin to query whether REM sleep really is a state of sleep, or a peculiar form of wakefulness within sleep!

8.11 Keeping cool

However, whilst many of the physiological changes in REM sleep do seem to resemble those of orienting responses, other changes seem quite unlike anything occurring during wakefulness. The REM sleep phenomena that come to mind are what seem to be impairments to homeostasis—particularly to thermoregulation, and blood flow to various organs. Nevertheless, Morrison still sees parallels with wakefulness, as for him these homeostatic changes are the result of the large number of orienting responses. He explains[47] that the physiological effects of orienting responses are often in opposition to those required by homeostasis. As the orienting actions take precedence, homeostasis seems to suffer somewhat. For example, the rise in blood flow in the skin during the orienting response leads to increased heat loss from the body, which would interfere with any need to conserve heat. The same applies to the phasic activities of REM sleep. Although such activities only occupy about one-third of REM sleep, Morrison believes that there are so many orienting responses here that the accompanying impairments to various aspects of homeostasis somehow spill over into the remaining REM sleep.

Changes in homeostatic control during REM sleep can be seen in blood flow to certain organs, especially to the brain where the effect is dramatic, often by as much as 50 per cent above non-REM sleep levels. Many people who believe that REM sleep has an important repair and consolidation role for the brain have taken this increase in blood flow as further evidence in support of this idea, in the same way as the rise in neural firing rates has been viewed (see Section 8.8). Similar interpretations have been used for the rises in brain metabolic rate and temperature during REM sleep, also found in many mammals. On the other hand, as I have already pointed out (Section 8.8), one could equally claim that heightened brain metabolism and neural activity would deter restitution etc, as these processes might well require a more restful brain, perhaps like that found in SWS (see Section 5.10).

Although the brain's metabolic rate rises in REM sleep to around that of aroused waking levels, the heightened blood flow to the brain is far greater than what is required. Some researchers simply dismiss this as another 'bizarre' peculiarity of REM sleep, associated with impaired homeostatic control of the blood supply to organs. A better-known example of this in humans is the increased blood flow to the penis, causing erection throughout most of REM sleep, which seems to have nothing to do with the sexual content of dreams. I have no idea why this strange event occurs, but in the case of the brain the large blood flow during REM sleep may have a purpose—to prevent the brain from overheating during the impaired thermoregulation.

One vital function of the blood concerns thermoregulation, as blood can distribute heat around the body, especially away from the brain. Overheating is a great risk for the brain, and its functioning is substantially impaired even with a small increase of 3°C. Damage occurs with a 5°C rise[48], which can lead to death. Brain cooling is not so harmful, as was evident in the case of shallow torpor (Section 7.5). Nevertheless, in humans at least, confused behaviour is apparent when brain temperature drops more than 3°C or so. The optimal working temperature of the mammalian brain varies somewhat from species to species, but is usually around 38.5°C, although humans are unusual in having a lower brain temperature of around 37.3°C. In sum, if brain temperature was to rise or even fall beyond a few degrees either way during REM sleep, as potentially might happen because of the apparent impairment to thermoregulation at this time, then for one reason or another the organism would be at risk.

The brain produces a considerable amount of 'waste' heat, as it is one of the most active of all organs even during the lowest state of sleep. For example, the comparatively large brain of adult humans makes up about 2.2 per cent of total body weight, but it accounts for about 20 per cent of our total resting metabolic rate. In SWS this latter proportion falls a few per cent, and rises in REM sleep. Although brain size varies across mammals, for all of them the brain still produces a lot of heat. Added to this is the problem that the brain is usually surrounded by fairly effective thermal insulation, of skull, scalp, and hair—also necessary to protect the brain from physical injury. So, to avoid the risk of overheating, the brain needs an effective method for removing excess heat. Just like many car engines, it has a good liquid cooling system and radiator.

The cooler the blood entering the brain, the greater is the removal of heat from the brain. Cooling can be further improved by increasing the blood flow. If the blood entering the brain happens to be warmer than usual, then to maintain its cooling effect the blood flow rate must increase in compensation. This latter situation seems to be what is happening in REM sleep, as the blood entering the brain is warmer than usual. But before explaining why this blood is warmer, I must first give a little background.

There are considerable differences between mammals in how they lose excess body heat. We humans increase blood flow through the skin capillaries, losing heat not only by convection and radiation, but most effectively by the evaporation of sweat. Obviously, sweating is of little use to most hairy and furry mammals, and alternative methods for cooling have been evolved. Any exposed skin surface usually evolves as a heat radiator, with the most common being the ears, especially where these are large, as in rabbits for example. A naked tail is particularly effective in rodents, and footpads are also useful. Horns make good radiators as they contain a rich blood supply. But perhaps the most intriguing method, used by the cat, dog, many carnivorous and hoofed mammals, is panting. This is not simply a method for 'cooling the blood in the lungs' as many people seem to think. Much of our knowledge about exactly how panting keeps mammals cool has come from the work of Drs James Hayward and Mary Anne Baker[49], carried out in the 1960s, at the Brain Research Institute, the University of California.

In these animals the main blood vessel supplying the brain, the carotid artery, divides up into a network (a 'rete') of small arterioles at the base of the brain. These re-unite, again as the carotid artery, before finally entering the brain. This network (the 'carotid rete') is a heat exchanger, and is surrounded by cool venous blood on route back to the heart, having drained from the cool and wet nasal membranes. Heat from the arterial blood within the rete passes to the surrounding venous blood. The cooled arterial blood leaving the rete now has more capacity for cooling the brain. The greater the air flow through the nose, the greater is the evaporative heat loss from the nasal membranes, the cooler the venous blood bathing the carotid rete, and the larger the potential cooling effect of the carotid blood on the brain. Panting is the method these animals use for producing a large nasal air flow.

For unaccountable reasons the nasal passages of these mammals dry up during REM sleep. So there is less cooling here, and warmer arterial blood enters the brain. To avoid the liability of the brain overheating, the most obvious countermeasure is to step up the blood flow into the brain, and this may account for the dramatic rise in the flow rate that is actually found. Nevertheless, brain temperature does rise slightly, but normally only to around waking levels, as there is usually a fall in this temperature during non-REM sleep. Such a rise may well be of benefit to the sleeping animal in preparing its brain for wakefulness.

Apart from the nose drying up in REM sleep, panting also ceases. This latter finding and other peculiarities of thermoregulation during REM sleep have been clearly demonstrated in a series of elegant studies by Parmeggiani and colleagues[50], whose earlier work on the cat I introduced in Section 7.2. These investigators have shown that when the part of the brain involved in detecting the brain's own temperature (the pre-optic area) is artificially warmed, to trick the brain into believing that it is overheating, the usual response of panting occurs during non-REM sleep—not quite to the extent found during wakefulness, but nevertheless panting is clearly present. But during REM sleep, all signs of panting cease with pre-optic warming.

Reductions in body heat loss during REM sleep are not just confined to animals with a carotid rete. In the rabbit, where the ear is the primary organ for thermoregulation, the skin capillaries constrict in REM sleep (this also happens in the cat[50]). During non-REM sleep, these capillaries regulate heat loss from the ear quite normally, but their constriction in REM sleep continues even in the most inappropriate circumstances, when the animal is sleeping in a high environmental temperature[51]. Potentially, this could lead to rapid brain overheating, but this does not happen. The rabbit's brain temperature still only rises by a fraction of a degree in REM sleep—something must be protecting the brain from overheating. Unfortunately, little is known about blood flow changes to the animal's brain at this time. The point I am making is that in an organ like the brain, where local thermoregulation really matters, such thermoregulation still seems to continue during REM sleep, albeit in a different way.

In humans, heat loss through the skin also falls in REM sleep, and sweating is reduced. Sweating is not blocked entirely though, and it returns if the environmental temperature continues to rise[52]. This important finding suggests that, for humans at least, the heat loss aspect of thermoregulation does not cease entirely in REM sleep. Instead, there is a greater tolerance of a warmer environment, with increased heat loss not occurring until a higher environmental temperature is reached. That is, there seems to be a rise in the 'set point' at which body temperature is regulated[52]. This is an important observation, and I shall return to it in Section 8.13. Human brain temperature alters very little during REM sleep, although there is a 30–50 per cent increase in blood flow. But it is unknown if, and to what extent, blood entering the human brain is warmer (because of a reduced heat loss from the skin and body).

To summarize so far, there is a fall in the ability of many mammals to lose body heat during REM sleep. But there is little evidence to show that at least for the brain, an organ where thermoregulation really matters, brain temperature alters by more than a fraction of a degree during REM sleep even in hot environments. Hitherto inexplicably large increases in the brain's blood flow during REM sleep may turn out be a countermeasure to protect its delicate workings from overheating. The small rises in brain temperature normally occurring in many mammals during REM sleep have the benefit of bringing this temperature up to that of wakefulness, allowing brain function and behaviour to be at their optimal readiness for wakefulness. If anything dangerous were to happen to brain temperature or to the animal in general during REM sleep, then all it has to do is wake up and thermoregulate properly, as REM sleep is a 'fragile' type of sleep. Certainly, thermoregulation is more loosely controlled during REM sleep, but, as will be seen, thermoregulation is not lost, and there may be an explanation for these peculiar changes.

8.12 Keeping warm

I mentioned in Sections 7.5 and 8.3 that REM sleep is commonly seen to be an ancestral form of sleep, as, for example, the parts of the mammalian brain involved in producing REM sleep are the more 'basic' areas in the hindbrain, also to be found in the less advanced animals such as reptiles and amphibia. This is a contentious view, as there is no clear sign of REM sleep in these animals, and instead I favour the ontogenetic hypothesis that REM sleep is a special development for the developing mammalian (and avian) fetus. But to continue the 'ancestral sleep' perspective for a little longer, reptiles have a primitive form of thermoregulation (i.e. poikilothermy—see Section 7.5), and it has been reasoned that, in mammals, thermoregulation reverts back to this primitive level during REM sleep.

But as I implied in the last section, I do not view thermoregulation in REM sleep to be poikilothermic. Bear in mind that poikilothermy means a virtual absence of thermoregulation—little ability to maintain a constant and warm body temperature under different environmental temperatures, and the inability to generate large quantities of body heat by metabolic means. However, it is clear that, for humans and other mammals, heat production (metabolic rate) during REM sleep remains about the same as for non-REM sleep, and despite the peculiarities of thermoregulation during REM sleep there is little sign that thermoregulation is seriously compromised at this time.

An excellent example of this in the case of humans comes from a study carried out by Dr Ed Haskell and colleagues[53], run jointly by the two laboratories in California (who did the work on shallow torpor I described in Section 7.5). They measured metabolic rate (oxygen consumption), skin and rectal temperatures, as well as sleep EEGs, in six near-naked subjects exposed to environmental temperatures ranging from 21°C to 34°C. There were no bed-clothes. At a thermoneutral temperature of 29°C, where the subjects felt neither warm nor cold but comfortable, oxygen consumption over the night fell by about 10–12 per cent from relaxed waking levels taken just prior to sleep. These changes during sleep can be seen for one subject in Fig. 8.4, where sleep stages, rectal temperature, and body movements are also shown. Rectal temperature fell by only a very small amount, around 0.5°C, mostly at the beginning of the night.

It should be remembered that because of our relatively large body size there is a 'thermal inertia' whereby rectal temperature is slow to respond to changes in metabolism. There can be a 15–30 minute lag in a temperature response to any alteration in oxygen consumption. On the other hand, for oxygen consumption itself the lag time for a potential change is very short.

Heat production (oxygen consumption) was at its lowest during SWS, at around 5 per cent below that during stage 2 sleep, and on average there was no difference in oxygen consumption between stage 2 and REM sleep. Skin temperature measurements are a good guide to heat loss (see Section 3.5)—the warmer the skin temperature, the more body heat that is being lost. These were also taken by Haskell and coworkers, and although skin temperatures altered according to the environmental conditions these showed no obvious changes (beyond a few tenths of a degree) from non-REM to REM sleep under any condition. Therefore, even taking into consideration the body's thermal inertia, there was little sign of any serious impairment to thermoregulation at any point over the night—even during 30–45 minutes of near-continuous REM sleep (see Fig. 8.4).

Dr Colin Shapiro and colleagues from Edinburgh University have also carefully measured oxygen consumption during human sleep stages[54], this time with subjects sleeping in an environment at 26°C (considered by them to be thermoneutral). These investigators particularly controlled for the effects that the circadian rhythm would have on heat production for each sleep stage over the night. Over the whole night, oxygen consumption fell by an average of 9 per cent from relaxed wakefulness levels. More specifically, oxygen consumption fell by about 5 per cent from stage 2 to stage 4 sleep, whereas REM sleep had the same level of heat production as stage 2 sleep.

Whilst thermoregulation seems virtually unaffected during human REM sleep in a thermoneutral environment, what happens in a cold sleeping environment, when there is a greater strain on thermoregulation? I have already mentioned that skin temperature seems to be unaffected[53]; however, there is a clear sign that something is awry, because shivering is blocked during REM sleep. Also, the levels of REM sleep fall, indicating that this sleep cannot cope with the cold. But as will be seen, such findings still do not lead me to revise my opinion that thermoregulation remains fairly intact during REM sleep not only in humans, but in several other species. Certainly though, thermoregulation does change in REM sleep. Let me begin by looking at the apparent fall in REM sleep in the cold.

Haskell and colleagues found that in an environmental temperature of 21°C, REM sleep levels dropped[55]. It has been reasoned that this may have been due to difficulties in thermoregulation during REM sleep, even though these investigators found little apparent sign of this. However, Haskell's study did not allow much time for their subjects to become more accustomed to sleeping in the cold, and a further experiment by Dr Jo Palca and

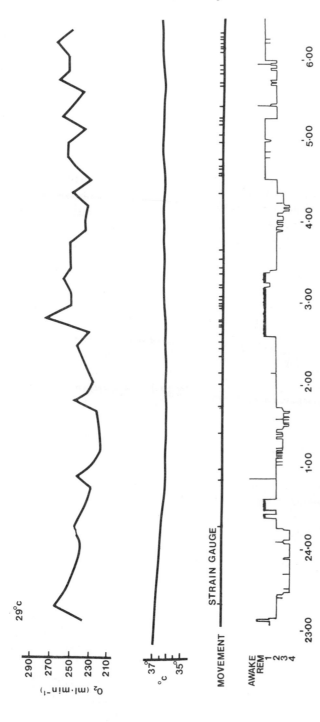

Fig. 8.4 Overnight changes in oxygen consumption (heat production), rectal temperature, body movements and sleep stages for a man sleeping in a thermoneutral environment of 29 °C. Note that the sleep hypnogram shows REM sleep uppermost, as a heavy line. Sleep was relatively uninterrupted. Oxygen consumption falls a little in SWS, but shows only small fluctuations in REM sleep. Rectal temperature is at its lowest during the first half of sleep, following SWS. See text for details. (From Haskell et al.[53]. Reproduced by permission of the American Physiological Society)

colleagues from the same laboratory[56] looked at this factor. Surprisingly, after 5 days of sleeping in the cold (21°C), subjects showed no reductions in REM sleep. The investigators concluded that the earlier findings of falls in REM sleep could have been largely due to psychological factors rather than to problems with thermoregulation.

It will be remembered (Section 7.2) that Parmeggiani's cats also showed falls in REM sleep when they had to sleep in the cold (with much of the lost REM sleep being the optional variety). Whilst it is not clear to what extent the animals were adapted to the situation, nevertheless the temperature was very cold, around 0°C—perhaps just too cold for REM sleep to cope with anyway. Recent work on the hamster[57], has shown that when animals used to a normal laboratory temperature had to live in an environment of 5°C, REM sleep fell at first. But by the fifth day levels began to increase noticeably, and within a few weeks REM sleep was virtually back to normal. We can assume that by then the animals must have been able to thermoregulate reasonably effectively during REM sleep in the cold, even if this was not the case to start with. Finally, I should add that the absence of REM sleep in animals entering shallow torpor (Section 7.5) is a different phenomenon to what I am describing here. If body temperature has to be regulated at a lower level, as in shallow torpor, then REM sleep is indeed poor at doing this. But it may be fairly good at regulating body temperature at near normal levels.

Both Haskell and Palca found that thermoregulation during REM sleep was intact in the cold[53, 56], despite an absence of shivering. As their findings were very similar, I shall concentrate on Haskell's, even though his subjects were less adapted (it was the amounts of REM sleep that differed between the studies, not thermoregulation). Comparing the cold with the thermoneutral environment, oxygen consumption during stage 2 sleep increased by 11 per cent, and also rose during REM sleep by 7 per cent. It will be remembered that heat loss from the skin showed little change from non-REM to REM sleep. Therefore, heat production and heat loss were largely unimpaired during REM sleep. But there is something else. The subjects shivered quite noticeably whilst awake, to a lesser extent in stage 2 sleep, and ceased shivering altogether in REM sleep. As oxygen consumption rose in stage 2 sleep in the cold it is likely that the cause was mainly through shivering. But this could not have been the reason for the smaller, but nevertheless noticeable increase in oxygen consumption during REM sleep. Where could this extra heat production have come from? The answer may be brown fat thermogenesis (see below), and is the topic of the next Section.

Humans may be unusual amongst mammals in their responses to cold during REM sleep, and much work has been done on the cat in this respect, mostly by Parmeggiani's group. Before describing these findings, let me first summarise the typical countermeasures against cold that are normally taken by mammals during wakefulness. These fall into two categories:

1. *Behavioural*—for example, the animal may move into a warmer environment, or curl up to cover the more exposed body areas.
2. *Physiological*—

   (a) Increase the production of body heat. This can be done either by shivering (the small but rapid contractions of voluntary muscles generate extra heat) or by the less common mechanism of 'non-shivering thermogenesis'. This is mostly found in newborn mammals, but only in certain adult mammals, particularly if they are adapted to living in the cold. This extra heat is mostly generated in deposits of special, dark-coloured fat, known as 'brown fat', that can produce heat rapidly. Brown fat contains a rich blood supply to transport the heat away.

   (b) Decrease heat loss. This can be done by reducing the blood supply to body surfaces (through constricting capillaries in the skin) and erecting body hair to create better insulation (goosepimples in humans are a vestige of this response).

Parmeggiani and his team have noted[58] that, normally, during relaxed wakefulness and non-REM sleep most cats will curl up and begin to shiver when the environmental temperature falls below 5°C. Shivering becomes very marked at 0°C, and will continue during non-REM sleep (without necessarily waking the animal up). At this temperature, shivering and curling up may even be greater during non-REM sleep than wakefulness[57]. However, around the onset of REM sleep shivering ceases, with the curling becoming more relaxed. This seemingly inappropriate response continues throughout REM sleep until the animal eventually awakens to begin violent shivering.

Now it might be thought that shivering is prevented during REM sleep because of the paralysis of voluntary muscles at this time. But this is not so, as destruction of the part of the locomotor centre underlying the paralysis does not lead to a return of shivering, even though the cat can now move about[59]. Morrison again argues[43] that this absence of shivering is because of priorities given to orienting responses (see Section 8.10). For example, a shivering human will momentarily stop shivering if his or her attention is suddenly distracted.

Parmeggiani reported[58] what seemed to be another inappropriate response to the cold (2°C) in cats during REM sleep, in addition to the lack of shivering—a small rise in ear temperature of about 1°C, indicating increased heat loss here. But as the area of bare skin on the ear is small, this level of response will not have much effect on overall body heat loss.

As a convenient rough guide to body temperature, Parmeggiani placed a thermocouple under the hairless skin of the cat's groin. However, this site does not reflect true core body temperature, and is still affected by blood flow to the skin. During REM sleep this temperature fell to a greater extent than during non-REM sleep. For example[58], in a cold environment of − 15°C the fall was about 0.5°C greater during a 9-minute period of REM sleep, compared with a similar period of non-REM sleep. Parmeggiani considered this to be another sign of impaired thermoregulation during REM sleep. But I believe this to be debatable point, as 0.5°C is a very small fall, especially as the animal may well have uncurled somewhat during REM sleep and exposed more of the skin of its groin. I must emphasize that Parmeggiani pursues a very difficult research area, and he has made some remarkable discoveries, only a few of which I will cover. Although I disagree with some of his interpretations, particularly that REM sleep is a poikilothermic state, this is in no way disrespectful of his work, as I hold it in great admiration.

The only true internal temperature site we have information about for REM sleep in cats sleeping in the cold is the brain (hypothalamus). Under these circumstances Parmeggiani has reported that this temperature still shows its usual rise during REM sleep, albeit only 0.2°C[58]. But I must point out that such episodes of REM sleep in the cold, lasting for only around 5–10 minutes, may be too short to allow potentially large changes in body or brain temperature to develop, especially as there will be some thermal inertia (less than that for humans, of course).

8.13 Increasing heat production without shivering

I mentioned just now that there are two forms of heat production in response to cold—shivering, and the non-shivering method within brown fat. Shivering ceases during REM sleep, but not much is known about what happens to the other form during REM sleep. Whilst brown fat is typically only found in any abundance in very young mammals, some remnants are left in adults, including humans, where it seems to be spread out more diffusely within muscle rather than gathered in distinct masses as in infants. However, if the adult acclimatizes to a cold environment and food is readily available, then the brown fat can become more active and be an important source of extra body heat. Most studies on thermoregulation during sleep use adult animals adapted only to the normal laboratory temperature, and under these circumstances non-shivering thermogenesis could not be expected to be present to any great extent in wakefulness or sleep.

I have some suspicion, and this is pure surmise, that the small further increase in oxygen consumption found by Haskell and colleagues in their human subjects during REM sleep in the cold (see last section), may have been partly due to non-shivering thermogenesis. Had the subjects been partly acclimatized to the cold, then we could have been more certain about this. Of the very few animal studies that have tried to look at this form of thermogenesis during sleep in the cold, the first used non-cold-adapted golden hamsters, and recorded the temperature of brown fat deposits[60]. No sign of this thermogenesis was found during REM sleep.

One of Parmeggiani's colleagues, Dr Carlo Franzini, has also started to look at the possibility of non-shivering thermogenesis in REM sleep, in young rabbits[61]. These animals were being used for other experiments, and although not ideal for work on non-shivering thermogenesis, as they only have small amounts of brown fat, there was an interesting outcome. Thermistors within this tissue showed that during REM sleep it became progressively warmer as the environmental temperature fell. When brown fat is activated blood flow through it rises substantially, to conduct the heat away to other parts of the body. Therefore, to establish fully that brown fat is firing, its blood flow needs to be measured. But this is an exceedingly difficult task, which still remains a problem for Franzini. So whilst these findings indicate that non-shivering thermogenesis was present during REM sleep, Franzini and colleagues remain cautious about this.

Unlike the rabbit, the rat is one animal that can develop sizeable deposits of brown fat even in adulthood. A recent investigation by Dr Werner Schmidek and colleagues from the Department of Physiology, at the University of Sao Paulo, Brazil[62], assessed thermoregulation in this animal throughout sleep. Although non-shivering thermogenesis was not looked at specifically, just heat production in general, some important findings can be gleaned. Two groups of adult rats were used, with one being previously partly acclimatized ('acclimated') for 5 weeks to living in a near-freezing environment of 1°C, and the other to living in a warmer environment at 23°C. It is highly likely that the former condition would have stimulated brown fat deposits to become more active, but the animals were not examined for this. Animals from each group then slept under various environmental temperatures ranging from 15°C ('cold') to 30°C ('warm'). Sleep EEGs were monitored, as were deep body temperature, oxygen consumption (to measure heat production), and body heat loss (determined from a calorimeter).

It was clear that for both groups of animals, and for all environmental sleeping conditions, heat production was greatest in wakefulness, less in non-REM sleep, and lowest in REM sleep (unlike humans—see Section 8.12). This can be seen in Fig. 8.5, which is a simplified version of the findings, only comparing heat production at the environmental temperatures of 15°C and 25°C. But the key point is that heat production during REM sleep obviously rose with the lower temperature—more so for the cold-adapted group, where heat production was about 40 per cent greater at 15°C than at 25°C. Shivering occurred at 15°C in both waking and non-REM sleep, and this would have made a substantial contribution to the rise in heat production at these times. However, there was no sign of shivering in REM sleep. But something was generating this extra heat, and, as the investigators pointed out, it is reasonable to conclude that non-shivering thermogenesis was mostly responsible.

In order to have a better perspective on thermoregulation, information

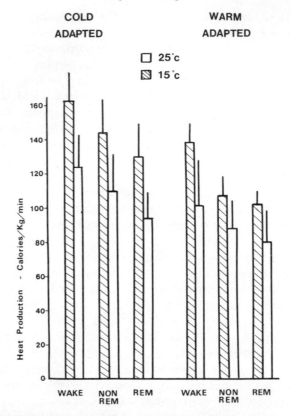

Fig. 8.5 Heat production is still evident in REM sleep in the laboratory rat.

Cold- and warm-adapted animals during wakefulness, non-REM sleep, and REM sleep, under two different environmental temperatures—15°C and 25°C. Vertical lines are standard deviations. Although heat production is lowest for REM sleep under each condition, it still rises by about 40 per cent in the cold-adapted animals and 25 per cent in the warm-adapted animals, as the temperature falls from 25°C to 15°C. This is probably due to non-shivering thermogenesis, which, unlike shivering thermogenesis, seems to continue during REM sleep. See text for details. (From Schmidek *et al.*[61]. Reproduced by permission of Elsvier Science Publishers BV)

about body heat loss is required. This increased in both groups of animals as the environmental temperature fell, with little difference between wakefulness, non-REM sleep, and REM sleep, until the 15°C condition, when there was a 10 per cent further increase in heat loss during REM sleep in both groups. However, the overall differences in heat storage between REM and non-REM sleep did not reach statistical significance for either group. To quote the authors, there was 'a diminished but persistent thermoregulatory control during REM sleep' (p. 269). By the way, deep body temperature was unchanged during REM sleep under all conditions, but it must be remembered that REM sleep episodes only lasted for 1–2 minutes under the coldest condition—probably too short for much to happen anyway.

To conclude, I believe that the evidence presented in both this section and the last one indicates that much of thermoregulation is maintained during REM sleep. Poikilothermy does not set in, but mammals do become more 'tolerant' of a wider range of both hot and cold environmental temperatures. Without doubt, something peculiar *is* going on, as thermoregulatory responses are more difficult to activate during REM sleep. There may be differences between species in this respect. For example, these responses seem to be more limited in the cat than in the rat and human. The level to which brown fat can be 'switched on' is a crucial factor with regard to the cold response, and usually several days of living in a cold environment are required to help prime this type of thermogenesis. There are good signs that non-shivering thermogenesis can persist during REM sleep, taking over from shivering, which is blocked. In sum, these findings refute the idea that thermoregulation during REM sleep is reptilian-like, but instead seem to support the ontogenetic hypothesis, as will be seen.

8.14 Thermoregulation in REM sleep reverts to the fetal level

Whilst the daily amounts of REM sleep fall dramatically from before birth to adulthood, most of its other characteristics change little, and are maintained in the adult. This is to a far greater extent than is the case for non-REM sleep. The EEG and rapid eye movement bursts of REM sleep in the human fetus at, say, 7 months gestation are similar to those of the adult, although, there are also some differences[63]. On the other hand, most of the characteristics of adult human non-REM sleep are not even developed by the time of birth.

Let me expand this last point by continuing to concentrate on human sleep. The prominent EEG features of adult human non-REM sleep such as spindles, delta waves, and K complexes (see Sections 1.3 and 6.9) do not appear until at least a few weeks after birth[63]. It is for this reason that the 'non-REM' sleep of the human fetus and newborn is usually called by other names such as 'quiet sleep' and 'transitional sleep', although these do form the beginnings of what later becomes non-REM sleep. In summary, non-REM sleep is essentially a postnatal development which is not really evident until about 2 to 3 months of age in the human. On the other hand, REM sleep seems to be more of a fetal-cum-neonatal state maintained into adulthood.

Before going any further, I would like to make two points of clarification. Firstly the concept that adult REM sleep is more fetal like than is non-REM sleep applies not only to humans but probably to most other mammals. Secondly it will be remembered from Section 7.10 that I proposed that human adult sleep (particularly its funtions) may be unusual amongst mammals in being generally more infant or fetal like anyway, in line with our tendency to be neotenous. Nevertheless, the first point still applies; adult human REM sleep is comparatively more more fetal like than is non-REM sleep.

Now for the real theme of this section—thermoregulation in mammalian adult REM sleep is also fetal like—that is thermoregulation during adult REM sleep reverts to the fetal level, and certainly not to a reptilian mode. Such a concept does not apply to mammalian adult non-REM sleep as by the time this form of sleep usually becomes established in the infant, particularly in the human baby, thermoregulation and most other homeostatic mechanisms are almost fully developed[64].

The status of thermoregulation in the mammalian fetus is very interesting, as to a large extent there is little point in the fetus needing to thermoregulate at all, unless a crisis occurs—the fetus is part of mother's body mass and comes under her thermoregulation. The metabolic rate of the fetus is similar to that of the mother[64] and at this stage the fetus cannot be considered as a typical small mammal with a relatively large surface area, having a high rate of body heat loss and needing a high level of heat production in compensation. Of course, this is the case as soon as it is born. Body temperature in the mammalian fetus is around 0.5°C higher than that of the mother. Within the uterus it lives in an environment of 100 per cent humidity, and very hot by adult standards at around 37–38°C (i.e. mother's own body temperature). This is much hotter than what it finds acceptable shortly after birth in the outside world. Therefore, about 37–38°C has to be the neutral ambient temperature for the fetus without it trying to invoke thermoregulatory countermeasures. This neutral ambient temperature range falls rapidly at birth, and, for example, in the 5-day-old naked full-size human infant it is about 33–34°C (at 50 per cent relative humidity), whereas for the naked adult it is about 27°C[64].

In the mammalian fetus just before birth, the main control centre for homeostasis, the hypothalamus, will be confronted with dual standards—one for the conditions that are going to be encountered in the cooler outside world as soon as birth occurs, requiring quick responses to a changing environmental temperature, and the other for the hot and wet internal world which it cannot or need not do much about. So, the thermoregulatory functions of the hypothalamus need to be dampened down or perhaps turned off in the fetus, but ready to switch on at birth.

Therefore, if REM sleep in the adult mammal is a throwback to that of the fetus, then the response by the hypothalamus to a change in environmental temperature during REM sleep may be affected in the same way. During adult REM sleep, and in response to any change in environmental temperature, the hypothalamus might do nothing at first, as it assumes that 'mother's thermoregulation is in control'. Also, the hypothalamus would be accepting as neutral a higher environmental temperature—similar to that encountered by the fetus. If this line of thinking is correct, then for example body and brain temperature will be allowed to rise a little (maybe not as high as fetal levels) before heat loss mechanisms are switched in. It will be remembered from Section 8.11 that the investigators studying sweating in human sleep concluded that the 'set point' for triggering sweating seemed to be raised during REM sleep[52], for reasons unknown to them.

From my perspective on the fetus, there is another angle to the 'impaired' sweating response during human adult REM sleep. How does the fetus increase its heat loss? Outside the mother the main method would be evaporative heat loss through sweating or panting in the case of 'panting' mammals (see Section 8.11), both of which are useless to the fetus. But it can still use its blood to transport away unwanted heat—down the umbilical artery to the placenta for the mother to dispose of through her blood and sweat. But of course, for the fetus this method is lost at birth, and, for example, could not be reverted to during adult REM sleep. Therefore, to lose excess body heat during adult REM sleep some form of sweating response would have to be re-instigated, albeit impaired.

What can the fetus do about increasing its heat production if it were to get cold? Little is known about what happens with the fetus *in utero*. What is certain, though, is that the warmth of the fetus is very much influenced by the mother and her relatively large surrounding body mass. But a lot more is known about heat production in the newborn. Of the two methods, shivering and brown fat thermogenesis, the latter is the first to develop in both the human[64] and rodent[65] for example. Shivering is a complex procedure involving the integration of brain, nerves, and muscle, and it seems that for many species the neuromuscular control of shivering needs additional time after birth to become fully organized. This is particularly evident in mammals not born in an advanced state of development, again like the rodent and human. It is also the usual explanation why so much brown fat is present at birth in many species, to compensate for the absence of shivering. The reader can now see why I suspect that non-shivering thermogenesis probably functions during REM sleep in the adult—it is the 'fetal mode of thermogenesis'.

Whether or not other physiological peculiarities during REM sleep in the adult may bear some semblance to the fetal condition, able to be explained in a similar way, are matters for a debate that I shall not pursue much further. Thermoregulation may be the only clear example, owing to the unusual restrictions placed on this process in the fetus by the mother.

There is little doubt that the control of thermoregulation by the hypothalamus is at least partly inactivated during REM sleep in the adult mammal. Two recent studies have clearly demonstrated this—one coming from Heller's laboratory, using the kangaroo rat[66], and the other from Parmeggiani's laboratory, using the cat[67]. For example, electrodes sited within the hypothalamus of this latter animal showed that certain neurones associated with thermoregulation, which are normally very responsive to warming in wakefulness and non-REM sleep, lose this responsivity almost entirely during REM sleep. But we do not know whether all the hypothalamic neurones associated with thermoregulation are affected in this way.

Of course, Parmeggiani believes that this inactivation of the hypothalamus is in line with REM sleep being a poikilothermic state. Morrison, though, explains such findings in terms of his orienting response hypothesis (ref. 47—see Section 8.11)—that the numerous orienting responses generated in the brain stem take priority over thermoregulation, and in effect override the hypothalamus's control of thermoregulation. This seems to be a plausible idea, and I see no reason why this state of affairs cannot run in parallel with my own views about thermoregulation during REM sleep; the two ideas do not exclude each other. Why should there only be one reason for the altered thermoregulation during REM sleep? In fact Morrison's ideas can easily be combined with the ontogenetic hypothesis—not that he would necessarily subscribe to such a union. So I take the responsibility for doing this, and these are my words:

'REM sleep is a special adaptation for the mammalian fetus, whereby the developing cerebrum is kept stimulated through bombardment by orienting responses. These emanate from the brain stem, and may wholly or partly override certain homeostatic events regulated by the hypothalamus. In many respects, REM sleep resembles exaggerated alert wakefulness, and for the fetus may, at least in part, act as a substitute for wakefulness.'

And to add my own perspective:

'Also, during REM sleep in the adult, thermoregulation, and maybe other aspects of homeostasis, revert to the fetal mode of control'.

8.15 Conclusions about REM sleep

Three related themes have emerged from this chapter:

1. In the absence of sound evidence that REM sleep is present in reptiles and other cold-blooded vertebrates, I have supported the argument that it is not a primitive form of sleep in the evolutionary sense, but a special development for the mammalian (and avian) fetus that continues in a reduced form in the adult. Certain physiological changes that occur during REM sleep in the adult, particularly in relation to thermoregulation, can reasonably be explained in terms of a reversal to the fetal level of control, and not to that of a reptilian state. The ontogenetic hypothesis provides one of the most plausible explanations for the function of REM sleep—that is in the developing fetus there is little sensory stimulation, and

so REM sleep acts as a substitute to stimulate and aid the development of the cerebrum. In adult life the diminished level of REM sleep continues to keep the sleeping cerebrum in a state of readiness so that it can react swiftly when awoken. Recent findings indicate that this stimulation seems to take the form of an exaggerated bombardment of the cerebrum by orienting responses that have no external cause.

2. It is remarkable how various neural events of REM sleep are so similar to those of alert wakefulness, and it might even be fairer to consider REM sleep to be more akin to wakefulness than to sleep. Wakefulness may be able to substitute for much of REM sleep, and seemingly for all of REM sleep in the dolphin. I have argued throughout this book that for the typical human adult at least half of REM sleep is 'optional'. The remaining 'core' REM sleep is so intertwined within the organization of sleep, counterbalancing the effects of the deeper forms of non-REM sleep, that it cannot be separated out. Dreaming may have evolved to assist this purpose—to help keep the cerebrum entertained, and to make some sense out of the the barrage of orienting responses. We do not know whether dreaming is only present in humans, but there is no reason to assume that it is unique to us. It may well occur throughout mammals and birds, although manifesting itself in different and simpler ways. Dreaming requires a cerebral cortex (or its equivalent in birds). Presumably, as the phylogenetic scale is descended, the simpler the cerebrum, and the simpler is the dream. But dreaming is only one phenomenon of REM sleep, and most of the brain centres controlling REM sleep lie in more basic parts of the brain. Thus, REM sleep can occur without a cerebrum, and consequently without dreaming. So it is unlikely that we have REM sleep just to dream. Besides, not all of dreaming is confined to REM sleep.

3. Findings from REM sleep deprivation studies are not convincing enough to warrant there being any vital association between REM sleep and memory or other aspects of the learning and forgetting process in the adult mammal. Although some of the experimental results may reach statistical significance, by far the majority of these effects are still relatively small, suggesting no more than a minor link with REM sleep. In view of the attention paid to REM sleep and dreaming, and the importance given to this form of sleep by many people, REM sleep deprivation in human adults is surprisingly uneventful—it can even be of benefit to people suffering from certain forms of depression. In some species, especially rodents, REM sleep deprivation seems to raise basic drive behaviours such as eating, exploration, aggression, etc. However, this is not really apparent when humans are deprived of REM sleep. In those animals showing this behaviour, at least part of the effect may well be due to the artificiality of the REM deprivation procedures and the presence of additional stresses.

References

1. Aserinsky, E., and Kleitman, N. (1955). Two types of ocular motility occurring in sleep. *Journal of Applied Physiology*, **8**, 1–10.

2. Aserinsky, E. and Kleitman, N. (1953). Regular occurring periods of eye motility and concomitant phenomena during sleep. *Science*, **118**, 273–274.

3. Dement, W. and Kleitman, N. (1957). Cyclic variations in EEG during sleep and their relation to eye movements, body motility and dreaming. *Electroencephalography and Clinical Neurophysiology*, **9**, 673–690.

4. Kleitman, N. (1963). *Sleep and Wakefulness* (second edition). Chicago University Press, Chicago.

5. Jacobson, E. (1938). *You Can Sleep Well. The ABC's of Restful Sleep for the Average Person*. Whittlesey House, New York.

6. Dement, W. and Kleitman, N. (1957). The relation of eye movements during sleep to dream activity: an objective method for the study of dreaming. *Journal of Experimental Psychology*, **53**, 339–346.

7. Foulkes, W.D. (1962). Dream reports from different stages of sleep. *Journal of Abnormal and Social Psychology*, **65**, 14–25.

8. Wolpert, E.A. and Trosman, H. (1958). Studies in psychophysiology of dreams. l. Experimental evocations of sequential dream studies. *AMA Archives of Neurology and Psychiatry*, **79**, 603–606.

9. Dement, W. and Wolpert, E.A. (1958). The relation of eye movements, body motility, and external stimuli to dream content. *Journal of Experimental Psychology*, **55**, 543–553.

10. Clavière, J. (1897). La rapidite de la pensee dans le reve. *Revue Philosophie*, **43**, 507–512.

11. Berger, R.J., Olley, P. and Oswald, l. (1962). The EEG, eye-movements and dreams of the blind. *Quarterly Journal of Experimental Psychology*, **14**, 183–187.

12. Freud, S. (1933). *New Introductory Lectures on Psychoanalysis*. Norton, New York.

13. Jung, C.G. (1933). *Modern Man In Search of a Soul*. Harcourt, Brace and World, New York.

14. Cohen, D.B. (1979). *Sleep and Dreaming*. Pergamon, New York.

15. Newman, E.A. and Evans, C.R. (1965). Human dream processes as analogous to computer programme clearance. *Nature*, **206**, 54.

16. Cartwright, R.D. (1977). *Night Life: Explorations in Dreaming*. Prentice Hall, New Jersey.

17. Hobson, J.A. and McCarley, R.W. (1977). The brain as a dream state generator: an activation-synthesis hypothesis of the dream process. *American Journal of Psychiatry*, **134**, 1335–1348.

18. Siegel, J.M., Nienhuis, R., Wheeler, R.L., McGinty, D.J. and Harper, R.M. (1981). Discharge patterns of reticular formation unit pairs in waking and REM sleep. *Experimental Neurology*, **74**, 875–981.

19. Vogel, G.W. (1978). An alternative view of the neurobiology of dreaming. *American Journal of Psychiatry*, **135**, 1531–1535.

20. Crick, F. and Mitchison, G. (1983). The function of dream sleep. *Nature*, **304**, 111–114.

21. Jouvet, M. (1980). Paradoxical sleep and the nature-nurture controversy. *Progress in Brain Research*, **53**, 331–346.
22. Gaarder, K. (1966). A conceptual model for sleep. *Archives of General Psychiatry*, **14**, 253–260.
23. Dewan, E. M. (1970). The programming 'P' hypothesis for REM sleep. In: Hartmann, E. (ed.) *Sleep and Dreaming*. Little, Brown, Boston. pp. 295–307.
24. Greenberg, R., Pearlman, C. A., Fingar, R., Kantrowitz, J. and Kawliche, S. (1970). The effects of dream deprivation: implications for a theory of the psychological function of dreaming. *British Journal of Medical Psychology*, **43**, 1–11.
25. Greenberg, R. and Pearlman, C. A. (1974). Cutting the REM nerve: an approach to the adaptive role of REM sleep. *Perspectives in Biology and Medicine*, **17**, 513–521.
26. Ephron, H. S. and Carrington, P. (1966). Rapid eye movement sleep and cortical homeostasis. *Psychological Review*, **73**, 500–526.
27. Snyder, F. (1966). Towards an evolutionary theory of dreaming. *American Journal of Psychiatry*. **123**, 121–136.
28. Vogel, G. W. (1979). A motivational function of REM sleep. In: Drucker-Colin, R., Shkurovich, M. and Sternman, M. B. (ed.) *The Functions of Sleep*. Academic Press, New York. pp. 233–50.
29. Horne, J. A. and McGrath, M. J. (1984). The consolidation hypothesis for REM sleep function: stress and other confounding factors—a review. *Biological Psychology*, **18**, 165–184.
30. Vogel, G. W. (1983). Evidence for REM sleep deprivation as the mechanisms of action of antidepressant drugs. *Progress in Neuropsychopharmacology and Biological Psychiatry*, **7**, 343–349.
31. Parmelee, A. H. and Stern, E. (1972). Development of states in infants. In: Clementine, C. D., Purpura, D. P. and Mayer, F. E. (ed.) *Sleep and the Maturing Nervous System*. Academic Press, New York. pp. 199–215.
32. Jouvet-Mounier, D., Astic, L. and Lacote, D. (1968). Ontogenesis of the states of sleep in the rat, cat and guinea pig during the first post-natal month. *Developmental Psychobiology*, **2**, 216–239.
33. Roffwarg, H. P., Muzio, J. and Dement, W. C. (1966). Ontogenetic development of the human sleep-dream cycle. *Science*, **152**, 604–619.
34. Denenberg, V. H. and Thoman, E. B. (1981). Evidence for a functional role for active (REM) sleep in infancy. *Sleep*, **4**, 185–192.
35. McGrath, M. J. and Cohen, D. B. (1978). REM sleep facilitation of adaptive waking behaviour: a review of the literature. *Psychological Bulletin*, **85**, 24–57.
36. Smith, C. (1985). Sleep states and learning: a review of the animal literature. *Neuroscience and Biobehavioural Reviews*, **9**, 157–168.
37. Maier, S. F. and Seligman, M. E. P. (1976). Learned helplessness: theory and evidence. *Journal of Experimental Psychology*, **105**, 3–46.
38. Van Luijtelaar, E. L. J. M. and Coenen, A. M. L. (1986). Electrophysiological evaluation of three paradoxical sleep deprivation techniques in rats. *Physiology and Behaviour*, **36**, 603–609.
39. Antelman, S. M. and Caggiula, A. R. (1980). Stress-induced behaviour: chemotherapy without drugs. In: Davidson, J. M. and Davidson, R. J. (ed.) *The Psychobiology of Consciousness*. Plenum Press, New York. pp. 65–104.

40. Cohen, D. B. (1980) The cognitive activity of sleep. *Progress in Brain Research*, **53**, 307–332.

41. Drucker-Colin, R. P. (1981). Neuroproteins, brain excitability and R E M sleep. In: Fishbein, W. (ed.) *Sleep, Dreams and Memory*. MTP Press, New York. pp. 73–94.

42. Guiditta, A., Rutigliano, B. and Vitale-Neugebauer, A. (1980). Influence of synchronised sleep on the biosynthesis of R N A in neuronal and mixed fractions isolated from rat cerebral cortex. *Journal of Neurochemistry*, **35**, 1267–1272.

43. Morrison, A. R. (1983). A window on the sleeping brain. *Scientific American*, **248** (April), 86–94.

44. Bowker, R. M. and Morrison, A. R. (1977). The P G O spike: an indicator of hyperalertness. In: Koella, W. P. and Levin, P. (ed.) *Sleep 1976*. Karger, Basel. 23–27.

45. Orem, J. and Keeling J. (1980). A compendium on the physiology of sleep. In: Orem, J. and Barnes, C. D. (ed.) *Physiology in Sleep*. Academic Press, New York. pp. 315–335.

46. Taylor, W. B., Moldofsky, H. and Furedy, J. J. (1985). Heart rate deceleration in R E M sleep: an orienting reaction interpretation. *Psychophysiology*, **22**, 110–115.

47. Morrison, A. R. and Reiner, P. B. (1985). A dissection of paradoxical sleep. In: McGinty, D. J., Drucker-Colin, R., Morrison, A. R. and Parmeggiani, P.-L. (ed.) *Brain Mechanisms of Sleep*. Raven Press, New York. pp. 97–110.

48. Burger, F. J. and Fuhrman, F. A. (1964). Evidence of injury by heat in mammalian tissues. *American Journal of Physiology*, **206**, 1057–1061.

49. Baker, M. A. (1979). A brain cooling system in mammals. *Scientific American*, **241**, 114–122.

50. Parmeggiani, P.-L., Franzini, C., Lenzi, P. and Zamboni, G. (1973). Threshold of respiratory responses to preoptic heating during sleep in freely moving cats. *Brain Research*, **52**, 189–201.

51. Baker, M. A. and Hayward, J. N. (1967). Autonomic basis for the rise in brain temperature during paradoxical sleep. *Science*, **157**, 1586–1588.

52. Libert, J.-P., Candas, V., Muzet, A. and Ehrhart, J. (1982). Thermoregulatory adjustments to thermal transients during slow wave sleep and R E M sleep in man. *Journal of Physiology (Paris)*, **78**, 251–257.

53. Haskell, E. H., Palca, J. W., Walker, J. M., Berger, R. J. and Heller, H. C. (1981). Metabolism and thermoregulation during stages of sleep in humans exposed to heat and cold. *Journal of Applied Physiology*, **51**, 948–954.

54. Shapiro, C. M., Goll, C. C., Cohen, G. R. and Oswald, l. (1984). Heat production during sleep. *Journal of Applied Physiology*, **56**, 671–677.

55. Haskell, E. H., Palca, J. W., Walker, J. M., Berger, R. J. and Heller, H. C. (1981). The effects of high and low ambient temperatures on human sleep stages. *Electroencephalography and Clinical Neurophysiology*, **51**, 494–501.

56. Palca, J. W., Walker, J. M. and Berger, R. J. (1986). Thermoregulation, metabolism, and sleep stages of sleep in cold-exposed men. *Journal of Applied Physiology*. **61**, 940–947.

57. Sichieri, R. and Schmidek, W. R. (1984). Influence of ambient temperature on the sleep wakefulness cycle in the hamster. *Physiology and Behaviour*, **33**, 871–877.

58. Parmeggiani, P-L. (1980). Temperature regulation during sleep: a study in homeostasis. In: Orem J. and Barnes, C. D. (ed.) *Physiology in Sleep*. Academic Press, New York. pp. 97–143.

59. Hendricks, J. C. (1982). Absence of shivering in the cat during paradoxical sleep without atonia. *Experimental Neurology*, **75**, 700–710.

60. Tegowska, E. and Narebski, J. (1980). The function of BAT in cold and after noradrenaline injection, dependence on size of animal and on integumental isolation value. In: Szelenyi, Z. and Szekely, M. (ed.) *Contributions to Thermal Physiology*, Pergamon Press, Oxford. pp. 531–533.

61. Franzini, C., Cianci, P., Lenzi, P., Libert, J-P., Horne, J. A. and Parmeggiani, P-L. (1986). Influence of brown adipose tissue on deep cervical temperature during sleep in the young rabbit. *Experientia*, **43**, 604–606.

62. Schmidek, W. R., Zachariassen, K. E. and Hammel, H. T. (1983). Total calorimetric measurements in the rat: influences of the sleep-wake cycle and of environmental temperature. *Brain Research*, **288**, 261–271.

63. Williams, R. L., Karacan, l. and Hursch, C. J. (1974). *Electroencephalography (EEG) of Human Sleep: Clinical Applications*. Wiley, New York.

64. Bruck, K. (1978). Heat production and temperature regulation. In: Stave, U. and Weech, A. A. (ed.) *Perinatal Physiology*. Plenum, New York. pp. 455–498.

65. Moore, R. E. and Donne, B. (1984). Nonshivering thermogenesis in the newborn mouse. In: Hales, J. R. S. (ed.) *Thermal Physiology*. Raven Press, New York. pp. 175–178.

66. Glotzbach, S. F. and Heller, H. C. (1984). Thermosensitivity of hypothalamic neurons during sleep and wakefulness. In: Hales, J. R. S. (ed.) *Thermal Physiology*. Raven Press, New York. pp. 91–94.

67. Parmeggiani, P-L., Azzaroni, A., Cevolani, D. and Ferrari, G. (1986). Polygraphic study of anterior hypothalamic-preoptic neuron thermosensitivity during sleep. *Electroencephalography and Clinical Neurophysiology*, **63**, 289–295.

Why do we sleep?

This book began with the dismal epitaph that, 'despite 50 years of research, many people feel that all that we can conclude about the function of sleep is that it overcomes sleepiness'. Such a hopeless notion is as helpful as the idea that we eat simply to stop the feeling of hunger, or drink just to overcome thirst. If the epitaph does turn out to be true, then as the doyen sleep researcher, Allan Rechtschaffen, has often remarked: 'sleep would have been one of the greatest mistakes Nature has made'. Other poignant remarks of his can be found in his well-known critique of theories about the function of sleep[1]. For example:

So many of them (my colleagues) have offered theories of sleep function which may be prophetic visions of the truth. But if they are, these prophesies have not rallied the faithful. None of these theories have compelled large numbers of sleep researchers to say—I believe. Yes, this is the function of sleep (p. 2) . . . The answer will not come from checking lists of possible misinterpretations, but from a new idea or result which possibly coalesces our facts and fantasies. It will probably come at four in the morning in a dingy laboratory in Minneapolis to a graduate student in biology who never read this paper. God bless him (p. 16).

I am neither a graduate student from Minneapolis, nor have I produced the answer. Some answers—yes maybe, the answer—no. This book has tried to look at the facts and coalesce them in various ways, with the result that several beliefs have been dispelled as fantasies. Most of the current issues relating to the function of sleep have been covered and the aim has been to try and weave some sort of overall picture about sleep. The picture shows that the epitaph is to say the least, premature. More likely, sleep research is still in its infancy.

The book has concentrated on humans, as this is the mammal I am most familiar with in my own studies. So I can be accused of being too anthropomorphic, of relying too much on what I understand to be the functions of human sleep as a basis for examining the sleep of other mammals. But this is as reasonable a starting point as any. Humans are particularly useful to study, as we can watch them in their natural environment, they can tell the researcher how they feel, how well they sleep, and whether they are worried by the experimental procedure, etc. These ends cannot be achieved when studying sleep in other mammals, where there are often unwanted factors concerning the experimental method, that seriously affect sleep itself. On the other hand, animal research has an advantage that

310

because various surgical procedures can be performed, great headway can still be made along other lines.

There is a well-known saying amongst biologists, from where I do not know, that 'teleology is the mistress with whom all biologists live, but none like to be seen in the company of'. My approach has been openly teleological as I believe that most of the phenomena of sleep have a purpose. There is no harm in such an outlook if it promotes enquiry, particularly in an area of research which many view to be near to a dead end. The harm in teleology comes when one assumes that one's own views are always correct.

There are many assumptions about human sleep that are often found in one form or another as pronouncements in general textbooks on biology, medicine, and psychology:

- We need 8 hours sleep a night.
- Sleep deprivation is harmful to health.
- Sleep is a state of enhanced tissue growth and repair (restitution)—more specifically:
    REM sleep is for brain (cerebral) restitution and for the consolidation of memories.
    Sleep stages 3 and 4 (SWS) are for body restitution.
- 'Sleepiness' takes a single form.
- We sleep primarily in order to dream and to have REM sleep. This is typified by the division of sleep into REM and non-REM sleep.
- The functions of sleep are universal across mammals—rat and human alike.
- REM sleep is a 'primitive' form of sleep, which for example accounts for the apparent loss of thermoregulation in this sleep state.

But these beliefs are not as clear-cut as they at first seem, and within this book I have argued that all either need qualifying, or are wrong. My main conclusions (together with the chapters from which they come) are as follows:

- Excluding the brain, sleep deprivation is uneventful, and does not cause physical or psychiatric illness. Even the behavioural and psychological changes are not dramatic, and there seems to be some reserve capacity for the brain to cope with limited sleep deprivation (Chapters 2 and 3).
- Again excluding the brain, human sleep is not a condition of heightened tissue repair (restitution). Food intake and physical rest play the key roles here. Evidence suggesting that tissue restitution is increased during human sleep (such as the sleep-related human growth hormone release, and increases in cell division during sleep) is misleading (Chapter 4).
- Mostly because of their inability to show relaxed wakefulness, small mammals such as rodents may have a rise in tissue restitution during sleep.

But sleep is not the stimulus for this restitution. Sleep is just the immobilizer, producing the rest to enable restitution. This is one of several ways in which the functions of sleep essentially differ between rodents and humans (Chapter 4).

- Unlike many organs, the brain, particularly the cerebral cortex, is unable to 'relax' outside sleep and is always in a state of readiness during wakefulness. This may be why the cerebrum seems to need sleep, perhaps for the recovery and restitution of neural and related tissues (Chapter 5). The more advanced the cerebrum, as in humans, the greater the role sleep has in this respect, and the lesser this role for rodents (Chapter 7).
- Even the human cerebrum does not need 8 hours sleep per night, but only a portion of sleep, which I have named *core* sleep. Core sleep typically occupies the first three sleep cycles (Chapter 6).
- Core sleep, which could well be associated with cerebral restitution, is mainly identified in humans as EEG delta activity, otherwise referred to as slow wave sleep (SWS) stages 3, and particularly stage 4. However, core sleep also includes the REM sleep within the first three sleep cycles. This makes up around half of a typical night's REM sleep (Chapter 6).
- The remaining half of REM sleep is dispensable, together with much of stage 2 sleep. This constitutes what I have called *optional* sleep, which is some sort of behavioural drive to sleep, having the function of occupying unproductive hours and in the case of small mammals of conserving energy. Unlike core sleep, it has a circadian rhythm (Chapter 6). The main EEG sign of optional sleep is stage 2 sleep (Chapter 6).
- After sleep deprivation, it is the lost core sleep that is reclaimed. Lost optional sleep is indeed lost. Human short sleepers have less optional sleep, but the usual amounts of core sleep. People who normally sleep 7–8 hours a night can successfully adapt to cutting their sleep down to around 5.5–6 hours with little difficulty. It is their optional sleep that is diminished. Optional sleep can also be extended (Chapter 6).
- The cerebrum has some spare capacity to cope with limited sleep loss. This is independent of its need for recovery (Chapter 2).
- Increased 'brain work' during wakefulness leads to rises in SWS, not in REM sleep, further indicating that it is SWS that is linked with cerebral recovery (Chapter 5).
- There may well be two forms of sleepiness: *core sleepiness*, associated with the loss of core sleep and reflected in impaired cerebral functioning, and *optional sleepiness*, associated with the loss of optional sleep and mostly affecting motivation (Chapter 2).
- Most standard psychological and behavioural tests of sleepiness would be unable to discriminate between core and optional sleepiness. In fact, such tests are generally unhelpful from the viewpoint of sleep function. The interesting tests in this respect are probably those involving high levels of

'cerebration' such as creativity and 'divergent' (rather than 'convergent') thinking (Chapter 2).

● Our sleep does not centre around REM sleep, but SWS instead. The division of sleep into core and optional sleep gives a better perspective to sleep function than does the REM/non-REM classification of sleep (Chapter 6).

● The core–optional perspective can be applied to the sleep of other mammals. Core sleep is influenced by cerebral advancement, and optional sleep by the energy conservation value of sleep, as well as by the safety of the sleeper, body size, and the degree to which the animal displays relaxed wakefulness. All these factors interact to produce different emphases on the functions of sleep, changing as the phylogenetic scale is ascended (Chapter 7).

● REM sleep is not essential to memory consolidation, and may have less restitutive benefit for the cerebrum than is commonly thought. Many of the findings with animals in this respect have probably been artefacts of the experimental techniques (Chapter 8).

● Dreaming is very much of an enigma. Whether or not it is largely confined to REM sleep is a matter for debate. Dreaming is usually pleasant and entertaining, and could even be viewed as the 'cinema of the mind', to keep the sleeping cerebrum occupied. Maybe it also helps mental conflicts to resolve themselves. There is no strong evidence to show that we sleep simply in order to dream, or that dreaming is really crucial to our mental wellbeing. Fantasy exists not only within the dream or for the dreamer, but often (but not always) for those people who 'interpret' dreams (Chapter 8).

● REM sleep is not a primitive form of sleep in the evolutionary sense, but is more likely to be a mammalian fetal state retained into adulthood. It is similar to wakefulness, and may, at least in part, be some sort of substitute for wakefulness, for keeping the cerebrum stimulated. This stimulation resembles orienting ('alarm') responses, which may account for some of the phenomena of REM sleep (Chapter 8).

● Thermoregulation during REM sleep is not absent or 'reptilian-like', but seems to be at the level of the mammalian fetus or neonate, and is more loosely controlled. Most aspects still function quite well, and for example heat production does not diminish (Chapter 8).

Some of these views may stand the test of time. However, like the majority of theories, most will fail or be superseded, but not without a fight I hope. What is very clear is that the eventual solutions to the function of sleep will not be straightforward, but will unravel with new developments in sleep research, in subtly different ways for various groups of mammals. I believe that exciting times still lie ahead for that graduate student in Minneapolis.

References

1. Rechtschaffen, A. (1979). The function of sleep: methodological issues. In: Drucker-Colin, R., Shkurovich, M. and Sterman, M.B. (ed.) *The Functions of Sleep*. Academic Press, New York. pp. 1–17.

Index